Imaging of the Lower Limb

Editors

ALBERTO BAZZOCCHI
GIUSEPPE GUGLIELMI

RADIOLOGIC CLINICS
OF NORTH AMERICA

www.radiologic.theclinics.com

Consulting Editor
FRANK H. MILLER

March 2023 • Volume 61 • Number 2

ELSEVIER

1600 John F. Kennedy Boulevard • Suite 1800 • Philadelphia, Pennsylvania, 19103-2899

http://www.theclinics.com

RADIOLOGIC CLINICS OF NORTH AMERICA Volume 61, Number 2
March 2023 ISSN 0033-8389, ISBN 13: 978-0-323-98783-7

Editor: John Vassallo (j.vassallo@elsevier.com)
Developmental Editor: Karen Solomon

Radiologic Clinics of North America (ISSN 0033-8389) is published bimonthly by Elsevier Inc., 360 Park Avenue South, New York, NY 10010-1710. Months of issue are January, March, May, July, September, and November. Periodicals postage paid at New York, NY and additional mailing offices. Subscription prices are USD 544 per year for US individuals, USD 1107 per year for US institutions, USD 100 per year for US students and residents, USD 643 per year for Canadian individuals, USD 1415 per year for Canadian institutions, USD 739 per year for international individuals, USD 1415 per year for international institutions, USD 100 per year for Canadian students/residents, and USD 315 per year for international students/residents. To receive student and resident rate, orders must be accompanied by name of affiliated institution, date of term and the signature of program/residency coordinatior on institution letterhead. Orders will be billed at individual rate until proof of status is received. Foreign air speed delivery is included in all *Clinics* subscription prices. All prices are subject to change without notice. **POSTMASTER:** Send address changes to *Radiologic Clinics of North America*, Elsevier Health Sciences Division, Subscription Customer Service, 3251 Riverport Lane, Maryland Heights, MO63043. **Customer Service: Telephone: 1-800-654-2452** (U.S. and Canada); **1-314-447-8871** (outside U.S. and Canada). **Fax: 1-314-447-8029. E-mail: journalscustomerservice-usa@elsevier.com (for print support); journalsonlinesupport-usa@elsevier.com (for online support)**.

Reprints. For copies of 100 or more of articles in this publication, please contact the Commercial Reprints Department, Elsevier Inc., 360 Park Avenue South, New York, New York 10010-1710. Tel.: +1-212-633-3874; Fax: +1-212-633-3820; E-mail: reprints@elsevier.com.

Radiologic Clinics of North America also published in Greek Paschalidis Medical Publications, Athens, Greece.

Radiologic Clinics of North America is covered in *MEDLINE/PubMed (Index Medicus), EMBASE/Excerpta Medica, Current Contents/Life Sciences, Current Contents/Clinical Medicine, RSNA Index to Imaging Literature, BIOSIS, Science Citation Index,* and *ISI/BIOMED.*

Contributors

CONSULTING EDITOR

FRANK H. MILLER, MD, FACR, FSAR, FSABI
Lee F. Rogers, MD Professor of Medical
Education, Chief, Body Imaging Section,
Medical Director, MRI, Professor, Department
of Radiology, Northwestern Memorial Hospital,
Northwestern University Feinberg School of
Medicine, Chicago, Illinois, USA

EDITORS

ALBERTO BAZZOCCHI, MD, PhD
Diagnostic and Interventional Radiology,
IRCCS Istituto Ortopedico Rizzoli, Bologna,
Italy

GIUSEPPE GUGLIELMI, MD
Department of Radiology, Hospital
San Giovanni Rotondo, Department of
Radiology, University of Foggia, Foggia, Italy

AUTHORS

DOMENICO ALBANO, MD, PhD
IRCCS Istituto Ortopedico Galeazzi, Milano,
Italy

SINAN AL-QASSAB, MBChB, MRCS, FRCR
Consultant Radiologist, Radiology
Department, Robert Jones and Agnes Hunt
Orthopaedic Hospital, Oswestry, United
Kingdom

FRANCISCO APARISI, MD, PhD
Department of Radiology, Hospital
Vithas Nueve de Octubre, Valencia,
Spain

**MARIA PILAR APARISI GÓMEZ, MBCHB,
FRANZCR**
Department of Radiology, Auckland City
Hospital, Grafton, Auckland, New Zealand;
Department of Radiology, IMSKE, Valencia,
Spain

FRANCESCO ARRIGONI, MD
Emergency Radiology, San Salvatore Hospital,
L'Aquila, Italy

JOE D. BAAL, MD
Department of Radiology and Biomedical
Imaging, University of California, San
Francisco, San Francisco, California, USA

ANTONIO BARILE, MD
Department of Biotechnological and Applied
Clinical Sciences, University of L'Aquila,
L'Aquila, Italy

ALBERTO BAZZOCCHI, MD, PhD
Diagnostic and Interventional Radiology,
IRCCS Istituto Ortopedico Rizzoli, Bologna,
Italy

KERENSA M. BEEKMAN, MD, PhD
Department of Radiology and Nuclear
Medicine, Amsterdam Movement Sciences,
Amsterdam UMC, Location AMC, University of
Amsterdam, Amsterdam, the Netherlands

LUIS S. BELTRAN, MD
Assistant Professor, Department of Radiology,
Harvard Medical School, Brigham and Women's
Hospital, Boston, Massachusetts, USA

JENNY T. BENCARDINO, MD
Professor of Radiology, Chief of
Musculoskeletal Imaging, Department of
Radiology, University of Pennsylvania Health
System, Philadelphia, Pennsylvania,
USA

FEDERICO BRUNO, MD
Emergency Radiology, San Salvatore Hospital,
L'Aquila, Italy

**DONAL G. CAHILL, BSc, BMBS, MRCPI,
FFRRCSI**
Department of Imaging and Interventional
Radiology, The Chinese University of Hong
Kong, The Prince of Wales Hospital, Shatin,
Hong Kong

KATHERINE L. CECIL, MD
Department of Radiology and Biomedical
Imaging, University of California, San
Francisco, San Francisco, California,
USA

CHRISTINE B. CHUNG, MD
Professor, Department of Radiology,
University of California, San Diego, VA Medical
Center, San Diego, La Jolla, California,
USA

MICHEL D. CREMA, MD
Institut d'Imagerie du Sport, Institut National du
Sport, de l'Expertise et de la Performance
(INSEP), Paris, France

JULIA DAFFINÀ, MD
Department of Biotechnological and Applied
Clinical Sciences, University of L'Aquila,
L'Aquila, Italy

ERNESTO DI CESARE, MD
Department of Life, Health and Environmental
Sciences, University of L'Aquila, L'Aquila, Italy

YOSHIMI ENDO, MD
Associate Attending Radiologist, Hospital for
Special Surgery, New York, New York,
USA; Associate Professor of Clinical
Radiology, Weill Medical College of Cornell
University

BENJAMIN FRITZ, MD
Department of Radiology, Balgrist University
Hospital, Faculty of Medicine, University of
Zurich, Zurich, Switzerland

JAN FRITZ, MD
Department of Radiology, Division of
Musculoskeletal Radiology, NYU Grossman
School of Medicine, New York, New York,
USA

**JAMES F. GRIFFITH, MB, BCh, BAO, FRCR,
MRCP (UK), FRCR (Edin), FHKAM
(Radiology)**
Professor and Chairman, Department of
Imaging and Interventional Radiology, The
Chinese University of Hong Kong, The
Prince of Wales Hospital, Shatin,
Hong Kong

SALVATORE GITTO, MD
Dipartimento di Scienze Biomediche per La
Salute, Università Degli Studi di Milano, Milan,
Italy

ALI GUERMAZI, MD, PhD
Department of Radiology, Boston University
School of Medicine, Boston, Massachusetts,
USA; Department of Radiology, VA Boston
Healthcare System, West Roxbury,
Massachusetts, USA

GIUSEPPE GUGLIELMI, MD
Department of Radiology, Hospital
San Giovanni Rotondo, Department of
Radiology, University of Foggia, Foggia,
Italy

DAICHI HAYASHI, MD, PhD
Department of Radiology, Stony Brook
University, Stony Brook, New York,
USA

MOHAMED JARRAYA, MD
Professor, Department of Radiology,
Massachusetts General Hospital, Harvard
Medical School, Boston, Massachusetts, USA

P. PAUL F.M. KUIJER, PhD
Department of Public and Occupational
Health, Amsterdam Movement Sciences,
Amsterdam Public Health, Amsterdam UMC,
University of Amsterdam, Amsterdam, the
Netherlands

RADHESH LALAM, MBBS, MRCS, FRCR
Consultant Radiologist, Radiology
Department, Robert Jones and Agnes Hunt
Orthopaedic Hospital, Oswestry, United
Kingdom

THOMAS M. LINK, MD, PhD
Department of Radiology and Biomedical Imaging, University of California, San Francisco, San Francisco, California, USA

MARIO MAAS, MD, PhD
Department of Radiology and Nuclear Medicine, Amsterdam Movement Sciences, Location AMC, University of Amsterdam, Academic Center for Evidence-Based Sports Medicine (ACES), Amsterdam Collaboration for Health and Safety in Sports (ACHSS), International Olympic Committee (IOC) Research Center, Amsterdam UMC, Amsterdam, the Netherlands

GIULIO MARIA MARCHEGGIANI MUCCIOLI, MD, PhD
2nd Orthopaedic and Traumatology Clinic, IRCCS Istituto Ortopedico Rizzoli, Dipartimento di Scienze Biomediche e Neuromotorie DIBINEM, University of Bologna, Bologna, Italy

CARLO MASCIOCCHI, MD
Department of Biotechnological and Applied Clinical Sciences, University of L'Aquila, L'Aquila, Italy

KEVIN McGILL, MD
Department of Radiology and Biomedical Imaging, University of California, San Francisco, San Francisco, California, USA

CARMELO MESSINA, MD
IRCCS Istituto Ortopedico Galeazzi, Dipartimento di Scienze Biomediche per La Salute, Università Degli Studi di Milano, Milan, Italy

THEODORE T. MILLER, MD
Attending Radiologist, Hospital for Special Surgery, New York, New York, USA; Professor of Radiology, Weill Medical College of Cornell University

AUREA VALERIA ROSA MOHANA-BORGES, MD
Post-Doctoral Fellow, Department of Radiology, University of California, San Diego, La Jolla, California, USA

RICCARDO MONTI, MD
Department of Biotechnological and Applied Clinical Sciences, University of L'Aquila, L'Aquila, Italy

MATTHEW O'BRIEN, MD
Diagnostic Radiology, Oregon Health & Science University, Portland, Oregon, USA

PIERPAOLO PALUMBO, MD
Emergency Radiology, San Salvatore Hospital, L'Aquila, Italy

RINA PATEL, MD
Department of Radiology and Biomedical Imaging, University of California, San Francisco, San Francisco, California, USA

FRANK W. ROEMER, MD
Department of Radiology, Boston University School of Medicine, Boston, Massachusetts, USA; Department of Radiology, Friedrich-Alexander University Erlangen-Nürnberg (FAU) and University Hospital Erlangen, Erlangen, Germany

LUCA MARIA SCONFIENZA, MD, PhD
IRCCS Istituto Ortopedico Galeazzi, Dipartimento di Scienze Biomediche per La Salute, Università Degli Studi di Milano, Milan, Italy

FRANCESCA SERPI, MD
Dipartimento di Scienze Biomediche per La Salute, Università Degli Studi di Milano, Milan, Italy

JASPREET SINGH, MRCP, FRCR
Consultant Radiologist, Robert Jones and Agnes Hunt Orthopaedic Hospital, Oswestry, United Kingdom

DARRYL B. SNEAG, MD
Associate Attending Radiologist, Hospital for Special Surgery, New York, New York, USA; Associate Professor of Radiology, Weill Medical College of Cornell University

ALESSANDRA SPLENDIANI, MD
Department of Biotechnological and Applied Clinical Sciences, University of L'Aquila, L'Aquila, Italy

PRUDENCIA N.M. TYRRELL, MBBCh, BAO, MRCPI, FRCR
Consultant Radiologist, Robert Jones and Agnes Hunt Orthopaedic Hospital, Oswestry, United Kingdom

ANNA VERBITSKIY, MD
Clinical Assistant Professor, Department of Radiology, NYU Grossman School of Medicine, New York, New York, USA

MAX K.H. YAM, MBChB, FRCR
Department of Radiology, North District
Hospital, Sheung Shui, Hong Kong

STEFANO ZAFFAGNINI, MD
2nd Orthopaedic and Traumatology Clinic,
IRCCS Istituto Ortopedico Rizzoli,
Dipartimento di Scienze Biomediche e
Neuromotorie DIBINEM, University of Bologna,
Bologna, Italy

NICOLAS ZULUAGA, MD
Clinical Research Fellow, Department of
Radiology, University of Pennsylvania Health
System, Philadelphia, Pennsylvania,
USA

Contents

> Detailed knowledge of anatomy helps to understand pathologic processes. This article focuses on the anatomy and functionality of the hip, with emphasis on recently studied concepts and anatomic features that have an association with the development of symptoms. The most common anatomic variants posing a challenge for diagnosis and other common findings in asymptomatic patients are reviewed. Good understanding of the different surgical procedures helps in providing as much information as possible to guarantee a favorable outcome, improving prognosis. We review what are the commonly expected postsurgical appearances and the most common postsurgical complications.

> Overuse injuries of the hip are common, and clinical diagnosis may be difficult because of overlapping and nonspecific clinical symptoms. Imaging can play an essential role in guiding diagnosis and management. Femoroacetabular joint structural abnormalities result in various conditions that can predispose patients to early development of osteoarthritis. Repetitive stress on the skeletally immature hip can result in apophyseal injuries. Notable nonosseous overuse hip pathologies include athletic pubalgia, trochanteric bursitis, and injuries involving the iliopsoas myotendinous unit. Timely diagnosis of overuse injuries of the hip can facilitate improved response to conservative measures and prevent irreversible damage.

> Acute hip pain following injury more commonly originates locally in and around the hip joint rather than being referred from the lumbar spine, sacroiliac joints, groin, or pelvis. Clinical assessment can usually localize the pain source to the hip region. Thereafter, imaging helps define the precise cause of acute hip pain. This review discusses the imaging of common causes of acute hip pain following injury in adults, addressing injuries in and around the hip joint. Pediatric and postsurgical causes of hip pain following injury are not discussed.

> Detailed knowledge of anatomy helps to understand pathologic processes. This article focuses on the anatomy and functionality of the knee, with emphasis on recently studied concepts and anatomic features that have an association with the development of pathology. The most common anatomic variants posing a challenge for diagnosis and other common findings in asymptomatic patients are reviewed. Good understanding of the different surgical procedures helps in

providing as much information as possible to guarantee a positive outcome, improving prognosis. We review what are the commonly expected postsurgical appearances and the most common postsurgical complications.

Mohamed Jarraya, Frank W. Roemer, Daichi Hayashi, Michel D. Crema, and Ali Guermazi

Overuse-related injuries of the knee joint and periarticular soft tissues include a heterogenous group of sports and nonsports-related injuries. These conditions include friction and impingement syndromes, bone stress injuries, bursitis, and tendon-related pathology such as tendinopathy and snapping. Traction apophysitis are also discussed as commonly seen in the pediatric population. Although multiple imaging modalities can be used, this review focuses on MR imaging, which is the most common and, often, the only modality used.

Benjamin Fritz and Jan Fritz

Acute knee injury ranges among the most common joint injuries in professional and recreational athletes. Radiographs can detect joint effusion, fractures, deformities, and malalignment; however, MR imaging is most accurate for radiographically occult fractures, chondral injury, and soft tissue injuries. Using a structured checklist approach for systematic MR imaging evaluation and reporting, this article reviews the MR imaging appearances of the spectrum of traumatic knee injuries, including osteochondral injuries, cruciate ligament tears, meniscus tears and ramp lesions, anterolateral complex and collateral ligament injuries, patellofemoral translation, extensor mechanism tears, and nerve and vascular injuries.

Maria Pilar Aparisi Gómez, Francisco Aparisi, Giuseppe Guglielmi, and Alberto Bazzocchi

The anatomy of the ankle and foot is complex, allowing for a wide range of functionality. The movements of the joints represent a complex dynamic interaction. A solid understanding of the characteristics and actions of the anatomic elements helps explain the mechanisms and patterns of injury. This article reviews the anatomy, with special focus on concepts that are the object of recent study and the features that favor the development of symptoms. Good understanding of the surgical procedures helps in providing information to guarantee a favorable outcome. We review the commonly expected postsurgical appearances and the most common postsurgical complications.

Kerensa M. Beekman, P. Paul F.M. Kuijer, and Mario Maas

Overuse injuries of the ankle and foot are common injuries both in sport and in a work-related context. After clinical assessment, imaging is key for early diagnosis. In this overview article, we focus on imaging techniques, protocols, and imaging findings of overuse injuries of the ankle and foot; we emphasize the important role of structured reporting; and we discuss clinical symptoms, epidemiology, and risk factors in sports and in a work-related context.

Luis S. Beltran, Nicolas Zuluaga, Anna Verbitskiy, and Jenny T. Bencardino

Ankle and foot injuries are very common injuries in the general population, and more so in athletes. MR imaging is the optimal modality to evaluate for ligamentous injuries of the ankle and associated conditions after ankle sprain. In this article, the authors discuss the epidemiology, biomechanics, normal anatomy, and pathology of the ankle as well as injuries of the hindfoot and midfoot that are often associated with ankle injuries.

Imaging methods capable of detecting inflammation, such as MR imaging and ultrasound, are of paramount importance in rheumatic disease management, not only for diagnostic purposes but also for monitoring disease activity and treatment response. However, more advanced stages of arthritis, characterized by findings of cumulative structural damage, have traditionally been accomplished by radiographs and computed tomography. The purpose of this review is to provide an overview of imaging of some of the most prevalent inflammatory rheumatic diseases affecting the lower limb (osteoarthritis, rheumatoid arthritis, and gout) and up-to-date recommendations regarding imaging diagnostic workup.

Bone and soft tissue lesions are frequently seen in the lower limbs. Many are non-neoplastic but may mimic tumours. In this article, we discuss a practical approach for the diagnosis and management of the most common tumours and tumour-like conditions seen in the lower limbs.

The purpose of this article is to discuss most common diagnostic pitfalls of the lower limb with specific attention to the knee, ankle, and foot joints. The knowledge of normal anatomic variants, correlation with age, symptoms, and medical history together with these potential MR imaging pitfalls is fundamental for an accurate interpretation of the imaging findings of the lower limb.

Continued advancements in magnetic resonance (MR) neurography and ultrasound have made both indispensable tools for the workup of peripheral neuropathy. Ultrasound provides high spatial resolution of superficial nerves, and techniques such as "sonopalpation" and dynamic maneuvers can improve accuracy. Superior soft tissue contrast, ability to evaluate both superficial and deep nerves with similar high resolution, and reliable characterization of denervation are strengths of MR neurography. Nevertheless, familiarity with normal anatomy, anatomic variants, and common sites of nerve entrapment is essential for radiologists to use both MR neurography and ultrasound effectively.

Imaging guidance is essential for musculoskeletal interventional procedures performed in the lower limb. A strong evidence supports the use of imaging guidance to improve safety, accuracy, and effectiveness of these interventions. Joints, tendons, bursae, and nerves can be effectively approached especially with ultrasound-guided injections. Here, we discuss evidence and technique of the most common image-guided musculoskeletal interventional procedures in the lower limb.

PROGRAM OBJECTIVE

The objective of the *Radiologic Clinics of North America* is to keep practicing radiologists and radiology residents up to date with current clinical practice in radiology by providing timely articles reviewing the state of the art in patient care.

TARGET AUDIENCE

Practicing radiologists, radiology residents, and other healthcare professionals who provide patient care utilizing radiologic findings.

LEARNING OBJECTIVES

Upon completion of this activity, participants will be able to:

1. Describe the common anatomical variants and other common findings in asymptomatic patients, together with the common pitfalls encountered with lower limb imaging.
2. Discuss the different imaging modalities and the benefits as a critical role in assessing, diagnosing, and treating disorders, injuries, and complications in the lower limbs.
3. Recognize MRI imaging as an excellent modality for assessing, diagnosing, and managing disorders and injuries, as well as complications of the lower limbs.

ACCREDITATION

The Elsevier Office of Continuing Medical Education (EOCME) is accredited by the Accreditation Council for Continuing Medical Education (ACCME) to provide continuing medical education for physicians.

The EOCME designates this journal-based CME activity for a maximum of 14 *AMA PRA Category 1 Credit*(s)™. Physicians should claim only the credit commensurate with the extent of their participation in the activity.

All other healthcare professionals requesting continuing education credit for this enduring material will be issued a certificate of participation.

DISCLOSURE OF CONFLICTS OF INTEREST

The EOCME assesses conflict of interest with its instructors, faculty, planners, and other individuals who are in a position to control the content of CME activities. All relevant conflicts of interest that are identified are thoroughly vetted by EOCME for fair balance, scientific objectivity, and patient care recommendations. EOCME is committed to providing its learners with CME activities that promote improvements or quality in healthcare and not a specific proprietary business or a commercial interest.

The planning committee, staff, authors, and editors listed below have identified no financial relationships or relationships to products or devices they or their spouse/life partner have with commercial interest related to the content of this CME activity:

Domenico Albano, MD; Sinan Al-Qassab, MBChB, MRCS, FRCR; Francisco Aparisi, MD, PhD; Maria Pilar Aparisi Gómez, MBChB, FRANZCR; Francesco Arrigoni, MD; Joe D. Baal, MD; Antonio Barile, MD; Alberto Bazzocchi, MD, PhD; Kerensa M. Beekman, MD, PhD; Luis S. Beltran, MD; Jenny T. Bencardino, MD; Federico Bruno, MD; Donal G. Cahill, BSc, BMBS, MRCPI, FFR RCSI; Katherine L. Cecil, MD; Christine B. Chung, MD; Julia Daffinà, MD; Ernesto Di Cesare, MD; Benjamin Fritz, MD; Salvatore Gitto, MD; James F. Griffith, MB, BCh, BAO, FRCR, MRCP (UK), FRCR (Edin), FHKAM (Radiology); Giuseppe Guglielmi, MD; Daichi Hayashi, MD, PhD; Mohamed Jarraya, MD; P. Paul F.M. Kuijer, PhD; Pradeep Kuttysankaran; Radhesh Lalam, MBBS, MRCS, FRCR; Thomas M. Link, MD, PhD; Mario Maas, MD, PhD; Giulio Maria Marcheggiani Muccioli, MD, PhD; Carlo Masciocchi, MD; Kevin McGill, MD; Carmelo Messina, MD; Aurea Valeria Rosa Mohana-Borges, MD; Riccardo Monti, MBA; Matthew O'Brien, MD; Pierpaolo Palumbo, MD; Rina Patel, MD; Luca Maria Sconfienza, MD, PhD; Francesca Serpi, MD; Jaspreet Singh, MRCP, FRCR; Alessandra Splendiani, MD; Doreen Thomas-Payne, MSN, BSN, RN, PMHNP-BC; Prudencia N.M. Tyrrell, MBBCh, BAO, MRCPI, FRCR; Anna Verbitskiy, MD; Max K.H. Yam, MBChB, FRCR; Stefano Zaffagnini, MD; Nicolas Zuluaga, MD

The planning committee, staff, authors, and editors listed below have identified financial relationships or relationships to products or devices they or their spouse/life partner have with commercial interest related to the content of this CME activity:

Michel D. Crema, MD: Shareholder: Boston Imaging Core Lab, LLC, Yoshimi Endo, MD: Research Support: GE Healthcare, Jan Fritz, MD: Research Support: Siemens AG, BTG International, Zimmer Biomed, DePuy Synthes, QED, SyntheticMR; Scientific Advisor: Siemens AG, SyntheticMR, GE Healthcare, QED, BTG, ImageBiopsy Lab, Boston Scientific, Mirata Pharma; Patent Beneficiary: Siemens Healthcare, Ali Guermazi, MD, PhD: Consultant: Pfizer, Regeneron, Merck Serono, TissueGene, AstraZeneca, Novartis; Shareholder: Boston Imaging Core Lab, LLC, Theodore T. Miller, MD: Research Support: GE Healthcare, Frank W. Roemer, MD: Consultant: Calibr; Shareholder: Boston Imaging Core Lab, LLC, Darryl B. Sneag, MD: Research Support: GE Healthcare

UNAPPROVED/OFF-LABEL USE DISCLOSURE

The EOCME requires CME faculty to disclose to the participants:

1. When products or procedures being discussed are off-label, unlabelled, experimental, and/or investigational (not US Food and Drug Administration [FDA] approved); and

2. Any limitations on the information presented, such as data that are preliminary or that represent ongoing research, interim analyses, and/or unsupported opinions. Faculty may discuss information about pharmaceutical agents that is outside of FDA-approved labelling. This information is intended solely for CME and is not intended to promote off-label use of these medications. If you have any questions, contact the medical affairs department of the manufacturer for the most recent prescribing information.

TO ENROLL

To enroll in the *Radiologic Clinics of North America* Continuing Medical Education program, call customer service at 1-800-654-2452 or sign up online at http://www.theclinics.com/home/cme. The CME program is available to subscribers for an additional annual fee of USD 356.00.

METHOD OF PARTICIPATION

In order to claim credit, participants must complete the following:
1. Complete enrolment as indicated above.
2. Read the activity.
3. Complete the CME Test and Evaluation. Participants must achieve a score of 70% on the test. All CME Tests and Evaluations must be completed online.

CME INQUIRIES/SPECIAL NEEDS

For all CME inquiries or special needs, please contact elsevierCME@elsevier.com.

RADIOLOGIC CLINICS OF NORTH AMERICA

SERIES OF RELATED INTEREST

Advances in Clinical Radiology
Available at: https://www.advancesinclinicalradiology.com/
Magnetic Resonance Imaging Clinics
Available at: https://www.mri.theclinics.com/
Neuroimaging Clinics
Available at: www.neuroimaging.theclinics.com
PET Clinics
Available at: www.pet.theclinics.com

THE CLINICS ARE AVAILABLE ONLINE!
Access your subscription at:
www.theclinics.com

Preface
Imaging of the Lower Limb

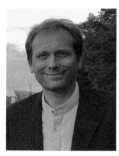   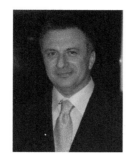

Alberto Bazzocchi, MD, PhD   Giuseppe Guglielmi, MD
Editors

The lower limbs support the weight of our bodies for our whole lives. The lower limbs have different biomechanical properties, sizes, proportions or symmetry, and vectors among individuals. Moreover, some of these features change with aging. The support offered by the lower limbs to the trunk (and to other parts of the body) implies a constant and diverse work for them, whether we are standing, walking, running, or practicing different kinds of sports and work-related activities. Joints and specific musculoskeletal structures of the lower limb are put under stress by a diversity of conditions, and this results in different prevalence of pathologic findings and diseases. Trauma of the lower limb is also very common, and imaging plays a fundamental role in the management of the patient.

The aim of this issue of *Radiologic Clinics of North America* is to provide the reader with a comprehensive and up-to-date imaging interpretation of disorders and hot topics related to the lower limb. This issue includes 14 review articles covering different aspects of imaging of the lower limb, with the invaluable contribution of several internationally acclaimed and credited authors.

The lower limb comprises different joints with completely different anatomy, therefore with significant differences in functions at different levels but still in a complex interaction. That is why it is so important to approach imaging diagnosis after reviewing the anatomy from a functional and surgical point of view. Several articles cover the different aspects of overuse pathology and traumatic injuries, joint by joint.

The incidence and features of specific rheumatic diseases and tumors, including the difficulties in differential diagnosis, are discussed in two different articles. Two special focus articles address tricks in MR imaging, and peripheral nerve imaging of the lower limb, respectively. At the end of the issue, a review of several interventional imaging-guided procedures on the lower limb is also included.

Alberto Bazzocchi, MD, PhD
Diagnostic and Interventional Radiology
IRCCS Istituto Ortopedico Rizzoli
Via G. C. Pupilli 1
40136 Bologna, Italy

Giuseppe Guglielmi, MD
Department of Radiology
University of Foggia
Viale L. Pinto 1
71100 Foggia, Italy

E-mail addresses:
abazzo@inwind.it (A. Bazzocchi)
giuseppe.guglielmi@unifg.it (G. Guglielmi)

https://doi.org/10.1016/j.rcl.2022.11.001

Particularities on Anatomy and Normal Postsurgical Appearances of the Hip

Maria Pilar Aparisi Gómez, MBChB, FRANZCR[a,b],*, Francisco Aparisi, MD, PhD[c],
Giuseppe Guglielmi, MD[d,e], Alberto Bazzocchi, MD, PhD[f]

KEYWORDS

• Hip • Anatomy • Postoperative period • Radiology • MR imaging

KEY POINTS

- A solid knowledge of the anatomy and biomechanics of the hip helps to understand the mechanisms of injury and provides a useful tool for accurate diagnosis and, with a positive impact on the selection of treatment and prognosis.
- A good understanding of the different surgical procedures used to treat hip pathology helps in providing as much information as possible to guarantee a favorable outcome of treatment, improving prognosis.
- Familiarity with the expected postsurgical appearances is mandatory, to be able to discern these from complications.

INTRODUCTION

Detailed knowledge of anatomy is necessary to understand the pathologic processes.

In this article, we focus on reviewing the components of the anatomy of the hip, with special attention to those concepts that have been the object of recent study or anatomic features that have a clear association with the development of symptoms or are a frequent location for injury, elucidating why this is the case.

We also describe the most common anatomic variants and other common findings in asymptomatic patients.

Finally, we highlight what are the commonly expected postsurgical appearances and the most common postsurgical complications.

THE HIP JOINT

The hip is a ball-and-socket type of joint, inherently stable, with a great range of motion. It is covered by a strong capsule and reinforced by the iliofemoral, pubofemoral, and ischiofemoral ligaments.

Despite its shape and inherent stability, the hip is a relatively incongruent joint, the acetabular diameter is slightly smaller than the femoral head. Added stability is provided by the labrum, which increases the socket surface.[1]

There are a variety of femoral head and acetabular morphologies. An alteration of the normal morphology resulting in impaired congruence is associated with conditions such as hip dysplasia and femoroacetabular impingement (FAI), of the cam, pincer, or mixed types (**Fig. 1**).

The authors have no funding information to disclose.
[a] Department of Radiology, Auckland City Hospital, 2 Park Road, Grafton, Auckland 1023, New Zealand;
[b] Department of Radiology. IMSKE, Calle Suiza, 11, Valencia 46024, Spain; [c] Department of Radiology, Hospital Vithas Nueve de Octubre, Calle Valle de la Ballestera, 59, Valencia 46015, Spain; [d] Department of Radiology, Hospital San Giovanni Rotondo, Italy; [e] Department of Radiology, University of Foggia, Viale Luigi Pinto 1, Foggia 71100, Italy; [f] Diagnostic and Interventional Radiology, IRCCS Istituto Ortopedico Rizzoli, Via G. C. Pupilli 1, Bologna 40136, Italy
* Corresponding author. Auckland City Hospital, 2 Park Road, Grafton, Auckland 1023, New Zealand
E-mail addresses: pilara@adhb.govt.nz; pilucaparisi193@gmail.com

Radiol Clin N Am 61 (2023) 167–190
https://doi.org/10.1016/j.rcl.2022.10.002

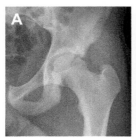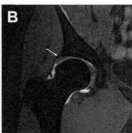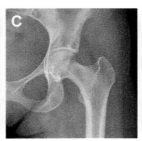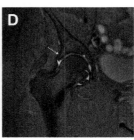

Fig. 1. Cam and pincer morphologies of the femoral head and acetabulum. (*A*) AP radiograph demonstrating the typical pistol grip deformity in the femoral head/neck junction. (*B*) coronal DP Fat sat in a different patient, demonstrating and increase in size of the acetabular labrum to compensate the deficient acetabular coverage, typical of the evolution of dysplasia. (*C*) AP radiograph in a 39-year-old woman demonstrates the typical features of excessive acetabular coverage seen in pincer deformity (crossover sign, larger lateral center angle, among others). (*D*) coronal DP fat sat in a different patient demonstrates a deep acetabulum, with a slightly overhanging acetabular rim surrounding the entirety of the head (*dotted arrow*)

It is important to mention that the existence of morphology alterations in the hip joint does not necessarily equate pathology. A systematic review[2] on the prevalence of radiographic findings suggestive of FAI in asymptomatic individuals analyzed 26 articles and found that the prevalence of asymptomatic cam deformity was 37%, and pincer deformity was found in up to 67% of asymptomatic hips, although the authors pointed out pincer deformity was poorly and not homogeneously defined across studies (diverse criteria), concluding that FAI morphologic features are common in asymptomatic patients. Decision-making needs to be based on a detailed clinical assessment, with an integration of patient history, physical examination, and imaging.[2] Nevertheless, comparative studies have found a significantly greater prevalence rate of structural bony abnormalities for symptomatic hips compared with asymptomatic.[3]

The hip is also intrinsically related to the pelvis and spine. Alterations at these levels will have a potential effect on hip biomechanics, which may lead to pathology. As an example, a recently published study by Kwon and colleagues[4] in 365 patients (449 hips) with hip pain, studied with MR imaging or MR arthrography (MRA) related the presence of a labral tear to the existence of high pelvic incidence, with or without FAI morphology.

Diving into the complex topic of the anatomic relation between hip—pelvis—spine is beyond the scope of this review article, which is focused on the lower limb.

Femur

The femoral head has an almost spherical shape (approximately two-third of a sphere).

The vascular supply is relatively scarce, the main suppliers are the medial and lateral circumflex arteries, branches of the profunda femoris. There is a small contribution to the artery of the ligamentum teres.

Morphologic variations of the proximal femur, especially related to the occurrence of FAI have been described. The most typical is the presence of a bony prominence in the junction of the femoral neck and head, known as pistol grip deformity, which is associated with cam-type FAI and labral tears.

However, other findings about the femoral head are also frequently seen, with different implications.

A circumscript osseous defect at the anteroinferior aspect of the femoral head, termed femoral head defect has been described as a nonpathological finding, normal variant, with no association with FAI, although it demonstrated a nonsignificant association with lower femoral antertorsion,[5] which may alter biomechanics with higher shear forces on the femoral neck-head junction.[6] This defect can present in three variants: type I is pointed, dent-like, type II is crate-like, like a depression and type III is round, cystic-like[5] (**Fig. 2**).

Herniation pits were described by Pitt and colleagues,[7] and are located in the proximal anterior an upper quadrant of the neck of the femur. These result from increased pressure of the adjacent capsule and synovium. In clinical practice, the herniation pit is normally asymptomatic, and reported to be present in 5% of the adult population. It is considered an incidental finding on examinations of patients with unexplained hip pain. Panzer and colleagues[8] evaluated the possibility of a correlation between the presence of herniation pits and morphologic abnormalities of the femoral head and acetabulum, as indicators of cam and pincer FAI. The authors found the pits were also present in the inferior portion (lower quadrant) of the proximal anterior femoral neck and that the alpha angle

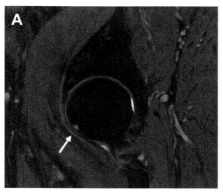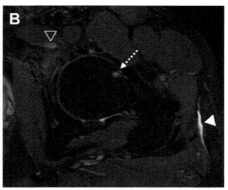

Fig. 2. Circumscript osseous defect at the anteroinferior aspect of the femoral head, known as femoral head defect, which is a normal variant. This defect can present in three types. Sagittal PD fat sat (*A*) demonstrates a type III defect, with round, cystic-like appearances (*white arrow*). Axial PD fat sat (*B*) demonstrates its lateralized position (*discontinuous white arrow*). Note the superior ramus fracture (*arrowhead*) and trochanteric bursitis (*solid arrowhead*) in this patient, scanned after trauma.

was significantly large (by 10%) in the group that had pits, but they did not find a correlation between the presence of herniation pits and morphologic indicators of pincer FAI.

In the frontal plane, the normal angle between the femoral neck and shaft ranges between 115 and 140° (average 135°). Coxa valga occurs when there is an increased femoral neck-shaft angle. Internal or external rotation can falsely simulate coxa valga. The femoral neck is normally anteverted relative to the femoral shaft, by approximately 15°. The femoral condyles are therefore internally rotated relative to the femoral neck.[9]

The lesser trochanter is located medially, in the inferior junction of the femoral neck and the femoral diaphysis and projects toward the posterior aspect. It is the site of insertion of the psoas and iliacus. The greater trochanter is lateral, located in the postero-superior junction of the neck and diaphysis, and has four different facets, for the insertion of the gluteus minimus and medius, and the origin of the obturator internus and piriformis (**Fig. 3**).

Acetabulum

The acetabulum is the confluence of the ischium (inferior and lateral), ilium (superiorly), and pubis (medially), at the triradiate cartilage. At the anteroinferior margin, the rim is not complete, with a gap known as the acetabular notch. The acetabulum provides coverage for 170° of the surface of the femoral head.

The three bones are sites of insertion of multiple muscles around the hip (as described in **Table 1**).

Joint Cartilage

The acetabulum is nearly circumferentially covered in cartilage, with the exception of the acetabular fossa. The appearances resemble a crescent moon, hence the name lunate cartilage. The femoral head is covered in cartilage, except for the fovea capitis. These points are the origin and insertion of the ligamentum teres.

The cartilage is thicker along the superior aspect of the joint, which represents the greater weight-bearing area for all range of movements of the hip.

Imaging the cartilage in the hip is challenging, due to its curvature, the fact it is globally thin and to the narrow joint space in normal anatomic circumstances. Fluid is what allows "contrast" to identify irregularities in the surface or defects. Normal cartilage has an intermediate-to-high signal on fluid-sensitive images. Sequences to analyze internal structure have been developed (T2 mapping) but the assessment is still challenging.

A supraacetabular fossa is a normal variant, located in the acetabular roof, at about 12 o'clock, which may be mistaken for an osteochondral defect. This is seen in up to 12.6% of the population.[10] A recent study has shown among pediatric patients, this is most frequent in adolescents, with a prevalence that declines with increasing age, supporting this could represent a developmental variant.[10] The supraacetabular fossa has smooth margins and does not display bone marrow edema or surrounding cartilage irregularity, characteristics that differentiate it from an osteochondral lesion (**Fig. 4**).

The stellate crease is another focal area that is not covered with hyaline cartilage, located in the inner margin of the acetabular cartilage, close to the superior aspect of the acetabular fossa[11] (**Fig. 5**).

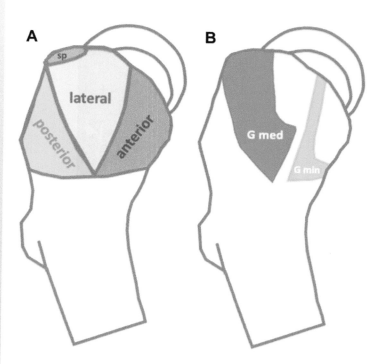

Fig. 3. The greater trochanter in a sagittal view. (*A*) Anatomy of the four facets (sp, superoposterior). (*B*) Footprints of the gluteus medius (G med) and gluteus minimus (G min).

The Labrum

The labrum is a fibrocartilaginous ring in continuity with the edge of the acetabulum, which blends inferiorly with the transverse acetabular ligament, that bridges through the acetabular notch, turning it into a foramen. The transverse ligament acts in fact as a functional part of the labrum, completing the circle with its strong flattened fibers.

The labrum increases in depth the socket (approximately by 21%),[12] with a larger area of joint surface (28% larger). This also reduces mechanical stress on the articular cartilage by absorbing shock. Without the labrum, the articular cartilage is subjected to increases in contact stress of up to 92%. The labrum also helps to enhance joint lubrication, by forming a seal about the femoral head that maintains a trace of joint fluid under negative pressure within the joint space.[13]

The configuration of the labrum is inhomogeneous[14] when it comes to shape, with variations in the thickness of up to 2 to 3 mm. In the anterior quadrant, it is the widest, in the posterosuperior is the thickest and it is the thinnest anteroinferiorly. Anatomically, it has a basal layer, a stratiform layer, and a superficial layer. There is a transition zone (1 to 2 mm) between the fibrocartilaginous labrum and the hyaline cartilage, at the chondrolabral junction. Normal cartilage may be interposed between the labrum and acetabular rim, seen as a smooth focus of intermediate to high signal intensity.[12]

The chondrolabral junction is the point from where delamination injuries progress.

The labrum is a poorly vascularized structure, the best-perfused region being the outer rim (0.5 mm, outer third), supplied by the capsule. This means healing capacity is low. The innervation is supplied by branches of the nerve to the quadratus femoris and the obturator nerve.

Labral injury may be the result of the detachment of the labrum from the adjacent acetabulum or represent intrinsic tears in the labral substance. Detachment is characteristic of cam-type FAI, and intrasubstance tears are common in pincer FAI and dysplasia.

In the case of detachment, MR imaging shows a fluid or contrast-filled (in MRA) cleft between the labral base and the acetabulum (chondrolabral junction) which may extend partially or fully through the labrum. These are the most common type. Intrinsic tears are more heterogeneous in MR imaging appearances, mainly appearing as irregularity in morphology and diverse patters of increased signal intensity or linear clefts.[15] Both types of tears may occur at the same time.

There is a strong association between perilabral abnormalities (chondral lesions, perilabral cysts) and labral tears. It has been reported that 73% of patients with labral tears also had chondral damage, which was also more severe than the damage seen in the context of no labral tear. In the case of a labral tear, 94% of times the chondral

Table 1
The muscles around the hip and their function

Muscle	Origin	Insertion	Function	Innervation	Particularities
A. Abductors					
Gluteus medius	Arises laterally from the wing of the ilium	Lateral and superoposterior facet of the greater trochanter	Abduction at hip joint Anterior portion assists in flexion and medial rotation. Posterior portion assists in extension and lateral rotation	Superior gluteal nerve (L4, L5, and S1)	Has three portions, anterior, middle, and posterior. Extremely important to maintain frontal plane stability.
Gluteus minimus	External surface of the ilium	Anterior facet of the greater trochanter	Abduction of the hip	Superior gluteal nerve	
Tensor fascia latae	Anterosuperior iliac spine (ASIS), anterior aspect iliac crest	Iliotibial band (with gluteus maximus), Gerdy tubercle	Stabilization of hip and knee. Abductor with gluteus medius and minimus. Accessory flexor of hip and knee	Superior gluteal nerve.	Involved in lateral snapping syndrome and IT band syndrome. Denervation in vitamin B12 deficiency.
B. Adductors					
Adductor longus	Anterior aspect of pubic body, inferior to pubic crest	Linea aspera femur, between brevis and magnus	Hip adductor External, lateral rotation, flexion	Obturator nerve	
Adductor brevis	Body of the pubis and inferior pubis rami	Linea aspera (above longus)	Hip adductor, flexor	Obturator nerve	In between anterior and posterior divisions of obturator nerve.
Adductor magnus	Adductor part: inferior ramus pubis and ischiatic ramus Hamstring part: ischial tuberosity	Adductor part: Posterior surface proximal femur, linea aspera, medial supracondylar line Hamstring part: adductor tubercle medial condyle femur	Thigh flexion, medial rotator. Extension and lateral rotation. Adductor of the thigh	Adductor part: Obturator nerve Hamstring part: sciatic nerve	Adductor and hamstring function

(continued on next page)

Table 1
(continued)

Muscle	Origin	Insertion	Function	Innervation	Particularities
Gracilis	Inferior ischiopubic ramus, body of the pubis	Medial tibia, pes anserinus	Adducts thigh, flexes the knee, medial rotation of femur and tibia	Obturator nerve	May be used in reconstruction surgery of the ACL. Smaller volume of the gracilis and sartorius in women and greater volume of vastus medialis predisposes to ACL injury, compared with men.
Pectineus	Pectineal line pubis	From base of the lesser trochanter to linea aspera	Adducts and flexes the thigh at the hip	Femoral and obturator nerve	
Obturator externus	Ramus of the surface of the pubis and ischium as well as from the external surface of the obturator membrane	Trochanteric fossa on the medial aspect of the greater trochanter.	Rotates hip during neutral and flexion. Stabilizer of the femoral head during flexion and internal rotation	Obturator nerve	Fibers pass laterally along the inferior margin of the acetabulum, acting like a sling at the inferior part of the neck. Hip joint stabilizer so preservation reduces risk of dislocation after total hip replacement (THR). There is an impingement syndrome related to transverse acetabular ligament release placing acetabular cup, happens at the inferior margin of the acetabulum.

C. Extensors and external rotators

Muscle	Origin	Insertion	Action	Innervation	Comment
Gluteus maximus	Posterior third of the iliac crest and the dorsum of the sacrum and coccyx	Iliotibial band and in the posterior margin of the femur just below the level opposite the lesser trochanter	Extensor, abductor and lateral rotator of thigh	Inferior gluteal nerve (L5, S1, and S2)	Paramount for standing from sitting position and to maintain erect position.
Piriformis	Anterior aspect of the sacrum S2 to S4. Sacrotuberous ligament, periphery of the greater sciatic notch	Superior and medial aspects of the greater trochanter	Lateral rotation of the hip abduction on flexion	Sacral plexus (L5, S1, and S2)	Divides the gluteal region into superior and inferior. Relationship with the sciatic nerve, this is normally inferior. (piriformis syndrome)
Obturator internus	Inferior margin of superior pubic ramus, pelvic surface of the obturator membrane	Greater trochanter of the femur	Lateral rotation, abduction. Stabilizes hip	Obturator internus nerve (L5, S1, and S2)	Goes through lesser sciatic foramen. Hip joint stabilizer so preservation reduces risk of dislocation after THR.
Superior gemellus	Outer surface of the spine of the ischium	Blends in with the obturator internus tendon	External rotation of the hip	Obturator internus	Deep stabilizer hip joint with inferior, obturator internus, and piriformis
Inferior gemellus	Ischial tuberosity	Blends in with the obturator internus tendon	External rotation of the hip. Dynamic stability to the hip joint	Nerve to Quadratus femoris (L4, L5, and S1)	Deep stabilizer hip joint with superior, obturator internus, and piriformis
Quadratus femoris	Lateral border ischial tuberosity	Quadrate tubercle on intertrochanteric crest	External rotation of the hip, assists in adduction. Stabilizes femoral head in acetabulum	Nerve to Quadratus femoris	Stabilizes femoral head in acetabulum. Closely related to the lesser trochanter, the femur and the ischium. Excessive friction might cause tears or impingement.

(continued on next page)

Table 1
(continued)

Muscle	Origin	Insertion	Function	Innervation	Particularities
D. Flexors					
Iliopsoas	Psoas major: Twelfth thoracic and five lumbar vertebrae Iliacus: iliac fossa of the ilium	Lesser trochanter	Flexion and external rotation of the thigh at the hip joint.	Iliacus: femoral nerve (L2 to L4) Psoas major: anterior rami of spinal nerves	Exits the pelvis and may be seen beneath the femoral vessels, medial to the iliacus. Closely related with the iliopectineal eminence, acetabular rim, anterior labrum, and femoral head. Repetitive movement may cause labral injury.
Sartorius	ASIS	Proximal tibia (pes anserinus)	At the hip it flexes, weakly abducts, rotates laterally. At the knee, flexor, with leg flexed rotates leg medially	Femoral nerve	Pelvic stabilizator, mainly in women, through constrictive effect on symphysis pubis
Rectus femoris	Direct anterior, or straight: anterior inferior iliac spine Indirect posterior, or reflected: lateral margin of the supra-acetabular surface and acetabular rim	Quadriceps tendon, superior pole of patella.	Hip flexion Knee extension	Femoral nerve	The tendon is anterolateral to the iliofemoral ligament and follows the lateral rim of the acetabulum

Muscle	Origin	Insertion	Action	Nerve	Comments
Pectineus	Iliopubic ramus, pectineal line	Distal to the lesser trochanter	Thigh adductor and flexor	Femoral nerve / Obturator nerve	
E. Hamstrings					
Semimembranosus	Superolateral aspect of the ischial tuberosity, beneath the proximal half of the semitendinosus muscle	Distal semimembranosas complex: Direct—posteromedial tibia, Anterior—medial collateral ligament, Oblique popliteal ligament, Capsular arm (toward posterior oblique ligament), Meniscal arm, Popliteus muscle	Hip extensors, Knee flexors, In knee flexion prevents external rotation, in knee extension prevents valgus	Tibial division sciatic nerve	Stabilizes knee (posterior capsule). Actively pulls the posterior horn of the medial meniscus, protects it from being crushed in flexion. Also traction effect over posterior horn external meniscus
Semitendinosus	Semitendinosus tendon and the long head of the biceps tendon form a conjoined tendon that arises from a medial impression on the superior aspect of the ischial tuberosity	Pes anserinus	Hip extensors, Knee flexors, Internal rotation when knee is flexed.	Tibial division sciatic nerve	More superficial than the semimembranosus. Used in ACL reconstructions (together with gracilis sometimes)
Biceps femoris	Long head: Medial impression on the superior aspect of the ischial tuberosity, conjoined tendon with semitendinosus. Short head: linea aspera, lateral supracondylar line of the femur	Fibular head, lateral aspect	Hip extensors, Knee flexors	Long head: tibial division sciatic nerve, Short head: peroneal division sciatic nerve	Contribution to arcuate ligament. (Posterolateral corner of the knee). Contributes to varus and rotatory stability of the knee.

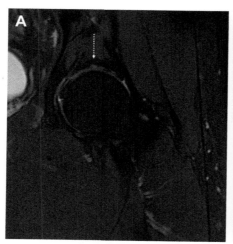
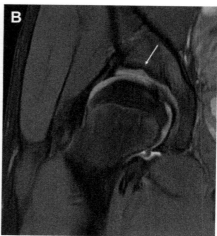

Fig. 4. A supraacetabular fossa is a normal variant, located in the acetabular roof, at about 12 o'clock depicted in a coronal PD fat sat image of the left hip of a 51-year-old (*A*). This may be mistaken with an osteochondral defect (*dotted arrow*). Coronal PD fat sat (*B*) in a 14-year-old boy demonstrates the supraacetabular fossa covered in normal cartilage (*bold arrow*).

damage occurred in the vicinity of the labral tear. The relative risk of a chondral lesion double if there is a labral lesion.[16] Isolated tears are more common in young people, with chondral lesions in association with labral tears are more common in the older population.

Labral Variation

The labrum may have variable shape, symmetry, and signal intensity on MR studies. The most common shape is triangular, reported in 66% to 69% of asymptomatic hips. Round (11%–16%) and flat (9% to 13%) configurations are not as common.[17] A systematic review of normal anatomic variation detected on MR imaging gave a similar rank of frequencies.[18] Absence of the labrum has been reported as high as 14%, but a study in a large group of asymptomatic patients suggested this was lower, approximately 3%.[17] It is likely some are mistaken by hypoplastic anterior labra (**Fig. 6**). The incidence of triangular labra decreases with increasing age, whereas the incidence of rounded, irregular margins increases with age.[19,20]

Fig. 5. The stellate crease is a focal area not covered with hyaline cartilage, located in the inner margin of the acetabular cartilage (coronal PD fat sat image), close to the superior aspect of the acetabular fossa (*arrow*).

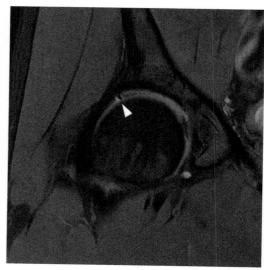

Fig. 6. Coronal PD fat sat depicting a hypoplastic anterosuperior labrum (*arrowhead*).

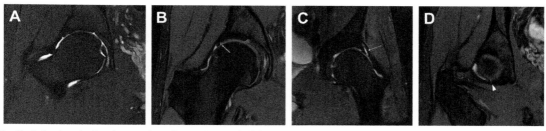

Fig. 7. Labral variation (coronal PD fat sat images). (*A*) Normal labrum. (*B*) Sublabral sulcus located posterosuperiorly (arrow). (*C*) Perilabral sulcus (*dotted arrow*). (*D*) The transverse ligament-labral junction sulcus is located in the anterior and posterior aspects where the transverse ligament is attached to the labrum. In this case it is showed in a posterior location (*arrowhead*)

When both hips in a patient without symptoms are compared, labral shape may differ between sides as much as 15%, and size 25%.[20]

The signal intensity of the labrum may also be variable.[17,19–21] In 44% to 56% of asymptomatic hips the labrum is hypointense in all sequences; however, the intermediate signal on T1 and proton density (PD)-weighted images was reported in 58% of asymptomatic hips, intermediate signal on T2 weighted images in 37% and high signal on T2 in 15%. This occurs more commonly in the superior and anterior aspects of the labrum, and may be due to the presence of small intralabral fibrovascular bundles or in the case of T1-weighted imaging, magic angle effect.[22] The region of increased signal may appear rounded, linear or curvilinear, and in some cases extend to the labral margins. This is more common with increasing age, and poses a challenge for differential diagnosis with a tear, which can be elucidated with intraarticular contrast.

A sulcus is located where the labrum meets the adjacent cartilage. In the asymptomatic hip there are several sulci that constitute normal variants. These are the sublabral sulcus, transverse ligament—labral junction sulcus and perilabral sulcus (**Fig. 7**).

Sublabral sulci may be present in as many as 25% of patients, and located in any anatomic position.[10] The systematic review by Kwee and colleagues, which included 24 studies in symptomatic patients reports a prevalence of 5% of sublabral sulci in these cases.[18] They are more frequent in the posterosuperior aspect (48%), anterosuperior (44%), and less common in the anteroinferior and posteroinferior (4%, respectively).[23] These sulci may be mistaken for tears, especially in the cases of the anteriorly located ones, which coincides with the most frequent location for a labral tear.

Sulci may be differentiated from tears based on their appearances, location, and the presence of perilabral abnormalities.

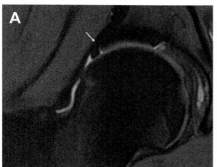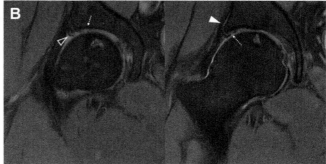

Fig. 8. Comparison of a sublabral sulcus with a labral tear. (*A*) Posterosuperior labral sulcus (*arrow*) in a coronal PD fat sat image (note there is a stellate crease also present). Sulci may be differentiated from tears based on their appearances, location and the presence of perilabral abnormalities. Note the smooth edges and absence of perilabral abnormalities. (*B*) Complex labral tear seen in coronal PD fat sat consecutive slices. In a more anterior plane (*left*) the labrum appears irregular and demonstrates increased signal intensity (*void arrowhead*). The adjacent acetabular cartilage demonstrates surface irregularity and thinning (*dotted arrows*). In a more posterior plane (*right*), a chondrolabral cleft is present with a slither of fluid signal tracking underneath the ligament attachment (bold arrowhead). The acetabular cartilage is noted to be irregular (dotted arrow). The patient had sequelae of an avascular necrosis (seen as foci of hyperintense bone marrow signal in the femoral head)

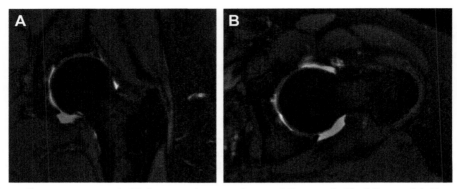

Fig. 9. Absent ligamentum teres in T1 fat sat arthrogram images (*A*) coronal, (*B*) oblique axial. Note the foveal indentation is not present in the head, there is only a mild foveal appearances in the cartilage in oblique axial. There is no synovial sheath present.

Sulci have smooth edges, whereas tears tend to be irregular. As described, most sulci are located anterosuperior or posterosuperiorly, and are less common in the inferior aspect. Most labral tears occur anteriorly or anterosuperiorly, the posterosuperior and anteroinferior are less common locations, and the posteroinferior rare.[24] The presence of perilabral abnormalities is seen in the context of tears and not sulci (**Fig. 8**).

The anterior labral sulcus, the most difficult to differentiate because of its location, is normally located at 4 o'clock (taking 3 o'clock as anterior, which is the most common nomenclature. The authors in this article take 9 o'clock as anterior and describe the sulcus as located at 4 o'clock), is linear and shows partial separation, with no perilabral abnormalities.[25]

The transverse ligament-labral junction sulcus is located in the anterior and posterior aspects where the transverse ligament is attached to the labrum. This may be seen in the anterior junction in 33% of asymptomatic hips and may be mistaken for a labral tear or detachment.[26] Labral tears are typically located slightly more superiorly (sulcus more inferior). An adjacent periligamentous recess anteromedial to the ligamentum teres is often seen with this normal sulcus.[26]

The perilabral sulcus is the space between the joint capsule and the labrum in the superior aspect. At this point the capsule inserts several millimeters above the labral base, whereas at the anterior and posterior margins, the capsule attaches directly at the base of the labrum. The presence of joint fluid in this space may mimic the existence of a perilabral cyst.[26,27]

The anterosuperior cleft is a partial extension of fluid into the undersurface of the anterior labrum on coronal and sagittal images. It has been seen as associated with mild developmental dysplasia of the hip.[10]

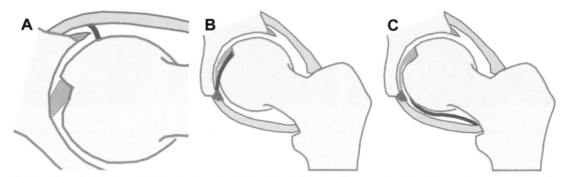

Fig. 10. Plicae in the hip. (*A*) Labral plica, located at the inferomedial aspect of the labrum (represented in the oblique axial plane). (*B*) Ligamentous plica located within the acetabular fossa at the acetabular attachment of the ligamentum teres. (*C*) Femoral neck plica, along the anterior joint capsule. The latter is the most commonly detected one, present in 95% of individuals.

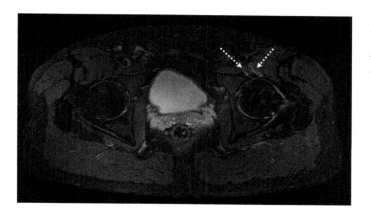

Fig. 11. Axial DP fat sat demonstrates fluid within the iliopsoas bursa on the left (*dotted arrows*). The bursa surrounds the tendon and may have a "U-shaped" configuration on axial images.

The Capsule and Ligaments

The joint capsule of the hip is different from capsules in other anatomic locations in the sense that is not elastic. Proximally, this is attached to the acetabulum, labrum, and transverse ligament, and covers the femoral head and most of the neck, to attach distally at the base of the trochanters.

The joint is externally reinforced by thickenings of the capsule, the iliofemoral (anteriorly), ischiofemoral (posteriorly) and pubofemoral (relatively weaker, also anterior) ligaments. These ligaments increase stability and restrict motion beyond normal range, protecting the joint from edge loading.[12,28]

A deep layer of circular fibers at the femoral neck, known as zona orbicularis constitutes a locking ring and aids to resist joint distraction.[28]

The acetabular ligament, the transverse acetabular ligament and the ligamentum teres, are intracapsular ligaments and provide extra support and function.

The ligamentum teres is intraarticular, and has a pyramidal morphology. Extends from its basal attachment as two bands on the acetabular notch and transverse ligament to the fovea capitis in the femoral head. It is covered by a synovial layer. The ligament has a smooth contour and on MR is homogenous in low signal intensity on all sequences, or mildly heterogenous with striations or bundles. Magic angle effect may be seen at the femoral insertion.[29]

The foveal artery runs with the ligament, and this contributes to vascularization of the head.

Sometimes, only the synovial sheath may be present, with no detectable ligament, ad in some cases neither of the structures is visible (**Fig. 9**).

The ligament is anatomically comparable to the anterior cruciate ligament of the knee, with two bands that have their origin in the acetabular

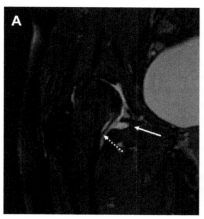
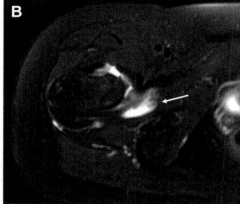

Fig. 12. The obturator externus bursa acts as a joint recess, a protrusion of the synovium. (*A*) Coronal PD fat sat showing fluid within the obturator externus bursa (*arrow*). Note the pectineofoveal fold (*dotted arrow*). (*B*) The bursa seen on the axial plane (axial PD fat sat) (*arrow*) It is located between the tendon of the obturator externus as it descends posterior to the femoral neck and the posterior hip capsule.

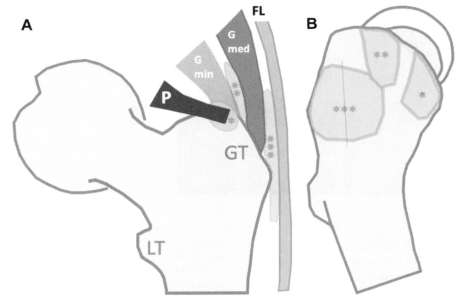

Fig. 13. Bursae around the hip. Seen in the coronal plane (*A*) the trochanteric (***) is the most superficial, located between the fascia lata (FL) and the gluteus medius (G med). The subgluteus medius bursa (**) is located deep to the gluteus medius tendon. The subgluteus minimus bursa (*) is located deep to the tendon of the gluteus minimus (G min), and posterior to the insertion of the pectineus (P). In the sagittal plane (*B*) the bursae approximately correspond to the trochanteric facets. GT, greater trocánter; LT, lesser trochanter.

transverse ligament and the pubic and ischial margins of the acetabular notch.

The function of the ligament is to stabilize the hip in adduction, flexion, and external rotation.[29]

Within the joint, there are several plicae. There is a ligamentous plica located within the acetabular fossa at the acetabular attachment of the ligamentum teres, a labral plica at the inferomedial margin of the labrum, and the femoral neck

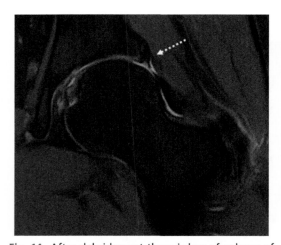

Fig. 14. After debridement there is loss of volume of the labrum, and the normal triangular morphology is lost, with the free margin appearing slightly irregular and blunted (*dotted arrow*). The chondrolabral junction should remain intact.

plica (pectinofoveal), along the anterior joint capsule. The pectineofoveal fold is the most commonly detected one, present in 95% of individuals, as a thickening of the medial capsule[30] (**Fig. 10**).

Bursae

There are several bursae around the hip.

The iliopsoas or iliopectineal bursa is intimately related to the anterior aspect of the hip joint, beneath the musculotendinous portion of the psoas. It has a communication with the hip joint in 10% to 15% of adults.[12] It is a very large bursa that extends to the iliac brim (**Fig. 11**).

The obturator externus bursa acts as a joint recess, a protrusion of the synovium. It is located between the tendon of the obturator externus as it descends posterior to the femoral neck and the posterior hip capsule (ischiofemoral ligament) (**Fig. 12**).

Around the greater trochanter, the trochanteric bursa is the most superficial. The subgluteus medius bursa lies underneath the gluteus medius tendon and the subgluteus minimus is located underneath the gluteus minimus tendon (**Fig. 13**).

Muscles

The muscles around the hip and their functions are summarized on **Table 1**.

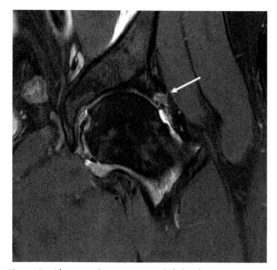

Fig. 15. Abnormal postsurgical labral appearances. The normal labral morphology cannot be defined, the presumed remnant appears hyperinense and irregular in shape (*arrow*). There is sinovitis in the medial joint recess. The presence of fluid signal within the labrum itself suggests recurrent tear or degeneration.

Neurovascular Bundle

The hip and thigh are vascularized by branches of the deep femoral artery, the gluteal and the obturator artery. The most important supply comes from the deep femoral artery, which are the medial circumflex and the lateral circumflex. In some cases, there is vascularity from the femoral artery.

The supply provided by the artery of the ligamentum teres is minimal.

The sciatic nerve is the largest nerve in the body, it may reach 2 cm in width.[31] It is a continuation of the sacral plexus and travels out of the pelvis through the sciatic notch, inferior to the piriformis.

POSTSURGICAL APPEARANCES
Postsurgical Labrum

After debridement, there is a loss of volume of the labrum, and the normal triangular morphology is lost, with the free margin appearing blunted.

The signal of the labrum should be low in T1- and T2-weighted images. The chondrolabral junction should remain intact in the residual labrum.

If suture banding o reattachment has been carried out, the volume of labral tissue should be similar to preoperative appearances. Morphology may not remain triangular and become irregular[32] (**Fig. 14**). The residual labral tissue should be closely attached to the acetabular rim. The suture material may have a mildly increased signal for up to months.

Complications include recurrent tears. The presence of interposed contrast or fluid signal between the labrum and the acetabulum or within the labrum itself suggests recurrent tear or detachment (**Figs. 15 and 16**). Occasionally, anchors may displace.

The development of adhesions may also occur. These appear as thin, fibrous lines between the labrum and capsule.

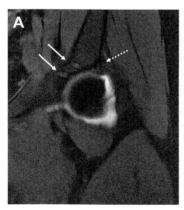
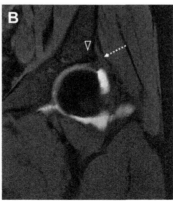
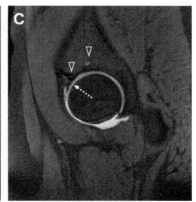

Fig. 16. Normal expected appearances of a reattached labrum on MR arthrogram. (*A*) Coronal T1 fat sat with intra articular gadolinium dilution at an anterior level demonstrates the tunnels for the anchors (*solid arrows*) and a portion of the labrum, which maintains the expected low signal (*dotted arrow*). There is no fluid cleft between the acetabular rim and the labrum. (*B*) Same sequence in a slightly more posterior plane demonstrates the end of the tunnel for a third anchor in the superior acetabular rim (*arrowhead*) and how there is continuity with no fluid cleft between the acetabular rim and the labrum (*dotted arrow*). An osteochondroplasty has also been performed (note notched appearance of femoral head and neck junction). (*C*) Sagittal coronal T1 fat sat with intra articular gadolinium dilution also demonstrates continuity in the chondrolabral junction with no interposed fluid (*dotted arrow*). The drilled tunnels of the anchors are partially visible (*arrowhead*).

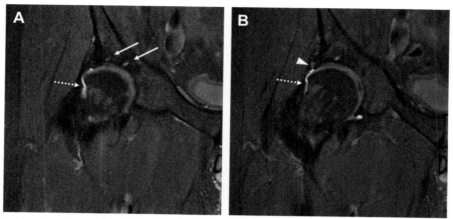

Fig. 17. Osteochondroplasty changes, shown in coronal DP fat sat. (*A*) On a more anterior plane, the acetabular anchors of labral reattachment are evident (*solid arrows*). After osteochondroplasty, the femur normally displays a focal notched defect at the site of cam deformity resection (*dotted arrow*). It has sharply demarcated contours. (*B*) a more posterior plane demonstrates continuity of the defect. The reinserted labrum is closely attached to the acetabular rim, with no interposed fluid signal intensity (expected appearances) (*arrowhead*).

Obliteration of the paralabral sulcus can be expected as a normal finding postsurgery.[33]

The mainstay for postsurgical labral evaluation is MR arthrography.

Postsurgical Changes after Treatment of Femoroacetabular Impingement

Impingement may be addressed through an open or arthroscopic approach.

Common surgical hip-preserving interventions are acetabuloplasty, osteochondroplasty, periacetabular osteotomy, and derotational femoral osteotomy.

Osteochondroplasty and acetabuloplasty are performed to address cam and pincer deformities. The goal is to restore normal morphology, by removing excess bone.[34]

In osteochondroplasty, the femur normally displays a focal notched defect at the site of bony prominence (cam deformity) resection. It has sharply demarcated contours. It has been established that in general, 30% of the diameter of the femur can be removed without risk of post intervention fracture (**Fig. 17**).

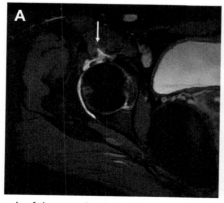
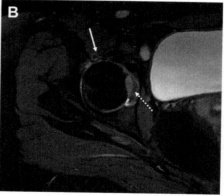

Fig. 18. Breach of the capsule after arthroscopy. (*A*) Axial DP fat sat image a week after arthroscopy and debridement of the ligamentum teres in the right hip demonstrates the presence of a small amount of fluid anteriorly in the joint, with indistinct margins to the capsule and fluid around the iliopsoas tendon (*solid arrow*). The ligament teres demonstrates mild thickening in increase in signal intensity. Recent postsurgical subcutaneous tissue edema is evident anteriorly. (*B*) Axial DP fat sat 4 months later demonstrates progressive healing of the anterior capsule, with slight residual thickening (*solid arrow*). The patient had ongoing pain after arthroscopy. Note the change in appearances of the ligamentum teres, which now appears thicker and more hyperintense, suggesting a partial tear (*dotted arrow*).

Table 2
Potential post arthroplasty complications

Potential Post Arthroplasty Complication	Expected Postsurgical Appearances	Pathologic Appearances
Loosening	• The flange of the femoral stem should sit flush with the cut surface of the femoral shaft • Stress shielding of the proximal femur refers to local bone demineralization due to the alleviation of normal weight-bearing stresses. Some degree of radiographically evident stress shielding is common and clinically acceptable; in advanced cases can increase the risk of periprosthetic fracture. • A distal femoral cement restrictor plug may be used, to prevent distal cement migration so that adequate contact with the prosthesis may be optimized. A small focus of entrapped gas may be visualized and should not be confused as the consequence of infection. • Bone scintigraphy with 99mTc-labeled methylene diphosphonate (99mTc-MDP) is a sensitive, although nonspecific, modality for determining aseptic loosening Increased tracer uptake, consistent with increased marginal osteoblastic activity, is considered physiologic for up to 12 mo after surgery.	• Alteration in component position when compared with prior radiographs. • Motion on stress views • Lucency adjacent to the femoral stem should be described with reference made to the standardized Gruen zones • Radiographic assessment of the acetabulum is difficult because of its shape, and loosening is best evaluated with CT • On bone scintigraphy with 99mTc-labeled methylene diphosphonate (99mTc-MDP) Uptake after 12 mo postsurgery is reflective of microinstability and therefore diagnostic of loosening, typically occurring medial to the inferior aspect of the femoral stem and at the greater trochanter (uptake may also be seen in infection)
Dislocation	More common using the traditional posterior approach, now minimized with the standard lateral (Hardinger) approach.	Immediate postsurgical: Due to lax pseudocapsule (inadequate pseudocapsule formation) Leak of contrast agent may be seen. After 3 mo: Generally due to acetabular malposition (excessive anteversion >20° or inclination >60°). After 5 y: Progressive pseudocapsule laxity, more common in elderly women. No leakage is seen, consistent with progressive, chronic stretching.

(*continued on next page*)

Table 2
(continued)

Potential Post Arthroplasty Complication	Expected Postsurgical Appearances	Pathologic Appearances
		Postoperative abductor muscle avulsion results in the loss of dynamic hip stability and is a risk factor for dislocation. MR imaging, US, and CT may be used to visualize the integrity of the abductor muscles and sequelae of avulsion.
Infection		• The radiographic signs of infection may be identical to those of mechanical aseptic loosening. • Radiographic abnormality developing rapidly and with an aggressive appearance favors the diagnosis of infection (rapidly developing osseous erosions and periosteal reaction) • MR imaging is useful to assess cellulitis, abscesses, sinus tracts, fistulas, periprosthetic collections, osteomyelitis, and signs of septic arthritis. • CT is also sensitive for similar pathology involving the soft tissues, including intrapelvic extension and psoas muscle involvement. • US also is particularly sensitive for evaluating soft tissue collections or joint effusions and may be used for guidance in performing arthrocentesis. It is reliable to distinguish a hematoma or abscess from a seroma. Power and color flow Doppler imaging enables the detection of hyperemia indicative of inflammation, which would favor an infected effusion or collection. • PET CT is sensitive but nonspecific in some cases. Abnormal increased glucose metabolism consistent with infection occurs in the prosthesis-bone interface along the femoral component. Increased glucose metabolism around the head and neck of the prosthesis is nonspecific, because it may be normal or seen in aseptic loosening or liner wear.

(continued on next page)

Table 2
(continued)

Potential Post Arthroplasty Complication	Expected Postsurgical Appearances	Pathologic Appearances
Acetabular liner wear Normally involves the superior, weight-bearing aspect	• The femoral head should be demonstrated radiographically to be equidistant between the superior and inferior margins of the acetabular cup on the anteroposterior radiograph.	• Eccentric positioning of the femoral head, resulting in a decrease in distance between the femoral head and superior margin of the acetabulum. • Increase in distance between the femoral head and inferior acetabular margin.
Particle disease Owing to shedding of submicron particles from the prosthetic component at the joint implant interfaces secondary to microscopic wear, with subsequent phagocytosis of particulate debris by macrophages stimulating a foreign body response and chronic, granulomatous inflammation. Occurs typically 1–5 y after arthroplasty.		• Osteolysis first occurs where joint fluid lies in contact with bone and may then progress around the cement-bone interfaces in cemented total hip arthroplasty and around the metal-bone interfaces in cementless total hip arthroplasty. • Early detection is critical, because the condition is asymptomatic until substantial bone loss has occurred, complicating future surgical options. • Presence of lucency at the prosthesis/bone (or bone/cement) interface, in the setting of acetabular liner wear, is consistent with the diagnosis. Lytic, expansile lesions with smooth endosteal scalloping (difference with mechanical loosening which is linear) • CT and MR imaging are sensitive modalities in detecting osteolytic foci due to particle disease, as well as associated local soft tissue collections (Extension to the pelvis or skin implies infection) • US can be used to guide diagnostic aspiration.
Metallosis and related conditions Abnormal buildup and deposition of metallic debris into the periprosthetic soft tissues and adjacent bone from the weight-bearing surface of metal on metal joint replacements Risk factors: • Female • Small prosthetic cup size • Small and large femoral head size	Range for acetabular component inclination: 35–55° Range for cup anteversion: 10–30°. Optimal valgus angle of the femoral component: 135–145° or within 15° of the anatomic neck.	• Positioning of the prosthesis along with acetabular inclination should be noted on plain radiographs may highlight patients at increased risk of complications. • The pathologic process primarily involves the soft tissues rather than bone. – Periprosthetic fluid collections – Pseudotumor formation – Soft tissue necrosis

(continued on next page)

Table 2
(continued)

Potential Post Arthroplasty Complication	Expected Postsurgical Appearances	Pathologic Appearances
• Poor positioning of components		– Aseptic lymphocytic vasculitis-associated lesions – Metallic debris may produce a radiodense line outlining the joint capsule or periprosthetic tissues in severe cases, producing the so-called metal bubble or metal line sign. CT: Periprosthetic collections or masses, along with high attenuation metallic debris. MR imaging: solid and cystic masses arising from anterior, posterior, and lateral aspects of the hip joint. Mild increased signal intensity in comparison to normal skeletal muscle on T1. The cystic lesions demonstrate fluid signal intensity on T2-weighted imaging; however, areas of reduced T2 signal intensity may be seen due to metal deposition. US: useful to guide arthrocentesis in patients with periprosthetic fluid collections. Aspiration of periprosthetic fluid typically reveals a thick black fluid.
Periprosthetic fracture May occur after prosthesis revision, or in uncemented prosthesis.		• Typically occur at the tip of the femoral stem, often preceded by an area of increased cortical thickening or "stress riser" • Periprosthetic fracture involvement of the acetabulum is uncommon.

Heterotopic bone formation
  Common
  Rarely clinically significant
Risk factors
• Ankylosing spondylitis
• Diffuse idiopathic skeletal hyperostosis
• Past history of heterotopic ossification
		• If extensive enough, heterotopic ossification may result in complete ankylosis
		• Confirmation of stability or maturation of the ossification is important, early surgery may worsen the extent of ossification. Radiological stability of 3 mo is consistent with quiescence.

Iliopsoas impingement occurs secondarily to an oversized acetabular cup	• Acetabulum should overhang for <12 mm on CT	• Overhanging of more than 12 mm on CT with compatible clinical presentation • MR imaging and US: Effusion, iliopsoas bursitis. Loss of normal tendon signal or fibrillar echogenicity. US allows dynamic assessment, with *(continued on next page)*

Table 2 (continued)		
Potential Post Arthroplasty Complication	**Expected Postsurgical Appearances**	**Pathologic Appearances**
		appearance of a snap or loss of normal movement over the margin of the acetabular component.

In acetabuloplasty, the acetabular rim trim may not be appreciated on radiographs, perhaps only noticeable as a mild change in contour.[35]

Radiographs and CT are useful to assess the degree of residual bony impingement, to assess the amount of bone removed.

Associated labral tears may be repaired, or the labrum may be resected.[32]

Complications include incomplete or excessive resection of bone. Incomplete resection will lead to persistent symptoms and excessive resection may lead to dislocation in the case of acetabuloplasty or fracture in the case of osteochondroplasty.[34]

Other potential complications are nonhealing (as always when there is an osteotomy), infection, and for arthroscopic approaches, avascular necrosis (AVN).[35]

Postsurgical Appearances after Ligamentus Teres, Chondral, and Capsular Repair

Ligament teres injuries are normally treated with debridement, with good results. Repair is an option that may be feasible. In a small subset of high-demand patients with hip instability that is refractory to standard arthroscopic management, reconstruction may be indicated.[36] may be debrided, repaired or reconstructed.

In the case of reconstruction, MR imaging has not yet been fully validated as means of assessment of the integrity of the graft, and arthroscopy is needed.[37] In general, if the ligamentum teres are repaired, there may be residual uniform decreased T2 signal intensity as a normal finding.[38] Recurrent tears may occur and will be better visualized with MR arthrography (**Fig. 18**).

Imaging of chondral repair is challenging, given MR arthrography does not correlate well with arthroscopy in the hip. Studies comparing MR arthrography to arthroscopic findings[39] open surgery[40] or the combination of both[41] found a sensitivity of 47% to 79% and specificity from 77% to

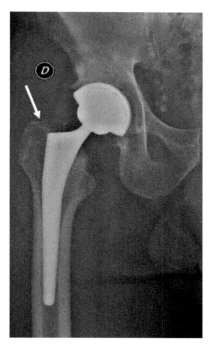

Fig. 19. Stress shielding of the proximal femur refers to local bone demineralization due to the alleviation of normal weight-bearing stresses (*arrow*). Some degree of radiographically evident stress shielding is common and clinically acceptable.

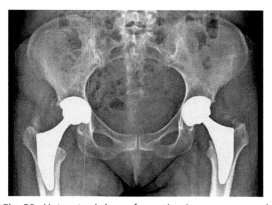

Fig. 20. Heterotopic bone formation is a common and rarely clinically significant situation after arthroplasty. Note the slightly asymmetrical radiolucency around the acetabular component of the left total hip replacement. Radiographic assessment of the acetabulum is difficult because of its shape, and loosening is best evaluated with CT.

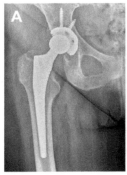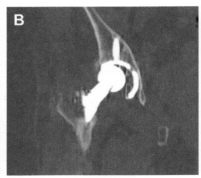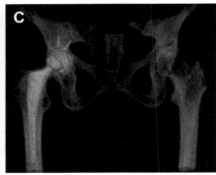

Fig. 21. Acetabular liner wear. This normally involves the superior, weight-bearing aspect. (*A*) AP radiograph. In normal circumstances, the femoral head should be demonstrated radiographically to be equidistant between the superior and inferior margins of the acetabular cup on the anteroposterior radiograph. In this case, it appears slightly eccentrical, closer to the superior margin of the acetabulum. (*B*) CT, coronal reconstruction and (*C*) 3D reconstruction highlighting the implants a year later shows wear of the acetabular liner, with progression of the eccentric location of the femoral head component, now in contact with the metallic cover at the superior aspect of the acetabular component.

89%. The negative predictive value is still 59%, so MR arthrography cannot rule out chondral lesions.[39]

If microfracture has been used, the presence of bone marrow edema in subchondral regions may be expected in the first few months. In general, it is important to assess for the integrity of cartilage and also compare it with presurgical imaging to assess potentially significant extra cartilage loss.[42]

After arthroscopic repair of the capsule (thermal capsulorrhaphy or plication with sutures), the capsule appears thicker and there may be foci of magnetic susceptibility artifact on MR imaging (see **Fig. 18**).

Postsurgical Appearances in Arthroplastic Hip Surgery

The evaluation with radiographs should be the first line in the postsurgical hip. It provides an overall assessment of the joint. Cross-sectional imaging is useful for disease confirmation and evaluation of severity and extent.

In the context of arthroplasty, mild changes in radiographs may be indicative of loosening/hardware failure. Radiologic assessment should include the entire prosthetic device in at least two planes, extending beyond the hardware by several centimeters, to cover adjacent soft tissues, bones, and cement restrictors.

Radiographs present the advantage of being able to show signs of most types of complications and allow serial comparison. In general, CT and MR imaging with metal artifact reduction sequences are reserved for more complex cases.

Loosening is the most common cause for revision of arthroplasty, followed by osteolysis (particle disease) and infection.

The imaging of complications of hip arthroplasty is summarized in **Table 2**[43–47] (**Figs. 19–21**).

SUMMARY

Detailed knowledge of anatomy helps to understand the pathologic processes and their expected findings around the hip. Familiarity with the most typical variants avoids misdiagnosis.

The correct understanding of the different types of surgical management approaches and the knowledge of the normal expected postsurgical appearances is extremely helpful in the assessment of potential postsurgical complications.

CLINICS CARE POINTS

- Knowledge of the anatomy and biomechanics of the hip, including its particularities, normal variation and frequency of pathologic associations allows to understand the mechanisms of injury and provides a useful tool for accurate diagnosis and indications for treatment.

- Familiarity with the surgical procedures and normal postsurgical appearances and findings related to potential complications allows to provide relevant information to surgeons to favor a positive outcome for the patient.

REFERENCES

1. Petersilge C. Imaging of the acetabular labrum. Magn Reson Imaging Clin N Am 2005;13(4): 641–52, vi.
2. Frank JM, Harris JD, Erickson BJ, et al. Prevalence of Femoroacetabular Impingement Imaging Findings in Asymptomatic Volunteers: A Systematic Review. Arthroscopy 2015;31(6):1199–204.
3. Lyu SH, Kwak YH, Lee YK, et al. Correlation of Structural Bony Abnormalities and Mechanical Symptoms of Hip Joints. Hip Pelvis 2014;26(2):115–23.
4. Kwon HM, Cho BW, Kim S, et al. Acetabular labral tear is associated with high pelvic incidence with or without femoroacetabular impingement morphology. Knee Surg Sports Traumatol Arthrosc 2022.
5. Boldt FK, Fritz B, Zingg PO, et al. Osseous defect of the anteroinferior femoral head: is it associated with femoroacetabular impingement (FAI)? Skeletal Radiol 2021;50(9):1781–90.
6. Scorcelletti M, Reeves ND, Rittweger J, et al. Femoral anteversion: significance and measurement. J Anat 2020;237(5):811–26.
7. Pitt MJ, Graham AR, Shipman JH, et al. Herniation pit of the femoral neck. AJR Am J Roentgenol 1982;138(6):1115–21.
8. Panzer S, Augat P, Esch U. CT assessment of herniation pits: prevalence, characteristics, and potential association with morphological predictors of femoroacetabular impingement. Eur Radiol 2008;18(9): 1869–75.
9. Urfali FE, Tok S, Kuyubaşi SN, et al. Is there a correlation between the femoral anteversion angle and the elasticity of the hip muscles in cases of intoeing gait due to increased femoral anteversion angle? J Ultrason 2022;22(88):e28–32.
10. Vaeth D, Dietrich TJ, Wildermuth S, et al. Age dependent prevalence of the supraacetabular fossa in children, adolescents and young adults. Insights Imaging 2022;13(1):91.
11. Chang CY, Huang AJ. MR imaging of normal hip anatomy. Magn Reson Imaging Clin N Am 2013; 21(1):1–19.
12. Nguyen MS, Kheyfits V, Giordano BD, et al. Hip anatomic variants that may mimic abnormalities at MRI: labral variants. AJR Am J Roentgenol 2013; 201(3):W394–400.
13. Agten CA, Sutter R, Buck FM, et al. Hip Imaging in Athletes: Sports Imaging Series. Radiology 2016; 280(2):351–69.
14. Bharam S. Labral tears, extra-articular injuries, and hip arthroscopy in the athlete. Clin Sports Med 2006;25(2):279–92, ix.
15. Blankenbaker DG, De Smet AA, Keene JS, et al. Classification and localization of acetabular labral tears. Skeletal Radiol 2007;36(5):391–7.
16. McCarthy JC, Noble PC, Schuck MR, et al. The Otto E. Aufranc Award: The role of labral lesions to development of early degenerative hip disease. Clin Orthop Relat Res 2001;393:25–37.
17. Lecouvet FE, Vande Berg BC, Malghem J, et al. MR imaging of the acetabular labrum: variations in 200 asymptomatic hips. AJR Am J Roentgenol 1996; 167(4):1025–8.
18. Kwee RM, Kavanagh EC, Adriaensen MEAPM. Normal anatomical variants of the labrum of the hip at magnetic resonance imaging: a systematic review. Eur Radiol 2013;23(6):1694–710.
19. Abe I, Harada Y, Oinuma K, et al. Acetabular labrum: abnormal findings at MR imaging in asymptomatic hips. Radiology 2000;216(2):576–81.
20. Aydingöz U, Oztürk MH. MR imaging of the acetabular labrum: a comparative study of both hips in 180 asymptomatic volunteers. Eur Radiol 2001;11(4): 567–74.
21. Cotten A, Boutry N, Demondion X, et al. Acetabular labrum: MRI in asymptomatic volunteers. J Comput Assist Tomogr 1998;22(1):1–7.
22. Blankenbaker DG, Tuite MJ. The painful hip: new concepts. Skeletal Radiol 2006;35(6):352–70.
23. Saddik D, Troupis J, Tirman P, et al. Prevalence and location of acetabular sublabral sulci at hip arthroscopy with retrospective MRI review. AJR Am J Roentgenol 2006;187(5):W507–11.
24. Groh MM, Herrera J. A comprehensive review of hip labral tears. Curr Rev Musculoskelet Med 2009;2(2): 105–17.
25. Studler U, Kalberer F, Leunig M, et al. MR arthrography of the hip: differentiation between an anterior sublabral recess as a normal variant and a labral tear. Radiology 2008;249(3):947–54.
26. DuBois DF, Omar IM. MR imaging of the hip: normal anatomic variants and imaging pitfalls. Magn Reson Imaging Clin N Am 2010;18(4):663–74.
27. Petersilge CA. MR arthrography for evaluation of the acetabular labrum. Skeletal Radiol 2001;30(8): 423–30.
28. Wagner FV, Negrão JR, Campos J, et al. Capsular ligaments of the hip: anatomic, histologic, and positional study in cadaveric specimens with MR arthrography. Radiology 2012;263(1):189–98.
29. Cerezal L, Kassarjian A, Canga A, et al. Anatomy, biomechanics, imaging, and management of ligamentum teres injuries. Radiographics 2010;30(6): 1637–51.
30. Mak MS, Teh J. Magnetic resonance imaging of the hip: anatomy and pathology. pjr 2020;85(1): 489–508.
31. Singh KP, Singh P, Gupta K. Reference values for the cross-sectional area of the normal sciatic nerve using high-resolution ultrasonography. J Ultrason 2021;21(85):e95–104.

32. Crim J. Imaging evaluation of the hip after arthroscopic surgery for femoroacetabular impingement. Skeletal Radiol 2017;46(10):1315–26.

33. Kim CHO, Dietrich TJ, Zingg PO, et al. Arthroscopic Hip Surgery: Frequency of Postoperative MR Arthrographic Findings in Asymptomatic and Symptomatic Patients. Radiology 2017;283(3):779–88.

34. Mills MK, Strickland CD, Jesse MK, et al. Postoperative Imaging in the Setting of Hip Preservation Surgery. Radiographics 2016;36(6):1746–58.

35. Li AE, Jawetz ST, Greditzer HG, et al. MRI Evaluation of Femoroacetabular Impingement After Hip Preservation Surgery. AJR Am J Roentgenol 2016;207(2): 392–400.

36. Simpson JM, Field RE, Villar RN. Arthroscopic reconstruction of the ligamentum teres. Arthroscopy 2011;27(3):436–41.

37. O'Donnell J, Klaber I, Takla A. Ligamentum teres reconstruction: indications, technique and minimum 1-year results in nine patients. J Hip Preservation Surg 2020;7(1):140–6.

38. Alam S, Yousaf A, Alborno Y, et al. Edema of the Ligamentum Teres as a Novel MRI Marker for Non-Traumatic Painful Hip Pathology: A Retrospective Observational Study. Cureus 2022. https://doi.org/10.7759/cureus.23388.

39. Keeney JA, Peelle MW, Jackson J, et al. Magnetic resonance arthrography versus arthroscopy in the evaluation of articular hip pathology. Clin Orthop Relat Res 2004;429:163–9.

40. Schmid MR, Nötzli HP, Zanetti M, et al. Cartilage lesions in the hip: diagnostic effectiveness of MR arthrography. Radiology 2003;226(2):382–6.

41. Smith TO, Simpson M, Ejindu V, et al. The diagnostic test accuracy of magnetic resonance imaging, magnetic resonance arthrography and computer tomography in the detection of chondral lesions of the hip. Eur J Orthop Surg Traumatol 2013;23(3):335–44.

42. Dallich AA, Rath E, Atzmon R, et al. Chondral lesions in the hip: a review of relevant anatomy, imaging and treatment modalities. J Hip Preservation Surg 2019; 6(1):3–15.

43. Mulcahy H, Chew FS. Current concepts of hip arthroplasty for radiologists: part 1, features and radiographic assessment. AJR Am J Roentgenol 2012; 199(3):559–69.

44. Mulcahy H, Chew FS. Current concepts of hip arthroplasty for radiologists: part 2, revisions and complications. AJR Am J Roentgenol 2012;199(3): 570–80.

45. Lombard C, Gillet P, Germain E, et al. Imaging in Hip Arthroplasty Management Part 2: Postoperative Diagnostic Imaging Strategy. J Clin Med 2022; 11(15):4416.

46. Deshmukh S, Omar IM. Imaging of Hip Arthroplasties: Normal Findings and Hardware Complications. Semin Musculoskelet Radiol 2019;23(2):162–76.

47. Fritz J, Lurie B, Miller TT, et al. MR imaging of hip arthroplasty implants. Radiographics 2014;34(4): E106–32.

Imaging of Overuse Injuries of the Hip

Joe D. Baal, MD[a], Katherine L. Cecil, MD[a], Rina Patel, MD[a], Matthew O'Brien, MD[b], Kevin McGill, MD[a], Thomas M. Link, MD, PhD[a],*

KEYWORDS

• Hip • Overuse • Injury

KEY POINTS

- Overuse injuries of the hip are common, and clinical diagnosis may be difficult because of overlapping and nonspecific clinical symptoms. Imaging can play an essential role in guiding diagnosis and subsequent management.
- Femoroacetabular joint structural abnormalities result in various conditions, including femoroacetabular impingement, which can predispose patients to early development of osteoarthritis.
- Repetitive stress on the skeletally immature hip can result in apophyseal injuries.
- Notable nonosseous overuse hip pathologies include athletic pubalgia, trochanteric bursitis, and injuries involving the iliopsoas myotendinous unit.
- Timely diagnosis of overuse injuries of the hip can facilitate improved response to conservative measures and can prevent irreversible damage.

INTRODUCTION

As one of the human body's largest weight bearing joints, the hip is subject to overuse injuries resulting from repetitive movements from daily and athletic activities. Overuse injuries of the hip commonly present with pain and encompass a broad differential diagnoses, ranging from osseous, cartilaginous/articular, and soft tissue-based etiologies. Although specific diagnoses may be ascertained from clinical signs and symptoms, these are oftentimes nonspecific. As such, imaging plays a significant role in differentiating the different types of overuse injuries of the hip. Timely diagnosis is essential in providing appropriate management and preventing exacerbation of injuries. This review aims to highlight the most up-to-date knowledge regarding the imaging of common overuse injuries of the hip through a discussion of hip anatomy, biomechanics, and associated imaging findings.

Normal Anatomy of the Hip

The hip is a ball-and-socket joint comprised of the femoral head and the acetabulum. Both the femoral head and acetabulum are lined by a thin layer of hyaline cartilage (1.5–5.0 mm in thickness).[1] The central surface of the femoral head has a focal depression termed the fovea capitis, from which the ligamentum teres arises and courses inferiorly to attach to the transverse ligament. A fibrocartilaginous labrum attaches to the bony rim of the acetabulum, providing further stability. The labrum encompasses the entire femoral head except along the inferomedial aspect, which is bordered by the transverse ligament. The hip joint capsule is comprised of 3 major ligaments: the ischiofemoral, iliofemoral, and pubofemoral ligaments.[2] Superiorly, the hip capsule arises above the labrum, which creates a perilabral recess. Synovium lines the inner surface of the

Disclosures: The authors have no conflicts of interest regarding this study.
[a] Department of Radiology and Biomedical Imaging, University of California, 400 Parnassus Avenue, Box 0628, San Francisco, CA 94143, USA; [b] Diagnostic Radiology, Oregon Health & Science University, L340, 3181 SW Sam Jackson Park Road Portland, OR 97239, USA
* Corresponding author. 400 Parnassus Avenue, A-367, San Francisco, CA 94143.
E-mail address: Thomas.Link@ucsf.edu

Radiol Clin N Am 61 (2023) 191–201
https://doi.org/10.1016/j.rcl.2022.10.003
0033-8389/23/© 2022 Elsevier Inc. All rights reserved.

joint capsule, encompassing the articular cartilage of the acetabulum and femoral head as well as the ligamentum teres, acetabular labrum, and transverse ligament.[3]

ABNORMALITIES OF THE HIP JOINT
Femoroacetabular Impingement

Femoroacetabular impingement (FAI) is a pathomechanical process that results from abnormal contact between the acetabular rim and the proximal femur. Cam-type FAI results from an aspherical morphology of the femoral head with a bony overgrowth at the anterior superior aspect of the femoral head-neck junction, which causes damage to the anterosuperior labrum and cartilage during hip flexion. Pincer-type FAI is secondary to a prominent acetabular rim providing overcoverage of the femoral head, resulting in damage to the posteroinferior acetabulum.[4,5] The most common type of FAI is the mixed-type, which is a combination of the pincer- and cam-type mechanisms. Chronic microtrauma that results from FAI predisposes patients to early development of hip osteoarthritis. Corrective surgeries to reshape the abnormal femoral head-neck junction morphology in cam-type FAI or the acetabular rim prominence in pincer-type FAI are performed and effective in reducing clinical symptoms.[6] Imaging plays an essential role in the early diagnosis of FAI and visualizing associated abnormalities including labral tears and cartilage delamination.

Initial assessment with radiographs can reveal certain structural abnormalities related to FAI. Some radiographic findings for cam-type FAI include asphericity of the femoral head, abnormal concavity of the femoral head-neck junction (pistol grip deformity), or cyst formation at the femoral head-neck junction (synovial herniation pit) (Fig. 1A). An alpha angle (measured between a line drawn at the center of the femoral head along the femoral neck and a line from the center of the femoral head to the femoral head/neck transition point) greater than 50° can also be used to support the diagnosis of cam-type FAI.[7] Radiographic findings for pincer-type FAI include posterior acetabular wall deficiency and acetabular retroversion (cross-over sign) (Fig. 1B). A lateral center edge angle (angle between a vertical line crossing the femoral head center with another line directed to the lateral edge of the acetabulum) of greater than 39° indicates acetabular overcoverage and is associated with pincer-type FAI.[8]

In addition to confirming morphologic abnormalities seen on radiography, MRI can reveal secondary signs of FAI and is useful in the evaluation for associated damage to the labrum and cartilage. Small cystic changes along the femoral head-neck junction, also called synovial herniation pit, can be seen in approximately 30% of patients with FAI. Labral tears can occur with both cam- and pincer-type FAI. Specifically, anterosuperior labral tears are most common in the setting of (cam-type) FAI (Fig. 2).[9] Paralabral cystic changes are useful markers for an underlying labral tear. For cartilage damage, cam-type FAI has a predilection for the anterosuperior cartilage, while pincer-type FAI more commonly affects the posteroinferior cartilage. Early chondral damage may appear as a focal delamination and can later progress as a flap tear (carpet lesion).[10] During arthroscopy, the surgeon may see the so-called wave sign.

Proximal Femur Stress Injuries

Stress injuries are common overuse injuries in athletes, representing 0.7% to 20% of injuries in sports medicine clinics.[11] Femoral stress injury is a relatively uncommon type of stress injury, accounting for less than 10% of all stress fractures in athletes.[12] These injuries result from an alteration in the bone remodeling process, where the rate of bone resorption caused by repetitive submaximal stress exceeds the rate of bone deposition. In competitive athletics, these injuries tend to occur in lean sports where maintaining a lower body weight is viewed as a competitive advantage, such as long distance running or diving. This is also a consideration in aesthetic lean sports, such as figure skating and ballet, where appearance is part of the judging process,[13] and thus participants in these sports are at a higher risk of developing an eating disorder leading to malnutrition and bone insufficiency.

The clinical presentation of stress injuries may have an insidious onset, often mimicking other causes of hip pain. Rapid diagnosis is crucial, especially for femoral neck stress injuries that can lead to devastating season- or career-ending injuries, if not properly treated. These can progress to complete fractures with nonunion or osteonecrosis with possible permanent disability.[14] Initial evaluation with radiographs is generally insensitive for identifying an acute stress injury. They are, however, helpful for identifying more subacute and chronic injuries that can exhibit linear sclerosis (Fig. 3) and/or periosteal thickening.

Nuclear medicine bone scan is another diagnostic examination that can be helpful by identifying a focus of hypermetabolism at the site of

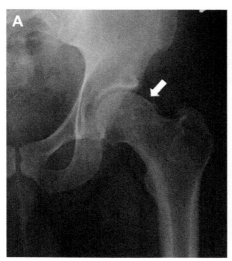
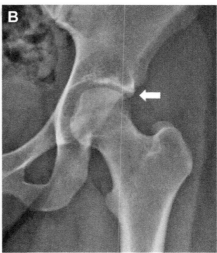

Fig. 1. (A) 30-year-old man with left hip pain. AP radiograph of the left hip demonstrating a mild pistol-grip morphology of the proximal femur (*arrow*), suggestive of cam-type FAI. (B) 24-year-old woman with left hip pain. AP radiograph of the left hip exhibiting acetabular retroversion with mild lateral acetabular overcoverage (*arrow*), suggesting underlying pincer-type FAI.

the stress injury. Although bone scans demonstrate high sensitivities of 74% to 84% for stress injuries, they also carry a considerable false-positive rate of over 30%.[15] The nuclear bone scan is also time-consuming and requires more

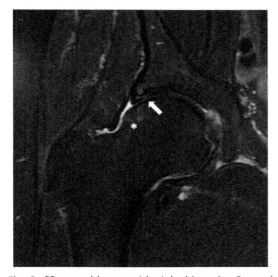

Fig. 2. 33-year-old man with right hip pain. Coronal T2-weighted fat-saturated MRI of the right hip showing osseous prominence of the lateral femoral head-neck junction (alpha angle 65°) with underlying bone marrow edema (*asterisk*). Degenerative antero-superior right labral tear and suggestion of cartilage delamination (*arrow*).

radiation than radiographs. There should be a low threshold for obtaining an MRI if a femoral neck stress injury is suspected. A standard hip MRI is highly sensitive for stress injuries and will also help by identifying additional underlying hip pathology. A grading system such as the one by Rohena-Quinquilla (**Table 1**)[16] can be used to help determine the time for return to activity. Other classification systems have been developed by Provencher[17] and Fullerton[18] to determine the role for surgical management. MRI will demonstrate edema on fluid-sensitive (fat saturated T2-weighted and STIR) sequences with a corresponding linear focus of low T1 signal. The medial aspect of the proximal femur is under compression, and the lateral aspect is under tension. Bone marrow edema pattern is seen on the compressive side in most cases but can also be present on the tension side. Compression side fractures involving less than 50% of the width and tension side stress changes without a fracture line can be managed conservatively with nonweightbearing and activity restrictions. Tension side stress injuries, compression injuries with greater than 50% involvement, or displaced fractures generally require surgical intervention.

Apophyseal Injuries

In the immature skeleton, the apophysis refers to a secondary ossification center that often forms an insertion point for a tendon or ligament. Given

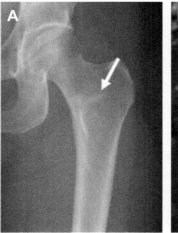 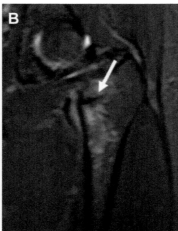 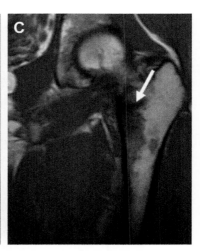

Fig. 3. 44-year-old woman recreational runner with left hip pain. (*A*) AP radiograph of the left hip demonstrates a focal area of linear sclerosis (*arrow*) at the medial base of the femoral neck suggestive of a stress injury. Coronal STIR (*B*) and T1 (*C*) weighted images of the left hip demonstrate a linear focus of hypointensity corresponding to the radiographic findings of the stress fracture (*arrow*) with adjacent bone marrow edema pattern.

the differential strength of the physeal cartilage compared with the attaching tendons and ligaments, the apophyses can be subject to injury from compounded stress from repetitive micro-trauma or overuse.[19]

Apophysitis refers to a traction injury and resultant inflammation of the physeal cartilage. On MRI, increased edema within the apophysis bone marrow and adjacent tendons can be seen on fluid-sensitive sequences. Slight widening of the associated physis can also be observed. In the pelvis, possible sites of apophysitis include the ischial tuberosity, the anterior inferior iliac spine, and the anterior superior iliac spine (**Fig. 4**). Although treatment for apophysitis is conservative, early diagnosis is essential to guide management and ensure preservation of the developing cartilage.[20]

Apophyseal avulsion injuries can occur in the setting of excessive forces from eccentric muscular contractions, often seen in adolescent patients who participate in organized sports.[21] Like apophysitis, avulsion injuries in the pelvis can occur at the ischial tuberosity, anterior superior/inferior iliac spine, greater trochanter, lesser trochanter and the iliac crest. Acute displaced avulsion injuries can be seen on radiographs as avulsed bone fragments. However, plain film diagnosis of avulsion injuries can be difficult in more chronic injuries where the injury can mimic aggressive pathology such as osteomyelitis or a bone tumor. Situations without a corresponding traumatic event may also present a diagnostic dilemma, such as in isolated avulsion fracture of the lesser trochanter in skeletally mature adults, which would be considered a pathologic fracture until proven otherwise.[22] In these situations, MRI can be useful in ruling out other pathologies and guiding appropriate management (**Fig. 5A, B**). On MRI, avulsion injuries will demonstrate osseous irregularity at the avulsion site. Reactive edema within the adjacent bone marrow and surrounding soft tissue may be visible on fluid-sensitive sequences (**Fig. 6A, B**).[23] Apophyseal avulsion fractures displaced less than 2 cm are treated conservatively, while those displaced greater than 2 cm are treated surgically.[24]

Table 1
MRI classification system for femoral neck stress injuries (FNSI) developed by Rohena-Quinquilla and colleagues[16]

FNSI Grade		MRI Findings
Low grade	1	Endosteal edema ≤ 6 mm
	2	Endosteal edema > 6 mm and no macroscopic fracture
High grade	3	Macroscopic fracture < 50% of femoral neck width
	4	Macroscopic fracture ≥ 50% of femoral neck width

Measurements are ideally performed in the coronal plane perpendicular to the long axis of the femoral neck and in the image that best displays the abnormality.

Reprinted from Femoral Neck Stress Injuries: Analysis of 156 Cases in a U.S. Military Population and Proposal of a New MRI Classification System, Rohena-Quinquilla IR, Rohena-Quinquilla FJ, Scully WF, Evanson JRL, AJR Am J Roentgenol. 2018;210(3):601–607. © 2018, the American Journal of Roentgenology.

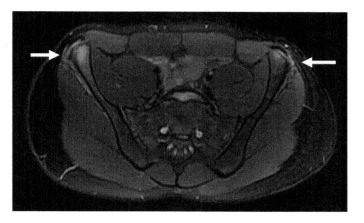

Fig. 4. 15-year-old boy with bilateral hip pain. Fat saturated T2-weighted axial MR image demonstrating fluid signal in the right greater than left anterior superior iliac spine at the insertion of the sartorius (*arrows*), compatible with apophysitis/apophyseal stress injury.

Athletic Pubalgia

Athletic pubalgia is a clinical term for lower abdominal and groin pain in athletes.[25–28] Many synonymous terms have been used with athletic pubalgia, including "sports or sportsman hernia." However, the term hernia should be avoided, as these are not true hernias.[27]

The definition of athletic pubalgia in the literature is not standardized and everchanging but encompasses a spectrum of pathology to the perisymphyseal structures ranging from chronic stress injury with bone inflammation (osteitis pubis) to injury to the musculotendinous structures of the lower abdomen and groin.[26] Many diagnoses may mimic or occur concomitantly with athletic pubalgia. Therefore, knowledge of the involved anatomy and subsequent imaging features is essential in timely diagnosis.

The anatomy at the pubis is complex with multiple muscle and tendon attachments. Of these structures, the rectus abdominis (RA) and adductor longus (AL) are the most important for stability. The RA and AL insertions merge with the periosteum to form a common RA-AL aponeurosis.[29]

Radiographs and large-field-of-view MRI (coronal T1, coronal STIR, axial FSE) identify pubic bone changes, concurrent findings of FAI, or alternate diagnoses like fractures. Small-field-of-view MR images in the plane of the pubic symphysis (axial/sagittal proton density, coronal T2 with fat saturation) are important to accurately assess complex pubic anatomy.[26,29] The small-field-of-view coronal oblique sequence is prescribed parallel to the anterior margin of the iliac crest (arcuate line) and is a sensitive sequence for evaluation of the RA-AL aponeurosis. Small-field-of-view sagittal oblique and axial oblique sequences based on the coronal oblique sequences are helpful for evaluating aponeurosis tears. Ultrasound is valuable in assessing soft tissue injuries, with the advantage of direct correlation with site of pain.[30] Dynamic evaluation with abduction and external rotation of the leg is also helpful in identifying tendon injuries on ultrasound.

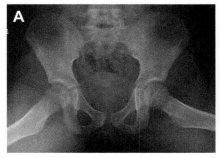
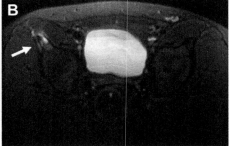

Fig. 5. 11-year-old boy with right hip pain. (*A*) Pelvic radiograph without definite evidence of acute osseous abnormalities in a patient with right hip pain. (*B*) Subsequent fat-saturated T2-weighted axial image of the pelvis reveals bone marrow edema pattern with increased signal along the right anterior inferior iliac spine, compatible with an apophyseal avulsion fracture at the insertion of the rectus femoris muscle (*arrow*).

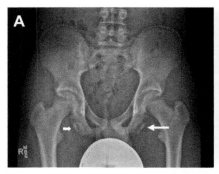
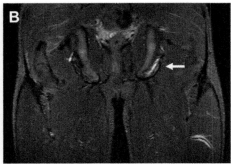

Fig. 6. (A) 14-year-old boy with left pelvic pain. Pelvic radiograph showing approximately 7 mm of separation of the left ischial tuberosity (*arrow*) and mild irregularity of the right ischial tuberosity (*smaller arrow*). (B) Subsequent STIR-weighted coronal image revealing fluid signal within the area of separation, compatible with acute minimally displaced avulsion fracture of the hamstring tendons (*arrow*). No abnormal T2 signal was observed on the right, indicating a more chronic process.

Imaging findings of athletic pubalgia include a range of musculotendinous injuries, such as muscle strain, tendinosis, calcification, tear, or avulsion (Fig. 7A–C).[26,29] Tears of the RA-AL aponeurosis appear as a superior cleft sign of fluid paralleling the inferior margin of the superior pubic ramus on MRI or ultrasound (Fig. 8).[30] Osseous changes, including bone marrow edema or bone productive changes, may be present. Given the wide range of pathology to the muscles/tendons, bone, and aponeurosis, the specific injury of each anatomic structure should be individually described.

Most injuries can be managed conservatively with rest, activity modification, or pain management.[25] If symptoms persist, ultrasound-guided interventions, such as fenestration for tendon pathology or corticosteroid injection for osteitis pubis, may be performed. Surgical intervention is usually reserved for tears of the RA-AL aponeurosis, and typically only in elite athletes.[26] Therefore, specific description of the integrity of the RA, AL, and aponeurosis is important to include in imaging reports.

Trochanteric Bursitis

Greater trochanteric pain syndrome, often clinically diagnosed as trochanteric bursitis, refers to chronic lateral hip pain that is exacerbated by active abduction and passive adduction of the hip, tenderness of the lateral hip on palpation, and pain when lying on the affected side at night.[31] Imaging findings encompass not only trochanteric bursitis but also the range of findings associated with tendinopathy and tear of the hip

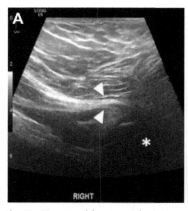
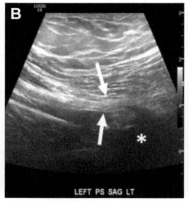
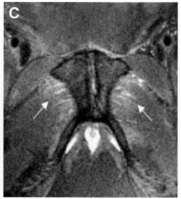

Fig. 7. 63-year-old man with right groin pain. Longitudinal ultrasound image of the right pubic bone (A) shows thin, uniformly hyperechoic rectus abdominis tendon insertion (*arrowheads*) at the pubic bone (*asterisk*) with no tendinosis or tear. Longitudinal ultrasound image of the left pubic bone (B) shows comparatively thickened, heterogeneously hypoechoic rectus abdominis tendon insertion (*thick arrows*), consistent with tendinosis. In the same patient, axial oblique T2 fat saturation MR image shows low grade strain of the adductor muscle insertion (*thin arrows*) without a tear.

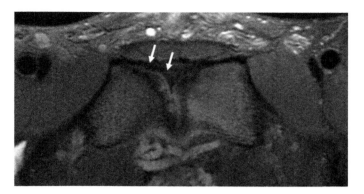

Fig. 8. 21-year-old male with right groin pain. Axial oblique T2 fat saturation MR image of the pubic symphysis shows a secondary cleft sign of linear T2 hyperintensity paralleling the right anterior pubic body (*arrows*), consistent with rectus abdominis-adductor longus aponeurosis tear.

abductors, gluteus minimus, and gluteus medius, in what has been described as rotator cuff tears of the hip. Of note, the gluteus minimus and gluteus medius inserts at the anterior and lateral aspects of the greater trochanter, while the gluteus maximus inserts along the gluteal tuberosity of the femur.[32]

The trochanteric bursal complex is comprised of the subgluteus maximus bursa, also known as the trochanteric bursa, and subgluteus medius bursa, with a minor subgluteus minimus bursa. These bursae are thought to act as cushions for the gluteal muscle tendons, the iliotibial band, and the tensor fascia latae, and play an important role in the progression of greater trochanteric pain syndrome commencing with bursitis secondary to impingement and progressing to gluteal tendinosis and tears.[32] Trochanteric bursitis can be described on ultrasound or MRI if there is fluid distension of the bursa (**Fig. 9**). Trochanteric bursitis most often coexists with gluteal tendinosis characterized by homogenous T2 hyperintensity and thickening, with possible

enhancement on MRI. Secondary features include calcification at the tendon insertion and bony cortical irregularity at the greater trochanter.[33] Ultrasound findings of tendinosis include thickening and hypoechogenicity within the gluteal tendons with loss of fibrillar architecture.

Focal and full-thickness gluteal tendon tears can also be evaluated on ultrasound and MRI. On ultrasound, a partial-thickness tear appears as intratendinous hypoechoic or anechoic foci or as tendinous contour defects, while a bald facet is suggestive of a full-thickness tear. MRI findings of a partial tear typically include circular or ovoid defects, most commonly in the gluteus minimus tendon extending to the adjacent part of the gluteus medius tendon and can involve the deep or superficial surfaces of the tendon or be seen as a longitudinal split or intrasubstance defect that may be filled with fluid (**Fig. 10**). Full-thickness tears can be diagnosed when complete tendon discontinuity or tendon retraction is apparent with a bald trochanter

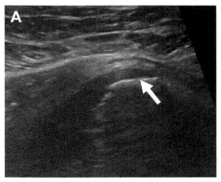
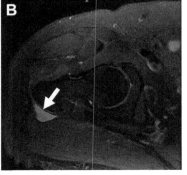

Fig. 9. 65-year-old male with right hip pain. (*A*) Coronal hip ultrasound showing anechoic fluid within the subgluteus medius bursa (*arrow*). (*B*) Axial oblique T2-weight image with fat saturation of the right hip shows large amount of trochanteric bursal fluid (*arrow*) compatible with trochanteric bursitis.

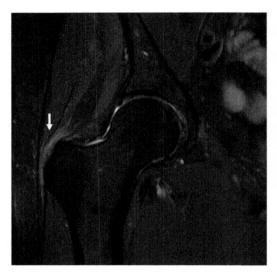

Fig. 10. 57-year-old woman with right hip pain. Coronal T2-weighted fat-saturated MRI of the right hip showing severe tendinosis and partial intrasubstance tear of the anterior fibers of the gluteus medius (*arrow*).

(Fig. 11).[34] Partial tears may occur in isolation but typically occur in a background of gluteal tendinosis.

These findings are important to identify in the work-up of lateral hip pain, as radiologists play a crucial role in conservative management by performing corticosteroid injections into the hip bursa.[35]

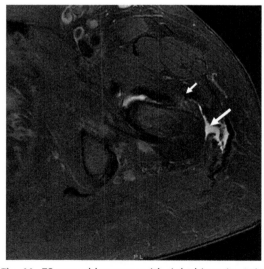

Fig. 11. 78-year-old woman with right hip pain. Axial T2-weighted fat-saturated MRI of the left hip showing complete tear of the gluteus medius tendon with retraction off the greater trochanter (bald trochanter) (*large arrow*). Additional partial tear of the gluteus minimus tendon (*small arrow*).

Iliopsoas Myotendinous Unit

The iliopsoas myotendinous unit consists of the iliacus muscle arising from the anterior iliac fossa and the psoas major muscle arising from the T5-L5 lateral elements.[36] The tendons often fuse at the acetabulum, although may remain bifid distally in up to 26% of patients.[37] These primary hip flexors are subject to elevated biomechanical stress as they glide over the anterior labrum and acetabulum, especially in various athletic activities.[38,39] The iliopsoas bursa tracks proximally from the hip between the tendon and bony undersurface and may communicate with the hip. Overuse-related pathologies of the iliopsoas myotendinous unity range from tendinopathy and tearing to bursitis, strain, snapping, and bursal distention from primary hip pathology.

Iliopsoas tendinopathy manifests clinically as pain with resisted hip flexion or passive stretching and can be challenging to diagnose.[40] MRI can show thickening with mildly hyperintense T1 and T2 tendon signal. The presence of internal T2 hyperintense fluid signal and frank tendon gapping suggests underlying tendon tear (Fig.12).[41] There is wide variance in return to activity depending on the type of tendon pathology.[38]

Iliopsoas bursal distention has colloquially been described as comma- or bubble-shaped on MRI and is seen as fluid tracking along the tendon (Fig. 13). Usually single, the bursa can be duplicate in patients with a distal bifid tendon. It may contain simple decompressed joint fluid, debris, hemorrhage, crystalline material, or synovitis depending on etiology. Iliopsoas bursal distention may be asymptomatic and does not necessarily imply active clinical bursitis.[42]

Snapping hip/coxa saltans is a clinical diagnosis but can be demonstrated with imaging, often coexisting with tendinopathy. The proposed pathophysiologic mechanism is related to the lateral position of the tendon during the FABER (flexion, abduction, external rotation) maneuver, with an interfering structure (eg, prominent anterior acetabular bony ridge, iliopsoas muscle bellies, bursal distention, arthroplasty hardware) preventing the hip from reaching a normal anatomic position. This results in growing tension on the tendon during reduction and subsequent abrupt release of this tension results in an audible, palpable, variably painful impaction of the tendon on the acetabulum. Although challenging, this can be shown with dynamic sonography, and historically with contrast

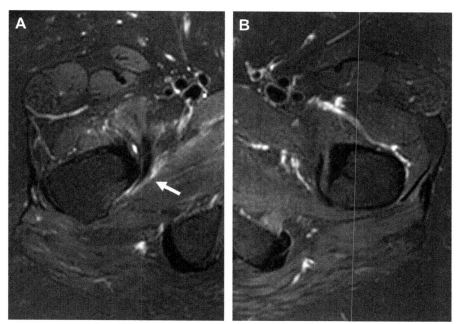

Fig. 12. 30-year-old woman with right hip pain. Axial T2-weighted fat-saturated MRI of both hips. (*A*) Mild thickening of the right distal iliopsoas tendon with isointense signal abnormality and peritendinous edema, compatible with iliopsoas tendinopathy/tendinosis (*arrow*). (*B*) Normal appearance of the left iliopsoas tendon.

fluoroscopy.[41] Conservative and definitive management options have shown success in long-term management, depending on patient population and underlying cause.

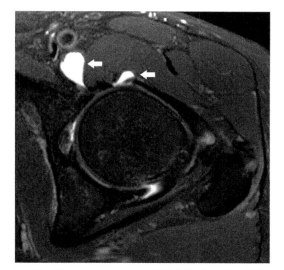

Fig. 13. 60-year-old woman with left hip pain. T2 fat-saturated axial image of the left hip with speech bubble appearance of iliopsoas bursal distention (*arrows*), which in this case was related to effusion from early osteoarthritis. Note the presence of medial and lateral lobules of bursal fluid, which is a somewhat uncommon bursal communication with the hip joint along both pubofemoral and iliofemoral ligaments, respectively.

SUMMARY

The hip is subject to overuse injuries from the many repetitive movements in daily life or athletic activities. A good understanding of the underlying anatomy of the hip and clinical presentation of the various overuse injuries of the hip can aid in diagnosis. However, given the nonspecific nature of symptoms that may present, imaging often plays a crucial role in recognizing these entities and guiding appropriate clinical management. Knowledge of the associated imaging signs and the appropriate use of different imaging modalities and protocols is essential for accurate diagnosis of overuse injuries of the hip.

CLINICS CARE POINTS

- In cases of FAI, MRI is useful for the assessment of secondary damage involving the labrum and the cartilage (predilection for the anterosuperior cartilage in CAM-type and posteroinferior cartilage in pincer-type FAI).
- Femoral stress injuries involving the tension side or greater than 50% involvement of the compression side generally warrant surgical evaluation.

- Apophyseal avulsion fractures displaced less than 2 cm are treated conservatively, while those displaced greater than 2 cm are treated surgically.
- Ultrasound is valuable in assessing soft tissue injuries with the advantage of direct correlation with the area of pain as well as dynamic evaluation of the involved structures.

REFERENCES

1. Hegazi TM, Belair JA, McCarthy EJ, et al. Sports injuries about the hip: what the radiologist should know. Radiographics 2016;36(6):1717–45.
2. Jesse MK, Petersen B, Strickland C, et al. Normal anatomy and imaging of the hip: emphasis on impingement assessment. Semin Musculoskelet Radiol 2013;17(3):229–47.
3. Chatha DS, Arora R. MR imaging of the normal hip. Magn Reson Imaging Clin N Am 2005;13(4):605–15.
4. Hodnett PA, Shelly MJ, MacMahon PJ, et al. MR imaging of overuse injuries of the hip. Magn Reson Imaging Clin N Am 2009;17(4):667–79, vi.
5. Banerjee P, Mclean CR. Femoroacetabular impingement: a review of diagnosis and management. Curr Rev Musculoskelet Med 2011;4(1):23–32.
6. Beaulé PE, Speirs AD, Anwander H, et al. Surgical correction of cam deformity in association with femoroacetabular impingement and its impact on the degenerative process within the hip joint. J Bone Joint Surg Am 2017;99(16):1373–81.
7. Rakhra KS, Sheikh AM, Allen D, et al. Comparison of MRI alpha angle measurement planes in femoroacetabular impingement. Clin Orthop 2009;467:660–5.
8. Tannast M, Siebenrock KA, Anderson SE. Femoroacetabular impingement: radiographic diagnosis-what the radiologist should know. AJR Am J Roentgenol 2007;188(6):1540–52.
9. Studler U, Kalberer F, Leunig M, et al. MR arthrography of the hip: differentiation between an anterior sublabral recess as a normal variant and a labral tear. Radiology 2008;249:947–54.
10. Pfirrmann CW, Mengiardi B, Dora C, et al. Cam and pincer femoroacetabular impingement: characteristic MR arthrographic findings in 50 patients. Radiology 2006;240:778–85.
11. Field AE, Gordon CM, Pierce LM, et al. Prospective study of physical activity and risk of developing a stress fracture among preadolescent and adolescent girls. Arch Pediatr Adolesc Med 2011;165(8):723–8.
12. Hulkko A, Orava S. Stress fractures in athletes. Int J Sports Med 1987;8:221–6.
13. Mancine RP, Gusfa DW, Moshrefi A, et al. Prevalence of disordered eating in athletes categorized by emphasis on leanness and activity type - a systematic review. J Eat Disord 2020;8:47.
14. Steele CE, Cochran G, Renninger C, et al. Femoral Neck Stress Fractures: MRI Risk Factors for Progression. J Bone Joint Surg Am 2018;100(17):1496–502.
15. Batt ME, Ugalde V, Anderson MW, et al. A prospective controlled study of diagnostic imaging for acute shin splints. Med Sci Sports Exerc 1998;30(11):1564–71.
16. Rohena-Quinquilla IR, Rohena-Quinquilla FJ, Scully WF, et al. Femoral neck stress injuries: analysis of 156 cases in a U.S. military population and proposal of a new MRI Classification System. AJR Am J Roentgenol 2018;210(3):601–7.
17. Provencher MT, Baldwin AJ, Gorman JD, et al. Atypical tensile-sided femoral neck stress fractures: the value of magnetic resonance imaging. Am J Sports Med 2004;32(6):1528–34.
18. Fullerton LR Jr, Snowdy HA. Femoral neck stress fractures. Am J Sports Med 1988;16(4):365–77.
19. Peck DM. Apophyseal injuries in the young athlete. Am Fam Physician 1995;51(8):1897–8, 1891-5.
20. Arnaiz J, Piedra T, de Lucas EM, et al. Imaging findings of lower limb apophysitis. AJR Am J Roentgenol 2011;196(3):W316–25.
21. Combs JA. Hip and pelvis avulsion fractures in adolescents. Phys Sportsmed 1994;22(7):41–9.
22. Bertin KC, Horstman J, Coleman SS. Isolated fracture of the lesser trochanter in adults: an initial manifestation of metastatic malignant disease. J Bone Joint Surg Am 1984;66(5):770–3.
23. Meyers AB, Laor T, Zbojniewicz AM, et al. MRI of radiographically occult ischial apophyseal avulsions. Pediatr Radiol 2012;42(11):1357–63.
24. Gidwani S, Jagiello J, Bircher M. Avulsion fracture of the ischial tuberosity in adolescents–an easily missed diagnosis. BMJ 2004;329(7457):99–100.
25. Kraeutler MJ, Mei-Dan O, Belk JW, et al. A systematic review shows high variation in terminology, surgical techniques, preoperative diagnostic measures, and geographic differences in the treatment of athletic pubalgia/sports hernia/core muscle injury/inguinal disruption. Arthroscopy 2021;37(7):2377–90.
26. Varada S, Moy MP, Wu F, et al. The prevalence of athletic pubalgia imaging findings on MRI in patients with femoracetabular impingement. Skeletal Radiol 2020;49:1249–58.
27. Zoga AC, Kavanagh EC, Omar IM, et al. Athletic pubalgia and the "sports hernia": MR imaging findings. Radiology 2008;247:797–807.
28. Omar IM, Zoga AC, Kavanagh EC, et al. Athletic pubalgia and "sports hernia": optimal MR imaging technique and findings. Radiographics 2008;28:1415–38.

29. Feeley BT, Powell JW, Muller MS, et al. Hip injuries and labral tears in the National Football League. Am J Sports Med 2008;36:2187–95.

30. Morley N, Grant T, Blount K, et al. Sonographic evaluation of athletic pubalgia. Skeletal Radiol 2016;45:689–99.

31. Segal NA, Felson DT, Torner JC, et al. Multicenter Osteoarthritis Study Group. Greater trochanteric pain syndrome: epidemiology and associated factors. Arch Phys Med Rehabil 2007;88:988–92.

32. Williams BS, Cohen SP. Greater trochanteric pain syndrome: a review of anatomy, diagnosis and treatment. Anesth Analg 2009;108:1662–70.

33. Chowdhury R, Naaser S, Lee J, et al. Imaging and management of greater trochanteric pain syndrome. Postgrad Med J 2014;90:576–81.

34. Cvitanic O, Henzie G, Skezas N, et al. MRI diagnosis of tears of the hip abductor tendons (gluteus medius and gluteus minimus). Am J Roentgenol 2004;182:137–43.

35. Lustenberger DP, Ng VY, Best TM, et al. Efficacy of treatment of trochanteric bursitis: a systematic review. Clin J Sport Med 2011;21:447–53.

36. Lifshitz L, Bar Sela S, Gal N, et al. Iliopsoas the hidden muscle: anatomy, diagnosis, and treatment. Curr Sports Med Rep 2020;19(6):235–43.

37. Crompton T, Lloyd C, Kokkinakis M, et al. The prevalence of bifid iliopsoas tendon on MRI in children. J Child Orthop 2014;8(4):333–6.

38. Tsukada S, Niga S, Nihei T, et al. Iliopsoas disorder in athletes with groin pain: prevalence in 638 consecutive patients assessed with MRI and clinical results in 134 patients with signal intensity changes in the iliopsoas. JB JS Open Access 2018;3(1):e0049.

39. Chopra A, Robinson P. Imaging athletic groin pain. Radiol Clin North Am 2016;54(5):865–73.

40. Haskel JD, Kaplan DJ, Fried JW, et al. The limited reliability of physical examination and imaging for diagnosis of iliopsoas tendinitis. Arthroscopy 2021;37(4):1170–8.

41. Bancroft LW, Blankenbaker DG. Imaging of the tendons about the pelvis. AJR Am J Roentgenol 2010;195(3):605–17.

42. Di Sante L, Paoloni M, De Benedittis S, et al. Groin pain and iliopsoas bursitis: always a cause-effect relationship? J Back Musculoskelet Rehabil 2014;27(1):103–6.

Imaging of the Acutely Injured Hip

Donal G. Cahill, BSc, BMBS, MRCPI, FFRRCSI[a], Max K.H. Yam, MBChB, FRCR[b],
James F. Griffith, MB, BCh, BAO, FRCR, MRCP (UK), FRCR (Edin), FHKAM (Radiology)[a],*

KEYWORDS

- Proximal femoral fracture • Insufficiency fracture • Pathological fracture • Atypical femoral fracture
- Gluteal tendon tear • muscle tear • Labral cyst leakage • Crystal desposition

KEY POINTS

- Clinical history and context are important when determining the likely cause of acute hip pain following an injury.
- Thereafter, assessment relies largely on imaging to isolate the specific cause of hip pain.
- A precise cause for hip pain can be identified in nearly all of the cases.
- Undertaking the most appropriate imaging test at the outset significantly increases efficiency in correctly identifying the cause of acute hip pain following an injury.

INTRODUCTION

Although some overlap exists, in general, the range of conditions resulting in acute hip pain following injury is different from that causing either acute hip pain in the absence of injury or chronic hip pain. In nearly all cases, imaging will precisely ascertain the cause and severity of acute hip pain following an injury, greatly assisting subsequent management. This imaging is discussed in this review.

Acetabular Fracture

Acetabular fracture is one of the most serious skeletal fractures and invariably follows severe trauma, irrespective of age. Although better management has improved patient outcomes, the mortality of pelviacatabular fracture is still approximately 10%, largely due to hemorrhage. Bleeding may be arterial or venous and from either direct vascular injury, oozing from the cut surface of bone, or soft-tissue injury. Arterial bleeding is treated by embolization, venous by pelvic ± retroperitoneal packing, and bone-cut surface oozing by fracture fixation.

Imaging. Computed tomography (CT) has greatly enhanced the diagnosis and assessment of pelvic fracture (**Fig. 1**). As time delay should be avoided, most severe trauma patients will proceed directly to contrast-enhanced CT examination following initial resuscitation.[1] Radiographs are less frequently performed during initial assessment nowadays. CT can, if necessary, provide a "radiographic view" similar to standard radiography.[2] CT allows accurate fracture detection and characterization as well as hematoma severity and concomitant visceral injury assessment. One commonly used classification system is the Judet–Letournel system (**Fig. 2, Table 1**). Examining the axial image at the level of the acetabular roof, determine if the acetabular component is a transverse, columnar, or wall fracture[1] (see **Fig. 1**). Thereafter, reformatted images will help more clearly determine the full fracture configuration[1] (see **Figs. 1** and **2**; **Fig. 3**). Active bleeding

The authors have nothing to disclose.
[a] Department of Imaging and Interventional Radiology, The Chinese University of Hong Kong, The Prince of Wales Hospital, Ngai Shing Street, Shatin, Hong Kong; [b] Department of Radiology, North District Hospital, 9 Po Kin Road, Sheung Shui, Hong Kong
* Corresponding author.
E-mail address: griffith@cuhk.edu.hk

Radiol Clin N Am 61 (2023) 203–217
https://doi.org/10.1016/j.rcl.2022.10.014

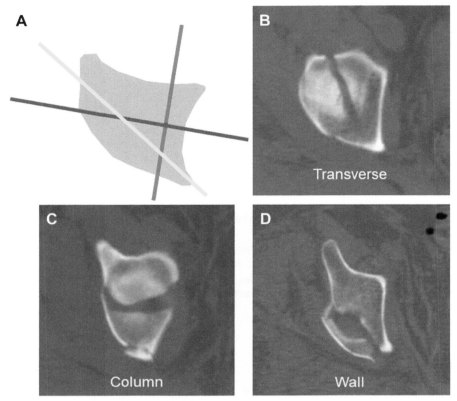

Fig. 1. At the level of the acetabular roof, determine if the elemental fracture is a transverse fracture (*red*), a column fracture (*blue*) or a wall fracture (*yellow*) (*A–D*).

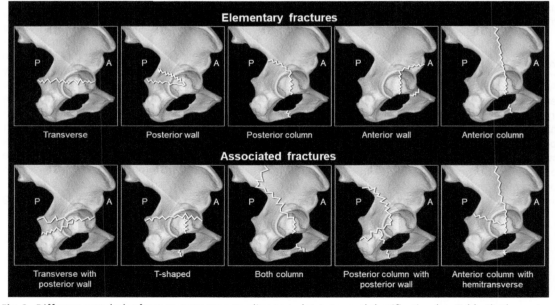

Fig. 2. Different acetabular fracture patterns according to Judet–Letournel classification (see Table 1). Elementary fractures are shown in the top row; associated fractures in the bottom row. A, anterior; P, posterior. Anterior column yellow, posterior column blue.

Table 1 Judet–Letournel classification of acetabular fractures	
Elementary fractures	A. Transverse
	B. Posterior wall
	C. Posterior column
	D. Anterior wall
	E. Anterior column
Associated fractures	A. Transverse with posterior wall
	B. T-shaped
	C. Both column
	D. Posterior column with posterior wall
	E. Anterior column with posterior wall
	F. Hemitransverse

Transverse (5%), posterior wall (20%), transverse with posterior wall (25%), T-shaped (10%), and both column (30%) account for 90% of fracture patterns encountered.

will not unusually be visible on CT due to tampo-nade, vasospasm, or hypotension. Embolization, with gelform or coils, is required in approximately 10% of patients with pelvic fracture to good effect. Hematoma location on pelvic CT provides a reliable indicator of the likely site of bleeding.[3]

Proximal Femoral Fracture

a. *Traumatic fracture of proximal femur.* Traumatic proximal femoral fractures tend to occur in two patient groups; younger patients with normal bone strength following high-energy trauma and older patients with reduced bone strength following either low-energy trauma or no

trauma.[4] The former are easy to identify clinically and radiographically, the latter (known as insufficiency or fatigue fracture) may be more problematic as a history of trauma is not invariably present.

Proximal femoral fractures are broadly classified as either intra- or extracapsular and displaced or non-displaced. Approximately 60% of proximal hip fractures are intracapsular and 80% of these are displaced.[5] As the main arteries supplying the femoral head, ascend from the medial and lateral femoral circumflex arteries along the femoral neck (**Fig. 4**), femoral head blood supply can be compromised by intracapsular fractures, particularly displaced fractures, potentially leading to avascular necrosis. Intracapsular fractures of the femoral neck may be sub-capital, transcervical, or basal (**Fig. 5**). Basal fractures do not typically lead to avascular necrosis and are often treated as extracapsular fractures.[6] Extracapsular fractures include intertrochanteric and subtrochanteric fractures (**Fig. 6**). Early fixation of intracapsular fractures in younger patients is warranted to minimize vascular compromise and the risk of non-displaced fractures becoming displaced.[6] Older patients are usually treated with total hip arthroplasty (THA), (when there is co-existent osteoarthritis) or hemi-arthroplasty.

Imaging. Frontal and lateral hip radiographs are usually adequate to identify proximal femoral fractures and classify the fracture subtype (see **Fig. 5** and see **6**). CT can help with more complex, comminuted fractures.

b. *Insufficiency (or fatigue) fracture of proximal femur.* Insufficiency fractures occur from normal

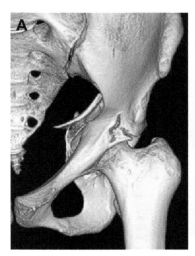
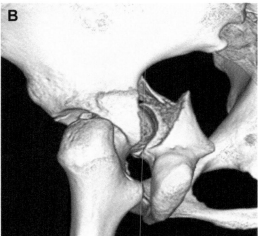

Fig. 3. DCT anterior (*A*) and posterior (*B*) views showing a transverse with posterior wall acetabular fracture.

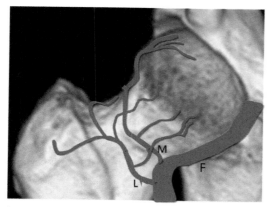

Fig. 4. Schematic diagram to represent that branches from the medial (M) and, to a lesser degree, the lateral circumflex arteries ascend on the surface of the femoral neck to supply the femoral head. The circumflex arteries usually arise from the profunda femoris artery (F).

stresses placed on bone of reduced bone strength. Insufficiency fractures are usually secondary to senile osteoporosis. Paget's disease, osteomalacia, renal osteodystrophy, hyperparathyroidism, and osteopetrosis are less common causes.

Imaging. Identification and classification of proximal femoral insufficiency fractures is primarily based on frontal and lateral hip radiographs (**Fig. 7**). Pertinent features to note are fracture location, displacement, comminution, as well as the degree of osteopenia. Approximately 5% of proximal femoral insufficiency fractures may be radiographically occult, that is, the fracture is not visible on radiographs (see **Fig. 7**A).[7] This radiographic nonvisibility is a result of reduced bone density, trabecular and cortical resorption, nondisplacement, and fracture impaction. In patients with clinically suspected proximal femoral fractures, and no fracture visible radiographically, MR imaging should be performed. MR imaging in this clinical setting will consistently reveal a proximal femoral fracture in approximately 40% of such patients (see **Fig. 7**C, D).[8] MR is also indicated in osteopenic patients with isolated greater trochanteric fractures on radiographs, as it will show radiographically occult intertrochanteric extension in a significant number of these fractures. If no proximal femoral fracture is present, MR imaging usually reveals another cause for hip pain, such as muscle strain or tear, unsuspected pubic rami, or acetabular fracture.[9] Only a limited MR imaging protocol comprising oblique coronal T1 spin echo and T2-fat-suppressed MR sequences is necessary.[10] Additional larger field-of-view (FOV) T2-fat suppressed axial imaging of the pelvis is helpful in identifying concomitant pelvic and sacral fractures. An alternative limited protocol is to undertake only large FOV T1- and T2-fat-suppressed coronal sequences of the pelvis and proximal femora.[11] This abbreviated sequence has no loss of accuracy for proximal femoral or pelvic fracture detection or classification, though is likely to compromise fracture depiction compared with smaller FOV imaging. MR sensitivity for the depiction of proximal femoral fractures is 100%. If access to MR imaging is limited, CT is a good alternative, with a sensitivity of 94% for occult femoral fractures.[12]

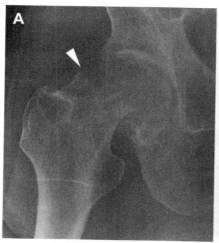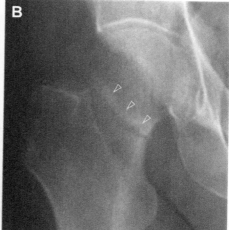

Fig. 5. Frontal hip radiographs demonstrating a moderately displaced subcapital fracture (*arrow*) (*A*) and a nondisplaced transcervical fracture (*arrowheads*) (*B*) of the femoral necks.

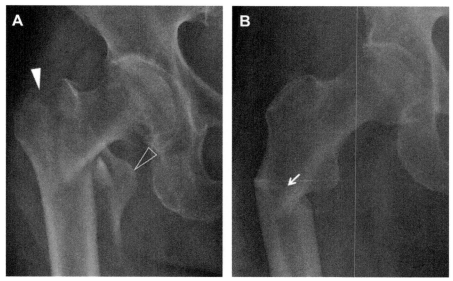

Fig. 6. Frontal hip radiographs showing a moderately displaced comminuted intertrochanteric fracture extending between the greater (*arrowhead*) and lesser trochanters (*open arrow*) (*A*) and a more distal moderately angulated subtrochanteric fracture (*arrow*) (*B*).

c. *Subchondral insufficiency fracture of femoral head.* Subchondral insufficiency fractures of the femoral head (SIFFH) often lead to the collapse of the articular surface.[13] This fracture is usually associated with osteoporosis.

Imaging. Subchondral insufficiency fractures are usually radiographically occult. Infrequently, a thin subarticular radiolucent line with a slight sclerotic rim ("crescent sign") may be seen though may also be a feature of osteonecrosis[14] (Fig. 8). Serial radiographs may show progressive femoral head flattening (Fig. 9A, B). Early MR imaging examination is very useful if SIFFH is clinically suspected. The earliest MR feature is pronounced subchondral bone marrow edema surrounding a thin, often subtle, serpiginous linear T1-hypointensity (see

Fig. 8B).[14] Histologically, this linear hypointensity is comprised of reparative callus and granulation tissue.[15] SIFFH can be confused with, and can co-exist with, osteonecrosis. Bone marrow edema is common in both conditions. Somewhat helpful distinguishing features are that (a) the linear T1-hypointensity in SIFFH tends to be incomplete and run more parallel to the articular surface, whereas the T1-linear hypointensity in osteonecrosis tends to be more complete, curvilinear, and convex to the articular surface and (b) SIFFH typically shows contrast enhancement both proximal and distal to the fracture line, whereas osteonecrosis will not show enhancement of devascularized tissue on the articular side of the fracture line. On T2-fat suppressed sequences, particular attention

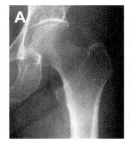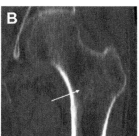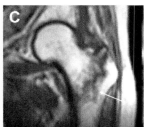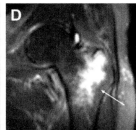

Fig. 7. Frontal radiograph of proximal femur shows osteopenia but no fracture in the elderly patient with clinically suspected proximal femoral fracture (*A*). Reformatted oblique coronal CT shows no fracture though hyperdense marrow signal suggestive of hemorrhage (*arrow*) (*B*). T1-weighted (*C*) and T2-weighted (*D*) fat-suppressed oblique coronal images clearly show a fracture line extending approximately 80% along the inter-trochanteric area with surrounding bone marrow edema (*arrows*). This was treated with screw fixation.

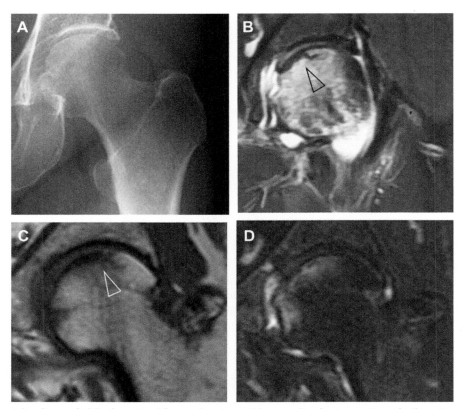

Fig. 8. Frontal radiograph (*A*) of proximal femur showing mild generalized osteopenia and otherwise normal appearances. T2-fat-suppressed oblique coronal MR image shows severe femoral head edema with hypointense subcortical fracture (*arrowhead*) (*B*). T1 oblique coronal (*C*) and T2-fat-suppressed oblique coronal MR images show that although the fracture is still apparent (*arrowhead*) (*D*), the bone marrow edema has nearly completely resolved indicative of a healing fracture.

should be paid to the marrow signal intensity between the linear hypointense line (seen on T1-weighted sequences) and the articular surface.[16] This marrow signal may be T2-hyperintense, heterogenous, or hypointense (see **Fig. 8**D). T2-hyperintense signal is associated with the shortest time between pain onset and MR imaging examination and indicates a good prognosis with a healing rate of approximately 85%.[16] If the T2-marrow signal is heterogenous, the healing rate is 75% and 20% if hypointense.[16] CT is more helpful with follow-up and prognostication rather than with initial diagnosis. CT may show a band of sclerosis or a radiolucent band in the area corresponding to the T1-hypointense line seen on MR (**Fig. 9**). Sclerosis is a good prognostic sign indicative of fracture healing, whereas an osteolucent band is a poor prognostic sign indicating peri-fracture osteolysis, which is likely to progress to articular surface collapse and possibly rapid destructive arthropathy (see **Fig. 9**B, C).[15] Early identification of SIFHH with MR imaging is key to a successful outcome.

d. *Atypical femoral fracture.* Atypical femoral fractures can occur anywhere along the femoral diaphysis from the lesser trochanter to the distal femoral metaphysis though most occur in the immediate subtrochanteric region (**Figs. 10** and **11**). Although atypical femoral fractures are most strongly associated with long-term (>3 years) bisphosphonate use, they can also be seen with denosumab treatment, with renal osteodystrophy, or occur de novo. Persons of Asian descent, those with inherent lateral femoral bowing, and varus hip geometry carry additional risk of atypical femoral fracture. Bisphosphonates bind to hydroxyapatite and induce osteoclast apoptosis leading to reduced bone remodeling ("adynamic bone disease"). This reduces the capacity of bone to repair day-to-day physiological microdamage. Even though the affected bone is hypermineralized (from osteoclastic inactivity), it is prone to fracture from microfracture accumulation and generalized increased bone brittleness.[17]

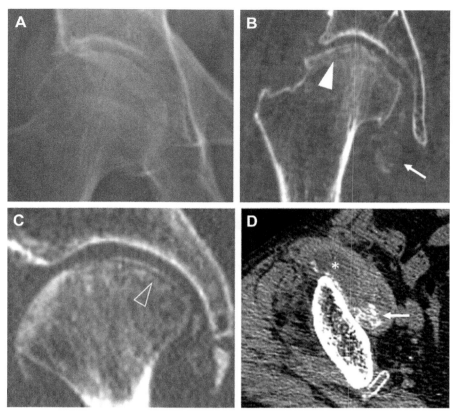

Fig. 9. Frontal radiograph of an 84-year-old man with hip pain. Frontal radiograph shows moderate osteopenia (*A*). There is no visible subchondral fracture of articular surface collapse. Oblique coronal reformatted CT image (*B*) 10 months later showing moderate diffuse articular surface collapse (*arrowhead*). There is calcific debris in the hip joint (*arrow*). Oblique sagittal reformatted CT showing subarticular crescent-shaped lucency (*arrowhead*) (*C*) Axial soft-tissue setting shows the distended iliopsoas bursa (*asterisk*) deep to the iliacus muscle containing calcific milieu (*arrow*). Ultrasound-guided hip joint aspiration (not shown) was negative for infection. This is compatible with rapid destructive arthropathy of the hip joint (*D*). The patient underwent THA soon after CT examination.

Imaging. Ideally, atypical femoral fractures should be detected at an early stage when only the lateral cortex is affected before a complete fracture occurs (see **Figs. 10A, B and 11A**). Patients may present with acute hip pain in the incomplete fracture stage, occasionally precipitated by injury. Bilateral involvement is common, so always examine the contralateral femur. Typically, one will see localized bony thickening ("beaking") of the lateral femoral cortex often with a radiolucent transversely orientated intracortical fracture.[18] The larger and sharper the beak, the greater the risk of imminent fracture. Also, fracture extension to >50% of the lateral cortical thickness increases fracture risk. The lateral femoral cortex is also diffusely thickened as a result of adynamic bone disease. Typically, the bone density is not osteopenic due to prolonged biphosphate therapy (see **Fig. 10**).

Complete atypical proximal femoral fractures usually occur either spontaneously or following even minimal trauma. They have a characteristic imaging appearance (see **Figs. 10C and 11B**). The lateral cortex is thickened. The sharp fracture line is orientated transversely or in a short oblique plane. The fracture is typically non-comminuted with a characteristic medial spike.[18]

Radiographic appearances are characteristic of both partial and complete fractures. Although additional imaging with either MR imaging or CT is not routinely indicated, they can be helpful in the incomplete fracture stage to assess fracture activity more closely. Specifically, CT will enable the lateral intracortical fracture to be appreciated more clearly to gauge healing once bisphosphonate therapy is discontinued. Similarly, the regression of peri-fracture edema on MR imaging provides a marker of fracture quiescence.

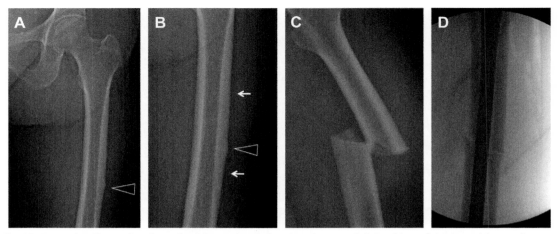

Fig. 10. Frontal radiographs of proximal femur (*A, B*) showing characteristic beaking of the lateral femoral cortex (*arrowhead*) with moderate thickening of the lateral femoral cortex (*arrows*) consistent with an incomplete atypical femoral fracture. Ten days later, a complete fracture occurred at this location (*C*). Fluoroscopic image on the following day shows surgical fixation with intramedullary rod (*D*).

e. *Pathological fracture.* Pathological fracture occurs at the site of weakened bone due to a focal bone abnormality such as a benign or malignant neoplasm or osteomyelitis.[17] Pathological fractures typically happen spontaneously or following minor trauma, which should be a red flag as to the likelihood of a pathological fracture. The highly vascularized subtrochanteric femur is a common site for pathologic metastatic fracture (**Fig. 12**). Although the hypervascularized acetabulum is another common site for metastases (see **Fig. 12**B), these metastases rarely fracture. Lytic metastases are more susceptible to fracture as bone loss has a greater negative impact on bone strength (see **Fig. 12**).

Imaging. The hallmark of a pathological fracture is the recognition of a pre-existing bone lesion at the site of fracture (see **Fig. 12**B). Review of any

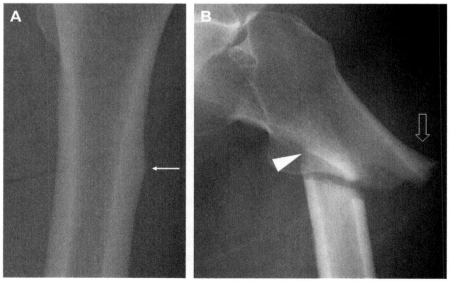

Fig. 11. Frontal radiographs of proximal femur showing focal cortical beaking with thin intracortical fracture (*arrow*) extending approximately 60% along the depth of the cortex (*A*). Three months later, a complete fracture is present, horizontally orientated with a medial spike (*arrowhead*) and thickening of the lateral femoral cortex (*open arrow*) (*B*).

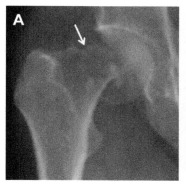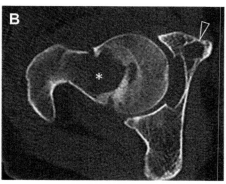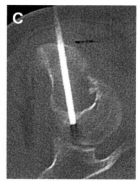

Fig. 12. Frontal radiograph showing a pathological fracture of the femoral neck (*arrow*) (*A*) with a large osteolytic area surrounding the transcervical fracture. Axial CT (*B*) of the same patient showing the osteolytic tumor (*asterisk*). There is another osteolytic lesion in the anterior acetabular pillar (*arrowhead*). CT-guided biopsy yielded tissue consistent with metastases (*C*).

previous radiographs or other imaging is helpful if available, as is a history of underlying malignancy. Radiographs are usually the key imaging modality. Particular attention should be paid to the fracture margins and immediate surrounding bone for evidence of bony replacement or infiltration, bony expansion, cortical scalloping, resorption or infiltration, or periosteal new bone formation. CT and MR imaging are helpful ancillary investigations if radiography is inconclusive (see **Fig. 12**B). On both CT and MR imaging, in addition to assessing the bony component, pay particular attention to replacement of marrow fat surrounding the fracture site and the presence of a peri-fracture soft-tissue mass, bearing in mind that peri-fracture hematoma and soft-tissue edema/inflammation may simulate tumor or infection to some degree. There are no hard and fast rules for making this distinction between tumor or infection and hematoma. The best indicator is to gauge if the perifracture marrow infiltration/inflammation is more extensive or the peri-fracture soft-tissue mass more severe than what you would generally expect. If out of proportion, you should consider the probability of a pathological fracture. Percutaneous biopsy under CT guidance is usually indicated and is generally definitive (see **Fig. 12**C).

PUBIC RAMI FRACTURE

Being stress risers, the pubic rami are susceptible to insufficiency fracture. Pubic rami fractures are the most common pelvic fracture in elderly patients. Fractures can occur at the medial, middle, or lateral one-third of the superior and inferior public rami and tend to be undisplaced or mild to moderately displaced (**Fig. 13**). Both superior and inferior rami fractures often occur concurrently. Approximately 60% of patients with pubic rami fractures will have a concurrent fracture of the pelvic ring comprising either a lateral compression fracture of the ilium or, more commonly, the sacral ala. Such additional pelvic ring fractures are usually not visible radiographically.[19]

Imaging. Most pubic rami fractures are readily seen on frontal pelvic radiographs. Approximately one-sixth may not be that clear radiographically, due to coexistent osteopenia.[19] As such, it is not uncommon to see radiographically occult or radiographically subtle pubic rami fractures on MR imaging examination performed for suspected proximal femoral fracture[8] (see **Fig. 13**). Some pubic rami fractures can undergo excessive osteolysis or excessive callus formation during healing simulating a bone tumor.[20]

GLUTEUS MEDIUS/MINIMUS TENDON TEAR

The gluteus minimus and medius tendons, known as "the rotator cuff tendons of the hip," are the most commonly injured hip tendons, usually related to preexistent tendinosis. Most gluteus minimus and medius tears are avulsion-type insertional tears with partial tears more common than complete tears (**Figs. 14** and **15**).[21] The gluteus minimus tendon inserts into the anterior facet of the greater trochanter, and is best seen on axial MR images. The gluteus medius tendon inserts into the lateral and superoposterior facets and is best seen on coronal and sagittal MR sequences. Most partial tears are avulsive-type tears, with a fluid-signal cleft partially separating the tendon from the bony insertional area though some tears may be a longitudinal split (ie, delamination) tear.

Although tendon tears may be a cause of acute hip pain following injury, they are also a cause of

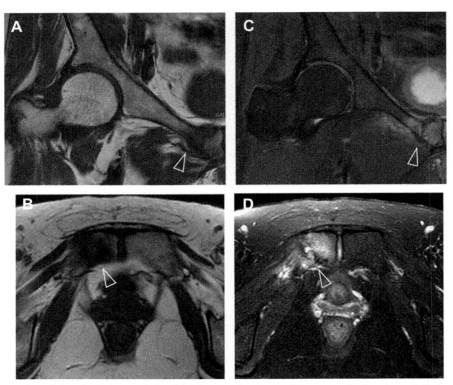

Fig. 13. Coronal T1- (*A*) and axial T1-weighted (*B*) images demonstrating a non-displaced medially located superior pubic ramus fracture (*arrowheads*). Note the hyperintense fluid signal surrounding the fracture on coronal T1- and axial T2-fat-suppressed coronal images (*arrowheads*) (*C, D*).

chronic pain or may be entirely asymptomatic. It is not uncommon to see hip abductor tendon tears on pelvic MR imaging examinations performed for unrelated reasons, usually isolated tears of the gluteus minimus followed by concurrent gluteus minimus and medius tears.[22–24] For the gluteus medius tendon, the lateral insertion tends to tear more frequently than the posterosuperior insertion.[22–24]

Imaging. Gluteus minimus and medius tendon tears are best seen on MR imaging examination, especially in the acute setting, as surrounding

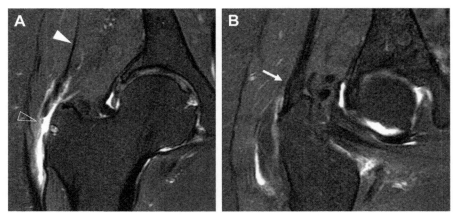

Fig. 14. T2-fat-saturated oblique coronal images of hip (*A, B*). There is a large avulsive-type partial tear of the gluteus medius tendon (*arrowhead*). All of the fibers are torn from their insertion on the lateral facet of the greater trochanter (*open arrowhead*), whereas the superoposterior fibers remain intact without tear (*arrow*). There seems to be mild underlying gluteus medius tendinosis.

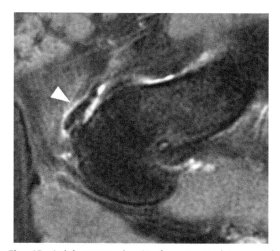

Fig. 15. Axial proton density fat-saturated image of hip. There is a partial thickness avulsive-type tear of the gluteus minimus tendon from the anterior facet of the greater trochanter. This tear mainly involves the more medially inserted fibers. Overall, approximately two-thirds of the tendon has been avulsed. There is mild gluteus minimus tendinosis and peritendinitis. No muscle fatty atrophy. This is most likely a quite recent tear.

soft issue edema and muscle sprain can be better appreciated on MR imaging than ultrasound (see **Figs. 14** and **15**). One should note whether the tear is partial or complete, insertional or intrasubstance, and provide an approximation as to the percentage of the tendon torn, and the degree of background tendinosis of the torn tendon.[21] The degree of tendon retraction and the presence of an avulsed bony fragment (very uncommon), if present, should be described as should the degree of surrounding peritendinitis.[21] Associated muscular changes can be helpful in estimating chronicity (eg, edema without fatty change implies a more recent tear, fatty infiltration, and atrophy a chronic tear). Prominent inflammation surrounding the tear site and the presence of a coexistent muscle sprain are the best markers of a recent tear.

RECTUS FEMORIS TENDON TEAR ± AVULSION FRACTURE

The rectus femoris has a direct head and an indirect head. The orientated longitudinally direct head arises more anteriorly from the anterior inferior iliac spine. The broader, transversely orientated triangular-shaped indirect head arises from the supra-acetabular sulcus and the lateral aspect of the hip capsule. The direct tendon (2 cm) is shorter than the indirect tendon (5.5 cm). Both tendons converge distally to form the "proximal tendinous complex." There is no dominant tear pattern. Tears may be partial or complete and involve either the direct or indirect heads or both heads simultaneously and may be located at the enthesis (± bony avulsion), within the tendon, or at the musculotendinous junction (**Fig. 16**). Conservative or surgical options are available with more severely (>2 cm) displaced tears tending to be surgically treated, particularly if there is a large bone avulsion.

Imaging. Radiographs are helpful to exclude a body avulsion with the addition of CT to help characterize this bony avulsion if surgical reattachment is being considered. Both ultrasound and MR imaging can help identify the presence and type of tear, though particularly in the acute setting, MR imaging is likely to be more accurate than ultrasound for detecting subtle tears (see **Figs. 15** and see **16**). If ultrasound shows a normal tendon, this effectively excludes a significant tear.

MUSCLE INJURY AROUND THE HIP

Acute muscle trauma around the hip is common due to eccentric (lengthening) contraction or blunt trauma. The biceps and rectus femoris muscles are commonly injured muscles.[25] Muscular tears tend to occur in young adults, mainly at the musculotendinous junction as opposed to the elderly where tendon tears are more common.[25]

Imaging MR imaging is ideally suited for imaging muscle Incomplete tears are more common and appear as localized areas of muscle hyperintensity on T2-fat-saturated MR sequences (**Fig. 17**) without discrete muscle fiber discontinuity. With more severe tears, muscle fiber retraction will be evident. One can report on the tear size, the approximate percentage of muscle fibers involved, and the location within the muscle, that is, proximal, middle, or distal within the muscle substance or at the myotendinous or myofascial junction (**Fig. 18**).

LABRAL CYST LEAKAGE

Acetabular labral tears are common and are often entirely asymptomatic. As there is often little or no peri-labral edema associated with even acute labral tears, it is usually not possible to ascertain whether a labral tear is related to a particular injury. Intra- or paralabral cysts are less common than labral tears, though still commonly seen on MR examinations (**Fig. 19**). The presence of edema and swelling around a paralabral cyst is, similar to ganglion cysts in the wrist, an indicator that the cyst is likely to be symptomatic and/or related to, or aggravated by, a recent injury.

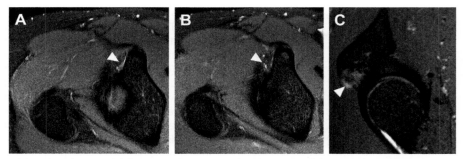

Fig. 16. Axial (*A*, *B*) and Sagittal (*C*) proton density-weighted images of the right hip demonstrating an incomplete avulsion of the indirect head of the rectus femoris muscle.

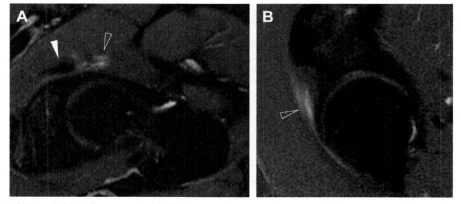

Fig. 17. Axial T2-weighted fat-suppressed MR image demonstrating a small iliopsoas muscle tear (*open arrowhead*) just posterior to the iliopsoas tendon (*arrowhead*) (*A*). Sagittal T2-weighted fat-suppressed MR image showing length of same small iliopasoas muscle tear (*open arrowhead*) (*B*).

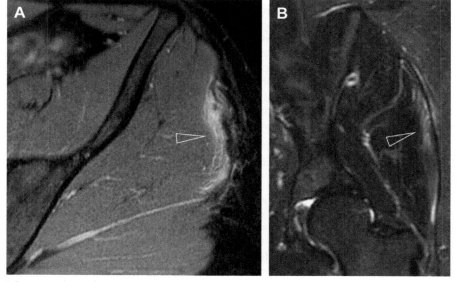

Fig. 18. Axial T2-weighted fat-suppressed MR image demonstrating a medium-sized myofascial tear of the gluteus maximus muscle laterally (*open arrowhead*) (*A*). Coronal T2-weighted fat-suppressed MR image showing length of same gluteus maximus myofascial tear (*open arrowhead*) (*B*).

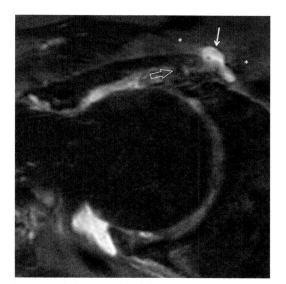

Fig. 19. Axial T2-weighted fat-suppressed MR image demonstrating a small anterior paralabral cyst (*arrow*) with mild pericystic edema (*asterisks*) indicating recent leakage or extension. There is severe degeneration of the anterior labrum, with multiple intrasubstance tears and a labrocapsular tear (*open arrow*).

Imaging. Paralabral cysts are readily identifiable by their location and configuration. The serpiginous tract leading to the labral area may be thin and interrupted. An associated labral tear is not invariably present as it may have healed or may be too small to resolve. As such MR imaging rather than ultrasound or CT is the best method to evaluate perilabral cysts. Percystic soft-tissue edema is also best appreciated on MR imaging.

Pain-Inducing Hip Pathology Highlighted by Injury

There are other conditions (notably crystal deposition, and transient osteoporosis of the hip) that can be uncovered by hip injury though the injury does not necessarily induce these conditions.

Hydroxyapatite crystal deposition

Hydroxyapatite crystals deposited in tendons, ligaments, and bursae around the hip joint can be activated by trauma, inducing severe hip pain that can mimic infection or other hip pathology. After the shoulder, the hip is the second most common site of hydroxyapatite deposition.[26] Minor trauma can cause preexistent crystal aggregates to move from the formative or resting stage to a resorptive stage inducing severe inflammation and pain.[26] The possibility of crystal inflammation should be considered in any patient with severe hip pain though no discernible bony injury.

Imaging. Radiographs may show dystrophic soft-tissue calcification, indicating that crystal deposition was present before recent injury (**Fig. 20A**). Absence of calcification does not exclude crystal deposition. Provided adequate transducer access can be achieved, ultrasound has high accuracy in depicting and localizing soft-tissue crystal deposition around the hip joint. Ultrasound can identify radiographically occult crystal aggregates (**Fig. 20B**).[26] Although ultrasound can also visualize associated soft-tissue inflammation as tissue swelling, edema and hyperemia, it is not as sensitive as MR imaging in this regard. Crystal deposition is usually the main differential diagnosis when moderate to severe soft-tissue inflammation is present around the hip joint (**Fig. 20C**). Pay particular attention to identifying, on MR imaging, the often small hypointense crystal aggregate foci, which are usually epicenter to the inflammation. As the ultrasound or MR imaging appearances are generally diagnostic, there is usually no need for histological or other correlation. Dual-energy CT helps exclude gouty tophi. As in the shoulder, ultrasound-guided

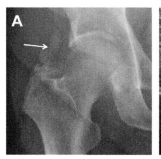
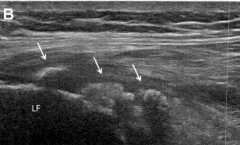
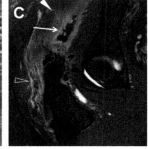

Fig. 20. Frontal hip radiograph showing calcific densities superior to the greater trochanter (*arrow*) in the region of the gluteus medius tendon (*A*). Longitudinal ultrasound showing crystal aggregates (*arrows*) in the region of the subgluteus medius bursa. LF, lateral facet greater trochanter (*B*). T2-weighted fat-suppressed oblique coronal MR image showing the hypointense calcific foci within the gluteus medius tendon (*arrow*) (*C*). There is quite severe surrounding soft-tissue (*open arrowhead*) and muscle (*arrowhead*) edema. This edema is better appreciated on MR imaging than ultrasound.

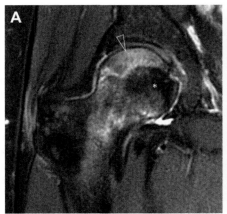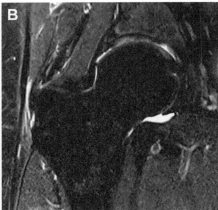

Fig. 21. Oblique coronal T2-weighted fat-suppressed MR image of a 32-year-old woman in the third trimester of pregnancy, demonstrating extensive bone marrow edema of the femoral head and neck (*open arrowhead*) (*A*). Note sparing of the medial aspect of the femoral head (***) and greater trochanter. Subsequent follow-up MR imaging in the same patient three months later, demonstrating complete resolution of the bone marrow edema (*B*).

barbotage and steroid injection can help alleviate symptoms.

Transient osteoporosis of the hip

Although the etiology of transient osteoporosis of the hip is unknown, it can be precipitated by minor trauma.[27] It is mostly seen in middle-aged men as well as women in the 3rd trimester of pregnancy or immediately post-partum. Histologically, increased osteoclastic activity unilaterally within the femoral head and neck is seen.[28] Patients develop mild to moderate-severity hip pain, aggravated by weightbearing, and restricted range of movement.[29] There are three stages characterized by (a) diffuse bone marrow edema; (b) demineralization; and (c) regression. Edema starts within 48 hours of pain onset, demineralization may be seen 1 to 2 months later though may not always be visible radiographically, whereas regression gradually occurs over the ensuing 6 to 9 months.[30] A successful outcome with either conservative treatment, ± assisted by antiresorptive agents such as alendronate, usually occurs.[27]

Imaging: In the initial stages, before demineralization, radiographs are normal. MR imaging is abnormal at the earliest stages showing diffuse bone marrow edema of the affected femoral head, sometimes sparing the medial portion of the femoral head as well as the greater trochanter, with variable extension into the femoral neck and proximal shaft (**Fig. 21**). Adjacent soft-tissue changes are minimal or absent.[29] Diffuse post-contrast enhancement is seen.[29] One can usually exclude confidently exclude other causes of diffuse femoral head edema such as SIFFH, osteoid osteoma, avascular necrosis, and osteomyelitis.

In conclusion, the causes of acute hip pain following trauma are many and varied. The clinical context enables one to choose the most appropriate imaging modality. Thereafter, imaging will be able to provide a specific diagnosis and assessment in most cases.

CLINICS CARE POINTS

- Computed tomography (CT) is extremely helpful in evaluating bony injury and soft-tissue abnormality in acetabular fractures.

- Early MR imaging should ideally be performed to detect radiographically occult proximal femoral fracture in osteoporotic patients with clinically suspected proximal femoral fracture. CT is the next best alternative.

- MR imaging is the only method to accurately detect both subchondral insufficiency fractures of the femoral head and transient osteoporosis of the hip (TOF) at an early stage.

- Ultrasound is helpful to detect muscle and tendon injury as well as crystal deposition, but MR imaging is more sensitive for identifying less severe injuries and showing the severity of soft-tissue inflammation.

REFERENCES

1. Lawrence DA, Menn K, Baumgaertner M, et al. Acetabular fractures: anatomic and clinical considerations. Am J Roentgenol 2013;201(3): W425–36.

2. Bishop JA, Rao AJ, Pouliot MA, et al. Conventional versus virtual radiographs of the injured pelvis and acetabulum. Skeletal Radiol 2015;44(9):1303–8.

3. Hallinan JTPD, Tan CH, Pua U. Emergency computed tomography for acute pelvic trauma: Where is the bleeder? Clin Radiol 2014;69(5): 529–37.

4. Grigoryan KV, Javedan H, Rudolph JL. Orthogeriatric care models and outcomes in hip fracture patients: a systematic review and meta-analysis. J Orthop Trauma 2014;28(3):e49–55.

5. Robertson GA, Wood AM. Hip hemi-arthroplasty for neck of femur fracture: what is the current evidence? World J Orthop 2018;9(11):235–44.

6. Sheehan SE, Shyu JY, Weaver MJ, et al. Proximal femoral fractures: what the orthopedic surgeon wants to know. Radiographics 2015;35(5):1563–84.

7. Deleanu B, Prejbeanu R, Tsiridis E, et al. Occult fractures of the proximal femur: imaging diagnosis and management of 82 cases in a regional trauma center. World J Emerg Surg 2015;10:55.

8. Dominguez S, Liu P, Roberts C, et al. Prevalence of traumatic hip and pelvic fractures in patients with suspected hip fracture and negative initial standard radiographs–a study of emergency department patients. Acad Emerg Med 2005;12(4):366–9.

9. Hampton M, Stevens R, Highland A, et al. Differential diagnosis of acute traumatic hip pain in the elderly. Acta Orthop Belg 2021;87:1–2021.

10. Wilson MP, Nobbee D, Murad MH, et al. Diagnostic accuracy of limited MRI protocols for detecting Radiographically occult hip fractures: a systematic review and meta-analysis. Am J Roentgenol 2020; 215(3):559–67.

11. Ross AB, Chan BY, Yi PH, et al. Diagnostic accuracy of an abbreviated MRI protocol for detecting radiographically occult hip and pelvis fractures in the elderly. Skeletal Radiol 2019;48(1):103–8.

12. Kellock TT, Khurana B, Mandell JC. Diagnostic performance of CT for occult proximal femoral fractures: a systematic review and meta-analysis. AJR Am J Roentgenol 2019;213(6):1324–30.

13. Bhimani R, Singh P, Bhimani F. Rapidly progressive hip disease-A rare entity in Korean population. Int J Surg Case Rep 2018;53:486–9.

14. Gaudiani MA, Samuel LT, Mahmood B, et al. Subchondral insufficiency fractures of the femoral head: systematic review of diagnosis, treatment and outcomes. J Hip Preserv Surg 2020;7(1):85–94.

15. Iwasaki K, Yamamoto T, Motomura G, et al. Computed tomography findings of subchondral insufficiency fractures of the femoral head. J Orthop 2018;15(1):173–6.

16. Sonoda K, Yamamoto T, Motomura G, et al. Fat-suppressed T2-weighted MRI appearance of subchondral insufficiency fracture of the femoral head. Skeletal Radiol 2016;45(11):1515–21.

17. Palmer W, Bancroft L, Bonar F, et al. Glossary of terms for musculoskeletal radiology. Skeletal Radiol 2020;49(Suppl 1):1–33.

18. Shane E, Burr D, Abrahamsen B, et al. Atypical subtrochanteric and diaphyseal femoral fractures: second report of a task force of the American Society for Bone and Mineral Research. J Bone Miner Res 2014;29(1):1–23.

19. van Berkel D, Herschkovich O, Taylor R, et al. The truth behind the pubic rami fracture: identification of pelvic fragility fractures at a university teaching hospital. Clin Med 2020;20(Suppl 2):s113.

20. Cheng X, Griffith JF, Chan WP. Top-ten pitfalls when imaging osteoporosis. Semin Musculoskelet Radiol 2019;23(4):453–64.

21. Cheung KK, Griffith JF. How to Report: Hip MRI. Semin Musculoskelet Radiol Oct 2021;25(5):681–9.

22. Zhu MF, Smith B, Krishna S, et al. The pathological features of hip abductor tendon tears - a cadaveric study. BMC Musculoskelet Disord 2020;21(1):778.

23. Tsutsumi M, Nimura A, Akita K. The gluteus medius tendon and its insertion sites: an anatomical study with possible implications for gluteus medius tears. J Bone Joint Surg Am 2019;101(2):177–84.

24. Chi AS, Long SS, Zoga AC, et al. Prevalence and pattern of gluteus medius and minimus tendon pathology and muscle atrophy in older individuals using MRI. Skeletal Radiol 2015;44(12):1727–33.

25. Flores DV, Gómez CM, Estrada-Castrillón M, et al. MR Imaging of muscle trauma: anatomy, biomechanics, pathophysiology, and imaging appearance. RadioGraphics 2018;38(1):124–48.

26. Reijnierse M, Schwabl C, Klauser A. Imaging of crystal disorders:: calcium pyrophosphate dihydrate crystal deposition disease, calcium hydroxyapatite crystal deposition disease and gout pathophysiology, imaging, and diagnosis. Radiologic Clin 2022;60(4): 641–56.

27. Emad Y, Ragab Y, Saad MA, et al. Transient regional osteoporosis of the hip with extensive bone marrow edema (BME): dramatic improvement after three months of Alendronate therapy. Radiol Case Rep 2021;16(9):2487–90.

28. McCarthy EF. The pathology of transient regional osteoporosis. Iowa Orthop J 1998;18:35–42.

29. Szwedowski D, Nitek Z, Walecki J. Evaluation of transient osteoporosis of the hip in magnetic resonance imaging. Pol J Radiol 2014;79:36–8.

30. Vaishya R, Agarwal AK, Kumar V, et al. Transient osteoporosis of the hip: a mysterious cause of hip pain in adults. Indian J Orthop 2017;51(4):455–60.

Particularities on Anatomy and Normal Postsurgical Appearances of the Knee

Maria Pilar Aparisi Gómez, MBChB, FRANZCR[a,b],
Giulio Maria Marcheggiani Muccioli, MD, PhD[c,d], Giuseppe Guglielmi, MD[e,f],
Stefano Zaffagnini, MD[c,d], Alberto Bazzocchi, MD, PhD[g,*]

KEYWORDS

• Knee • Anatomy • Postoperative period • Radiology • MR imaging

KEY POINTS

- The knee is a complex anatomic structure. A solid knowledge of the anatomy and biomechanics helps to understand the mechanisms of injury and provides a useful tool for accurate diagnosis, with a positive impact on management and prognosis.
- A good understanding of the different surgical procedures used to treat pathology helps in providing as much information as possible to guarantee a favorable outcome, improving levels of care and prognosis.
- Familiarity with the expected postsurgical appearances is mandatory to be able to discern these from complications.

INTRODUCTION

A detailed knowledge of the anatomy is necessary to understand the mechanisms of injury or the occurrence of certain pathologic processes. This is especially significant in the knee.

In this article, the authors focus on reviewing the components of the complex anatomy of the knee, with special attention to those concepts that have been the object of recent study as well as the anatomic features that have a clear association with the development of symptoms or are a frequent location for injury, elucidating why this is the case.

Frequently encountered anatomic variants and other common findings in asymptomatic patients are also described.

Finally, the authors highlight what are the commonly expected postsurgical appearances (postsurgical anatomy) and the most common postsurgical complications.

THE KNEE JOINT

The knee is the largest, most stressed and therefore most frequently imaged joint in the body. The knee is a synovial joint connecting femur, tibia, and patella. Its configuration is of a complex hinge, with two articulations: the tibiofemoral and the patellofemoral.

The anatomic disposition of the bones in these two joints provides a fulcrum for the extensor and flexor muscles. The multiple ligaments (intracapsular and extracapsular) as well as extensions

[a] Department of Radiology, Auckland City Hospital, 2 Park Road, Grafton, Auckland 1023, New Zealand; [b] Department of Radiology, IMSKE, Calle Suiza, 11, Valencia 46024, Spain; [c] 2nd Orthopaedic and Traumatology Clinic, IRCCS Istituto Ortopedico Rizzoli, Via G. C. Pupilli 1, Bologna 40136, Italy; [d] Dipartimento di Scienze Biomediche e Neuromotorie DIBINEM, University of Bologna, Via San Vitale, Bologna 40125, Italy; [e] Department of Radiology, Hospital San Giovanni Rotondo, Italy; [f] Department of Radiology, University of Foggia, Viale Luigi Pinto 1, Foggia 71100, Italy; [g] Diagnostic and Interventional Radiology, IRCCS Istituto Ortopedico Rizzoli, Via G. C. Pupilli 1, Bologna 40136, Italy
* Corresponding author.
E-mail address: abazzo@inwind.it

Radiol Clin N Am 61 (2023) 219–247
https://doi.org/10.1016/j.rcl.2022.10.009
0033-8389/23/© 2022 Elsevier Inc. All rights reserved.

of muscles crossing the joint are the stabilizers, balancing the biomechanical stress. Being a hinged joint, movement occurs along one axis (flexion and extension, in the sagittal plane), with a minimal degree of medial and lateral rotation.

Tibiofemoral Joint

The lateral and medial condyles have a smooth convex surface, separated by the deep groove of the intercondylar fossa. The medial condyle is larger, narrower, and projected slightly further than the lateral. The outer surfaces of the condyles are defined as medial and lateral epicondyles. In the posterior aspect, the elevations above the medial and lateral epicondyles are the supracondylar ridges.

The tibial plateaus are the slightly concave superior surfaces of the proximal tibia, which are separated by a bony ridge, the intercondylar eminence. The medial tibial articular surface is oval-shaped, and the lateral is more circular-shaped.

The joint surfaces are covered by thick articular cartilage, but yet are nor congruent. Congruency is facilitated by the menisci, which are more or less crescent-shaped.[1]

Patellofemoral Joint

The patellofemoral joint is a saddle joint.

Its components are the trochlear groove of the femur and the posterior surface of the patella.

The trochlear groove is located anteriorly in the femur, as vertical groove, which extends into the intercondylar fossa posteriorly. The shape of the trochlear groove allows for variation, which in some cases is related to patellar maltracking.

The patella is grossly triangular in shape, with a curved proximal base and pointed distal apex. The articular surface with the femur has a medial and a lateral facet, slightly concave, and is covered by a thick hyaline cartilage. Medial to the medial facet there is a third tiny facet, known as the odd facet, which is not covered in cartilage.

The patella is a sesamoid bone, included in the quadriceps tendon.[1] The extension of the quadriceps distal to the patella is the patellar ligament, which extends from the patellar apex into the tibial tuberosity.

A bipartite patella is an anatomic variation. This usually occurs in the superolateral aspect. This is connected to the patella through a synchondrosis. Eventually, abnormal mobility may occur, with development of symptoms, which translates into mechanical changes about the synchondrosis (**Fig. 1**).

Joint Capsule

The capsule is mainly formed by tendons and their expansions that together with ligaments form a thick sheath.[1]

The capsule is though relatively weak. It has two openings: an anterior one for the patella, attached to its margins, and a posterolateral one, for the popliteus tendon.

The capsule has different layers. There is an outer one, fibrous, in continuity with the adjacent tendons, and an inner synovial membrane, which reduces friction and nourishes the joint.

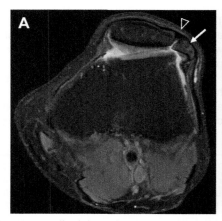 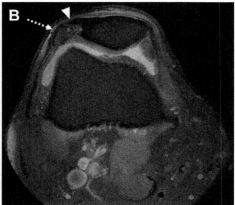

Fig. 1. Bipartite patella. (*A*) Axial proton density (PD) fat sat demonstrating a bipartite patella (*solid arrow*). This usually occurs in the superolateral aspect. This is connected to the patella through a synchondrosis and in continuity wih fibers of the quadriceps tendon (*hollow arrowhead*). Note there are signs of advanced chondropathy in the patellar cartilage. Eventually, abnormal mobility may occur, with development of symptoms, which translates into mechanical changes about the synchondrosis. (*B*) Axial PD fat sat demonstrates mild edema in the bipartite patella (*arrow*) and irregularity in the facets of the synchondrosis, with tiny subchondral cysts (*bold arrowhead*). Note there is mild chondropathy in the medial patellar aspect and a joint effusion.

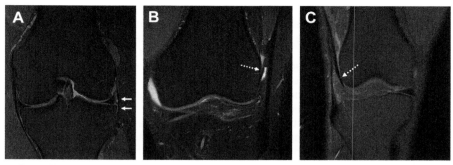

Fig. 2. Anterolateral ligament and Kaplan fibers. Coronal PD fat sat images demonstrating (*A*) the anterolateral ligament (*bold arrows*) here shown distally, close to the insertion just posterior to the iliotibial band in the tibia and (*B*) the Kaplan fibers (*dotted arrow*). (*C*) Prominent Kaplan fibers in a different patient (*dotted arrow*).

LIGAMENT COMPLEXES

Ligaments in the knee are extracapsular or intracapsular.

Extracapsular Ligaments

Patellar ligament
The connection between the patella and tibia could actually be considered a ligament, on the basis that it connects two bones. It is a thick fibrous band in continuity with the quadriceps tendon. However, if the patella is considered as sesamoid bone, this fibrous band is functionally in continuity with the quadriceps tendon and on this basis, may be considered a tendon. It extends from the apex of the patella to the tibial tuberosity. The ligament or tendon blends with the medial and lateral patellar retinacula, which are extensions of the vastus medialis and vastus lateralis and their fasciae.

Lateral aspect
The function of the collateral ligaments is to restrict excessive sideways movement.

The anterolateral corner The anterolateral corner (ALC) consists of the superficial and the deep aspects of the iliotibial tract, with the Kaplan fiber attachments to the distal femur, and the anterolateral ligament (ALL), a capsular thickening within the anterolateral capsule. The Kaplan fibers are noted to have two variations, either as a single or a double limb. They average between 30 and 40 mm from the lateral condyle.[2] The ALC provides anterolateral rotatory instability as a secondary stabilizer of the anterior cruciate ligament (ACL) (**Fig. 2**).

The ALL extends from the lateral epicondyle of the femur, closely related to the origin of the lateral collateral ligament (LCL) to insert onto the proximal anterolateral tibia, posterior to the insertion of the iliotibial band on Gerdy's tubercle[3] (**Fig. 3**).

Segond fractures have been reported by some groups to represent bony avulsions of the ALL.[4,5] The ALC consensus group[6] concluded that several structures attach to the region where Segond fractures occur, including the capsule-osseus layer of the iliotibial band, the ALL, and the anterior arm of the short head of the biceps, which means it not completely clear which one is the responsible structure for this lesion.

The ALL is an important stabilizer of internal rotation at flexion angles greater than 35°, complementing the function of the ACL (stabilizer of

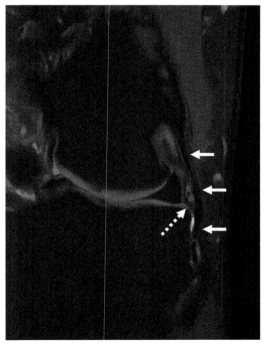

Fig. 3. Coronal PD fat sat image showing the anterolateral ligament in detail in its proximal course, closely related to the LCL (*arrows*). Deep to this, the coronary meniscotibial ligament is visible (*dotted arrow*).

internal rotation at angles <35° and resistance to anterior tibial translation/hyperextension) and injury to the ligament could result in knee instability at high angles of flexion.[7]

Biomechanical studies have confirmed that the ALC structures play an important role in controlling stability at the time of ACL reconstruction, but the optimal surgical procedure has not been determined clinically. Clinical evidence is still insufficient to support the indication of lateral extra-articular procedures as augmentation of ACL reconstruction.[6]

The posterolateral corner The structures in the posterolateral corner (PLC) are responsible for resisting varus angulation (or rotation) and external tibial rotation. They are secondary stabilizers with the cruciate ligaments, preventing anterior and posterior translation during the early phase of flexion (from 0° to 30°).[8]

Although the PLC has a very complex anatomy, the main structures are the LCL, the popliteus tendon, and the popliteofibular ligament (PFL) (**Fig. 4**).

The LCL has its origin in the lateral epicondyle of the femur, posterior to the insertion of the popliteus tendon, and immediately anterior to the origin of the lateral gastrocnemius. Its course is superficial to the popliteus tendon. Distally, it inserts into the lateral surface of the fibular head. The ligament splits the tendon of the biceps femoris in two at the insertion. The LCL is the primary static restraint to varus stress and also limits external rotation, especially in the early phase of flexion (0°–30°).[8]

The popliteus musculotendinous complex (popliteus tendon, muscle, and PFL) has a role as dynamic and static stabilizer in knee flexion at higher degrees, acting as a restraint to posterior translation, secondary to the posterior cruciate ligament (PCL).

The popliteus muscle arises from the posteromedial aspect of the proximal tibia. The tendon has an oblique lateral course under the arcuate, fabellofibular, and LCL and enters the joint through the popliteal hiatus, inserting in the popliteal sulcus of the lateral condyle. The tendon has two bundles, an anterior one, taut in flexion, and a posterior one, taut in extension.[9] A trifurcate appearance has also been described, as an anatomic variant.[10] Specific injuries occur in the myotendinous junction.

The popliteus tendon is connected to the posterior horn of the meniscus through the popliteomeniscal fascicles. These limit the movement of the meniscus during flexion, and also form the popliteal hiatus. There are two: a posterosuperior and an anteroinferior one (**Fig. 5**).

The PFL is one of the strongest lateral stabilizers, which extends from the popliteus, at the level of the musculotendinous junction (superficial) to the fibula. It runs just beneath the geniculate vessels. The ligament is difficult to visualize on Magnetic Resonance Imaging (MRI), better seen in coronal and sagittal (**Fig. 6**).[8]

There is a predictable pattern of sequential failure of the three major stabilizers of the PLC, starting with the LCL, followed by the PFL and finally the popliteus tendon.

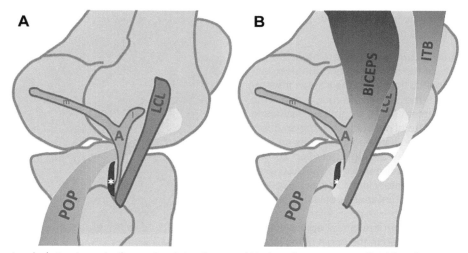

Fig. 4. Anatomical structures in the posterolateral corner (4A deep layer, 4B superficial layer) LCL, lateral collateral ligament; A, arcuate ligament, with its medial (M) and lateral (L) limbs; POP, popliteal tendon (and myotendinous junction). The popliteofibular (*asterisk*) is one of the strongest lateral stabilizers.

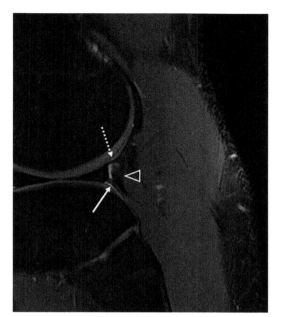

Fig. 5. Popliteomeniscal fascicles. Sagittal PD fat sat demonstrates the posterosuperior (*dotted arrow*) and anteroinferior (*solid arrow*) fascicles. These limit the movement of the meniscus during flexion, and also form the popliteal hiatus, through which the popliteal tendon (*arrowhead*) runs.

The arcuate ligament is a reinforcement of the capsule. It is a fibrous, "Y-shaped" band that arises from the posterior aspect (styloid process) of the fibular head, lateral to the PFL. The lateral limb runs superiorly along the capsule to insert in the lateral condyle, and the medial limb crosses medially, over the popliteus tendon, and attaches on the posterior side of the capsule. This ligament is a reinforcement for the posterolateral aspect of the knee, and although it may not be directly visible, disruption of the capsule is a reliable indicator of injury to it. The two limbs may not be present.[11] With a fabella, it is more common to identify the medial limb. Without it, the lateral limb is more commonly identified.[11]

The arcuate ligament, together with the oblique popliteal ligament (OPL), which is reinforced by an expansion of the semimebranosus insertion, prevent overextension of the knee.

The fabellofibular ligament runs from the lateral margin of the fabella or posterior aspect of the supracondylar process of the femur to insert in onto the tip of the fibular styloid process, posterior to the attachment of the biceps femoris.

The arcuate and fabellofibular ligaments are difficult to see on MR imaging. Non-fat-suppressed images are better to identify them,

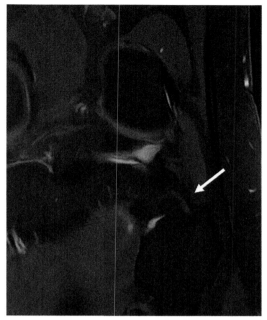

Fig. 6. Popliteofibular ligament. Coronal PD fat sat image demonstrating the popliteofibular ligament (*solid arrow*).

because there is a small amount of fat around them.

The biceps femoris has two heads. The long head has its origin in the ischial tuberosity, and the short in the mid-portion of the femur. Distally, both heads are composed by two tendinous structures, a direct and an anterior arm, visible on MR imaging in a large number of cases (71%).[12] On MR imaging, the tendon components merge with the LCL to insert forming a conjoined structure, in many cases.

Medial aspect
The medial complex The medial collateral ligament (MCL) is a strong, flat, and long ligament.

It has a superficial and a deep component.

The superficial component originates just proximal to the medial epicondyle and extends into the tibia, with two attachments, one in the medial tibial plateau and another one in the medial shaft. Anteriorly, this superficial fibers blend in with the medial patellofemoral ligament.[1]

The deep part is a vertical thickening of the joint capsule, located underneath the superficial ligament. It consists of meniscofemoral and meniscotibial fibers. This means that the medial meniscus is directly attached to the capsule and the MCL[13] (**Fig. 7**).

Meniscocapsular separations constitute injuries that may lead to instability. They can be diagnosed

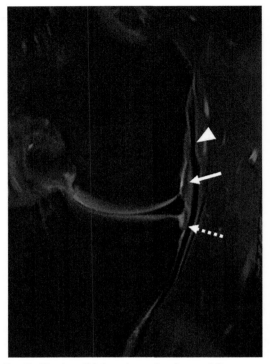

Fig. 7. Meniscotibial and meniscofemoral ligaments. Coronal PD fat sat image showing in detail the meniscofemoral (*bold arrow*) and meniscotibial (*dotted arrow*) fibers at the deep aspect of the MCL (*arrowhead*). The medial meniscus is directly attached to the capsule and the MCL.

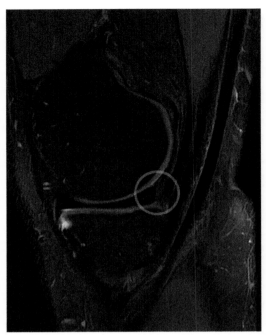

Fig. 8. Sagittal PD fat sat image, in the medial aspect of the knee, shows the region of meniscocapsular attachment in the posterior meniscal horn. A meniscocapsular separation that extends posteriorly is normally more significant in terms of stability. After trauma, the occurrence of a cleft filled with fluid in this location is indicative of meniscocapsular separation. A vertical tear in the peripheral aspect of the posterior horn has the same effect, resulting in instability.

in fluid sensitive sequences, easily missed in all other ones. If missed or untreated with immobilization or surgery, the interface between the capsule and meniscus may become avascular and reparative reattachment not occurs, resulting in instability. If the meniscocapsular separation is isolated to the segment of the MCL, it may be considered a tear of the deep fibers. Anterior and medial meniscocapsular separations normally have less significance. A meniscocapsular separation that extends posteriorly, involving the posterior oblique ligament (POL) is normally more significant in terms of stability[13] (**Fig. 8**).

The posteromedial corner The posteromedial corner (PMC) contains the structures lying between the posterior margin of the fibers of the MCL and the medial margin of the PCL.

The components of the PMC are the semimembranosus tendon, the OPL, the POL, the capsule, and the posterior horn of the medial meniscus. The MCL and coronary ligament, although related functionally, are not part of the PMC.

The semimembranosus tendon has five major insertional expansions, although as many as eight

have been described.[14] The principal one is the direct arm, but there is a capsular arm, an extension to the OPL, an anterior arm (tibial or reflected), and the inferior (popliteal) arm.

The direct arm inserts on the postero medial aspect of the medial tibial plateau. It has connections with the posterior aspect of the coronary ligament (meniscotibial ligament) of the posterior horn of the medial meniscus (**Fig. 9**).The medial meniscus may share innervation with the semimembranosus.[15] The capsular arm blends with the posteromedial capsule, together with the capsular arms of the OPL and POL. The extension to the OPL blends in with the OPL. The anterior arm passes under the POL and inserts into the medial proximal tibia, superior to the insertion of the MCL. The inferior arm also passes under the POL and inserts onto the tibia just above the MCL insertion.[13]

The direct and anterior arms are difficult to differentiate (**Fig. 10**).

The POL has its origin in the posterior margin of the MCL. Posteriorly, it blends with the capsule,

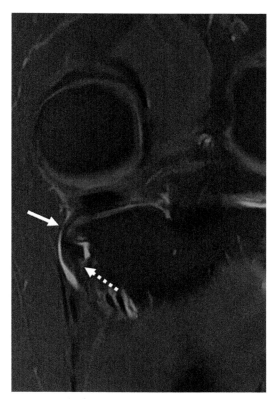

Fig. 9. Detail of the insertion of the semimembranosus. Coronal PD fat sat. The direct arm (*dotted arrow*) inserts on the posteromedial aspect of the medial tibial plateau and has connections with the posterior aspect of the coronary ligament (meniscotibial) of the posterior horn of the medial meniscus (*arrow*).

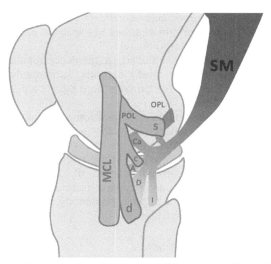

Fig. 10. Posteromedial corner. MCL, medial collateral ligament; POL, posterior oblique ligament, with its superior (S), central (c), and distal (d) arms. The semimembranosus (SM) has five insertional expansions, the main one is the direct one (D). There is a capsular arm (Ca), an extension to the OPL (OPL), an anterior arm (A), and the inferior (I) arm.

through three arms that are difficult to discern on MR imaging.[14] The central or tibial one is the most important, attaching into the posteromedial aspect of the medial meniscus and the posteromedial aspect of the tibia, passing deep to the anterior arm of the semimembranosus, merging with it (**Fig. 11**). The superior arm is seen superior to the joint line, and merges with the capsular

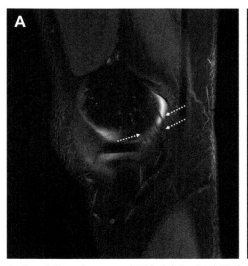

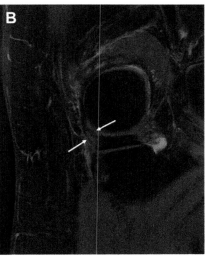

Fig. 11. Posterior oblique ligament (POL). (*A*) Sagittal PD fat sat image demonstrates the proximal fibers (*dotted arrows*), with some fluid interposed because of a partial volume effect. The POL has its origin in the posterior margin of the MCL. It blends with the capsule, through three arms that are difficult to discern on MR imaging. The central or tibial one is the most important, attaching into the posteromedial aspect of the medial meniscus and the posteromedial aspect of the tibia. (*B*) Detail of a coronal PD fat sat image demonstrates segments of this central arm related to the posterior meniscal horn (*arrows*). They are visible because of the existence of edema in the region, separating the planes. The edema is contiguous to an MCL lesion (not shown).

arm of the semimembranosus insertion to form the OPL. The inferior arm attaches to the direct insertion of the semimembranosus.

As previously mentioned, a meniscocapsular separation injury that extends posteriorly, involving the POL is normally more significant in terms of stability.

The OPL represents an expansion of the semimembranosus tendon and the superior POL, which extends posterior to the medial tibial condyle and then superiorly and laterally to attach on the meniscofemoral portion of the lateral capsule, the fabella and plantaris muscle. This ligament reinforces the capsule posteriorly, blending in with its central portion.

Intracapsular Ligaments

The cruciate ligaments are intracapsular extrasynovial structures that have a crossing disposition.

Anterior cruciate ligament

The ACL arises from the anterior intercondylar region of the tibia, in vicinity to the anterior meniscal root of the medial meniscus, and courses posterolaterally to insert in the medial surface of the lateral femoral condyle. At its tibial origin, the ACL is closely related to the anterior attachment of the lateral meniscus.

The ligament has two bundles: an anteromedial and a posterolateral one. The anteromedial bundle is slightly thicker than the posterolateral and longer (**Fig. 12**). The anteromedial attaches in the roof of the intercondylar notch, and the posterolateral, that is more vertical (and slightly shorter), in the wall of the notch.[16] The ACL is weaker than the PCL.

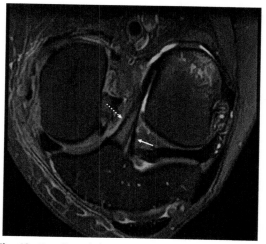

Fig. 12. Bundles of the ACL in an oblique coronal PD fat sat image. The anteromedial (*dotted arrow*) and a posterolateral (*solid arrow*).

The ACL prevents anterior displacement of the tibia (posterior translation of the femur), during flexion and extension.[17] The anteromedial bundle is responsible for the posterior translation of the femur at 30° of flexion, and the posterolateral prevents posterior translation in extension, besides from resisting hyperextension.

The ACL looks heterogeneous on MR imaging, with fluid quite often seen between bundles.

Posterior cruciate ligament

The PCL arises from the posterior intercondylar region of the tibia and has an anteromedial and superior course to insert in the anterior part of the lateral surface of the medial femoral condyle. It is stronger than the ACL, thicker and better vascularized. It is also shorter.[16]

The ligament prevents anterior rolling and displacement of the femur during extension as well as preventing hyperflexion.

The ligament also has two fiber bundles: an anterolateral and a posteromedial.[18]

When the knee flexes, the anterolateral band becomes tight, and the posteromedial bundle tightens during extension. The PCL as whole acts to resists anterior translation of the femur. When in flexion and weight bearing, the PCL stabilizes the femur.[19]

The two bundles are usually not clearly differentiated on MR imaging.

At the apex of the ligament, there may be magic angle effect, as a pitfall.

Menisci

The menisci are fibrocartilaginous structures that have a typical longitudinal-wedge configuration, with a crescent shape. They serve as facilitators of congruence and shock absorbers. They have two distinctive anatomic regions; in the peripheral one-third, they are thick and vascularized, and the collagen fibers are arranged circumferentially, ready to resist tensional forces, and in the inner two-thirds, they are thin and avascular centrally, with the collagen fiber bundles arranged radially, adapted for weight-bearing.[20]

The medial meniscus is C-shaped. Its anterior horn attaches to the anterior intercondylar area of the tibia and blends with the ACL. The posterior horn attaches to the posterior intercondylar area of the tibia, between the attachments of the lateral meniscus and the PCL.

The lateral meniscus is almost circular. Its anterior horn attaches to the anterior intercondylar area of the tibia and blends with the ACL. The posterior horn attaches to the posterior intercondylar area of the tibia, anterior to the posterior horn of the medial meniscus. The anterior horn of the lateral

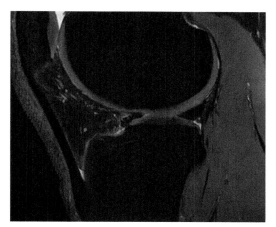

Fig. 13. Striated appearances of the anterior horn of the lateral meniscus in a sagittal PD fat sat image. This is caused by the ACL fibers that insert into the meniscus and has been reported in 60% of patients.

meniscus may sometimes have a speckled or striated appearance, which may resemble degeneration or a tear (**Fig. 13**). This is caused by the ACL fibers that insert into the meniscus, and has been reported in 60% of patients.[21]

On sagittal MR images, the posterior horn of the meniscus should never be smaller than the anterior, otherwise, there has been a meniscectomy or a tear (**Fig. 14**).The posterior horn of the medial meniscus is larger than the anterior; in the lateral meniscus, they have a more similar size.

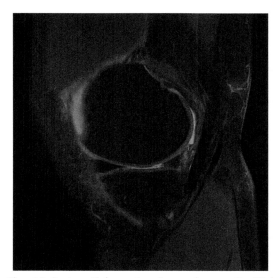

Fig. 14. Post-partial meniscectomy change. Sagittal PD fat sat demonstrates a posterior medial meniscal horn that is smaller than the anterior and has slightly irregular contours.

The normal meniscus lacks signal in all sequences.[22] However, increased signal is normal in children and young adults, especially in the posterior horns, in vicinity to the capsular attachment. This represents normal vascularity.

Meniscal ligaments

The menisci are stabilized by several ligaments.[23]

The transverse ligament is a band that connects the menisci anteriorly, extending from the anterior margin of the lateral meniscus to the anterior horn of the medial meniscus. This is not present in every knee (estimated to be present in 55%), and its exact role is uncertain, possibly vestigial.[24] The hypothesis is that it stabilizes during knee movements and decreases tensions generated in the longitudinal circumferential fibers. This ligament can cause an interpretation pitfall. At its insertion on the anterior horns, it may appear as a meniscal tear (more common laterally) (**Fig. 15**), but this can be easily ruled out by following the ligament across Hoffa's fat pad in sagittal.[21] Recently, an arthroscopic technique suggested the ligament as point of fixation for allograft meniscal transplant as an alternative to bone plug methods.[25]

The meniscofemoral ligaments (MFLs) are present in about 70.8% of knees, according to a recent systematic review.[26] These originate from the posterior medial condyle and run obliquely across the intercondylar notch, to insert into the posterior horn of the lateral meniscus. There is an anterior MFL (aMFL, also called Humphrey) and a posterior one (pMFL or Wrisberg ligament). Both of them are present in 17.6% of individuals[26] (**Fig. 16**).

The ligaments contribute to the complex biomechanics of the knee to provide stability synergistically. They may play a role helping the lateral meniscus to increase femorotibial congruency and reducing meniscal contact pressure in flexion and extension.[27]

The aMFL runs posterior to the ACL and anterior to the PCL. The presence of an aMFL contributes to the stabilization of the lateral compartment of the knee. Results in frequency from a systematic review (which includes MR imaging and cadaveric findings) report it as present in 55.5% of cases. The aMFL functions to support a torn PCL.[28]

The pMFL runs posterior to the PCL. This ligament plays a role in the recovery after PCL injuries and offers stability to the lateral meniscus, contributing to normal knee function. In a systematic review, the pooled prevalence was 70.4%. The shared features of the ligament with the PCL suggest that this needs to be considered when planning and performing arthroscopy.[29]

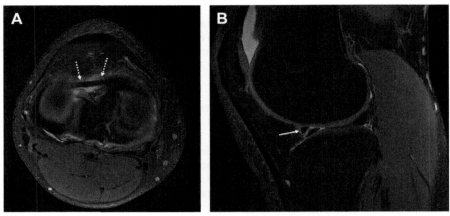

Fig. 15. Transverse ligament. (*A*) Axial PD fat sat demonstrates the ligament joining both anterior horns (*dotted arrows*). The ligament can cause an interpretation pitfall. At its insertion on the anterior horns, it may appear as a meniscal tear. (*B*) Sagittal PD fat sat demonstrating the ligament in close vicinity to the anterior horn of the lateral meniscus (*arrow*).

The insertions of the MFLs may give the appearances of a meniscal tear. When considering a pseudotear, it is important to follow the ligament to its attachments. This should not be mistaken with a meniscal tear progressing from the distal insertion of the MFLs through the lateral meniscus (typically associated with an ACL rupture, due to anterior tibial translation and traction against the PCL). Savoye and colleagues[30] described the "zip" sign, as a straight line from the distal insertion of the MFL seen on axial MR imaging (thin sections) that is visible in five sagittal images lateral to the PCL. This sign was reported to have a sensitivity of 87.5% to detect tears. Some investigators have reported that the average attachment lies approximately 14 mm laterally from the lateral edge of the PCL and therefore clefts extending further represent tears.[31]

The coronary ligaments are meniscotibial ligaments. In the medial aspect, they are part of the fibers of the deep component of the MCL, which is a vertical thickening of the joint capsule. The medial meniscus is directly attached to the capsule and the MCL. In the lateral aspect, the ligament extends from the inferior margin of the meniscus to the peripheral area of the tibial plateau.

The patellomeniscal ligaments are medial and lateral. These extend from the inferior third of the patella to insert in the anterior portion of the medial and lateral meniscus.

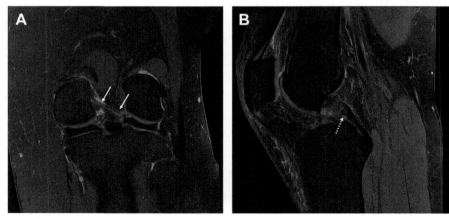

Fig. 16. Meniscofemoral ligaments. (*A*) Coronal PD fat sat demonstrates the ligament of Wrisberg (pMFL), extending from the posterior medial condyle across the intercondylar notch, to insert into the posterior horn of the lateral meniscus (*arrows*). (*B*) Sagittal PD fat sat in a different patient demonstrates the ligament of Humphrey (aMFL), seen transversally, anterior to the PCL (*dotted arrow*).

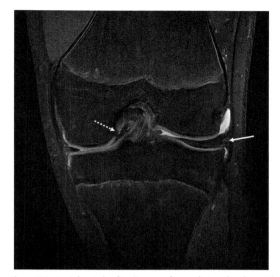

Fig. 17. Incidental finding of a lateral discoid meniscus in an adolescent after trauma. Coronal PD fat sat demonstrates the meniscus is normally attached to the capsule (*solid arrows*). Note there is a bucket handle tear of the medial meniscus, with the bucket handle fragment laterally displaced, in the intercondylar notch (*dotted arrow*).

Discoid meniscus

A discoid meniscus is a congenital malformation in which the meniscus is disk-shaped, instead of C-shaped. This is more frequent involving the lateral meniscus. Incidence has been reported as 0.8% to 3%.[32] The medial meniscus is less commonly discoid in shape.

Discoid menisci are often an incidental finding. They are at a higher risk of degeneration, with subsequent tear. Discoid menisci can cause symptoms without being torn.

Discoid meniscus constitutes a spectrum. Most discoid menisci are not completely disk-shaped, but the body is wider than expected, with a larger anterior or posterior horn (**Fig. 17**).

Discoid menisci have been grouped in complete, incomplete, depending on tibial plateau coverage, and Wrisberg variant.

The Wrisberg variant of the lateral discoid meniscus[33] consists of a discoid meniscus that lacks attachments to the capsule through the normal fascicles and attachment to the tibia through the coronary ligaments. This is normally seen in children. The only attachment of the posterior horn is in this case the Wrisberg ligament. The posterior horn is then mobile, subluxing into the joint with knee flexion.[34]

At the incidental finding of a discoid meniscus, it is important to carefully inspect capsular attachments, fascicles to the popliteus tendon (popliteomeniscal fascicles) and coronary ligaments. If the meniscus is a Wrisberg meniscus, this may be fixated to the capsule instead of performing a meniscectomy, thus reducing the risk of premature osteoarthritis.

The popliteomeniscal fascicles are normally visible on MR imaging, but the coronary ligaments are usually not visible in healthy knees. In general, on MR imaging, the lack of this normal fascicles and coronary ligaments shows as high T2 signal

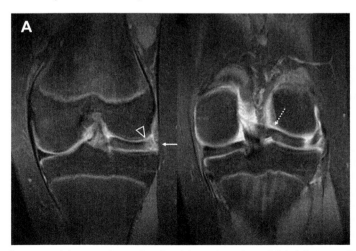
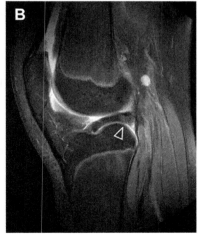

Fig. 18. Wrisberg variant of a discoid meniscus in a child. (*A*) Coronal PD fat sat (slices at different levels, more anterior on the left and posterior on the right) demonstrate there is no normal attachment of the meniscus to the capsule (*arrow*) and how the posterior meniscus is attached to the meniscofemoral ligament of Wrisberg (*dotted arrow*). The posterior horn is abnormally mobile, subluxing into the joint with knee flexion. In this case, the posterior meniscal horn demonstrates increased signal intensity (*arrowheads*) in the lateral and posterior aspects, in keeping with an intrasubstance tear/degeneration. (*B*) Sagittal PD fat sat demonstrating increased signal in the posterior aspect.

interposed between the lateral meniscus and the joint capsule, simulating a peripheral tear or a fascicle lesion[33] (**Fig. 18**).

Patellar Retinacula

Medial

The medial patellar retinaculum has a superficial and a deep layer. The superficial layer is composed by fibers of the vastus medialis, sartorius, and the MCL. The deep layer is formed by the proper medial patellofemoral ligament and fascial thickenings.

The medial patellofemoral ligament is the main structure that prevents the patella from lateral displacement (Krebs) (50%–60%) of restraining force. Together with the other components of the medial retinaculum and the vastus medialis, it is one of the medial stabilizers of the patella. The ligament has two origins,[35] one of them superior, superior to the femoral origin of the MCL, and another one that arises from the anterior edge of the proximal 3 cm of the superficial MCL. It inserts at the superomedial aspect of the patella.[36]

The medial retinaculum inserts onto the medial aspect of the patellar ligament/tendon, the patella and the quadriceps tendon, and extends medially to blend with the medial capsule and the medial tibial plateau. The retinaculum is an important stabilizer of the patella, resisting lateral dislocation.[36]

Lateral

The superficial layer arises from the iliotibial band and an extension of the vastus lateralis fascia. The deep layer is the lateral patellofemoral ligament proper, the patellotibial band, and transverse ligament.[37]

The lateral retinaculum inserts onto the quadriceps tendon, lateral border of the patella and patellar ligament/tendon, and extends laterally to blend with the lateral capsule and the lateral tibial plateau.

Plicae

During fetal development, the knee is divided into three compartments by synovial septa. If these fail to completely regress, they appear as folds within the joint and constitute the plicae. The common ones are the superior, inferior, and medial. More than half of the knees demonstrate one or more plicae on MR imaging (**Fig. 19**).

The suprapatellar plica runs from the posterior aspect of the quadriceps tendon, to the femoral metaphysis, located at the margin between the suprapatellar bursa and the joint cavity.[38]

The infrapatellar plica or ligamentum mucosum is the most common plica of the knee. Shape and size depend on the degree of regression. It has its origin in the anterior part of the intercondylar notch and traverses the infrapatellar fat pad to attach in the inferior pole of the patella. The infrapatellar plica may be very thick and is sometimes mistaken for the ACL in ACL-deficient knees. It may also represent a pitfall for focal nodular synovitis and a loose body in the infrapatellar fat pad.[38]

The medial patellar plica originates from the medial retinaculum and runs obliquely downward inserting onto the synovium in the inferior fat pad. Sometimes it is connected to the suprapatellar plica, but it is more frequent to see it separately. If large, it can be interposed in the medial aspect of the patellofemoral joint.[39]

The lateral patellar plica is very rare. It is very thin and originates in the lateral wall above the popliteal hiatus and inserts onto the synovium in the inferior fat pad.[39]

Bursae

Several bursae are present around the knee.

The most common one is the presence of a Baker's cyst. This is actually a joint recess that extends from the hiatus between medial gastrocnemius and semimembranosus tendon. It can get quite large and contain hemorrhagic debris. It can also leak or tear causing adjacent inflammation, and sometimes mimic a deep vein thrombosis.[40]

The prepatellar bursa is located anterior to the patella and patellar tendon.

The pes anserinus bursa is located in the anteromedial aspect of the tibia, below the joint line, beneath the tendons forming the pes anserinus, superficial to the MCL. If distended it extends toward the joint.

The semimembranosus—tibial collateral bursa is seen along the posteromedial joint, wrapping like a horseshoe around the semimembranosus tendon. It may be confused with a meniscal cyst.

The MCL bursa lies deep to the MCL, and when distended has a cyst-like configuration, between MCL layers. It may be a confused with meniscocapsular separation or a meniscal cyst.[41]

Muscles

The muscles crossing the knee and their functions are summarized on **Table 1**.

POSTSURGICAL APPEARANCES

The postoperative knee may present multiple challenges. Besides from the specifics of postsurgical complications, other pathology may appear

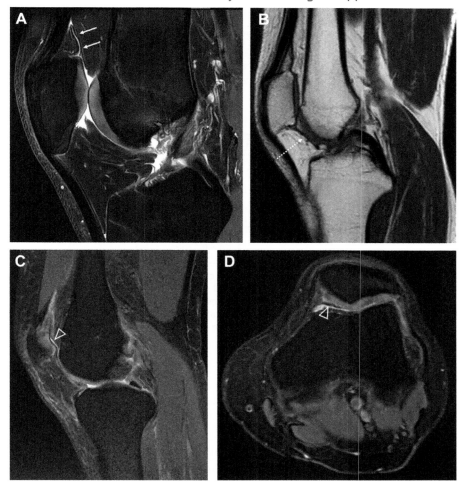

Fig. 19. Knee plicae. (*A*) Sagittal PD fat sat demonstrating a thin, normal suprapatellar plica (*arrows*). (*B*) Sagittal T1 demonstrating an infrapatellar plica (*dotted arrow*). (C) Sagittal PD fat sat demonstrating a medial plica (*arrowhead*). (*D*) Axial PD fat sat demonstrating the plica medial to the patella (same patient as in C).

Table 1 Muscles crossing the knee and their functions		
Action	**Primary**	**Assisting**
Flexors	Biceps femoris Semitendinosus semimembranosus	Popliteus Gracilis Sartorius
Extensor	Quadriceps	Tensor fascia latae
Internal Rotation (mainly last stage of extension, but also in flexion)	Popliteus Semitendinosus Semimembranosus	Gracilis Sartorius
External Rotation (flexion)	Biceps femoris	

superimposed. Imaging may be artifact and difficult to interpret.

Knowledge and familiarity with the surgical procedures as well as interaction with the referring surgeons are paramount to provide good answers to clinical questions.

Every imaging method is useful for the assessment of the postsurgical knee, but it is common to refer postsurgical complications to MR imaging. This is the modality more frequently performed, because it is the one yielding more information.

Ligament procedures

Anterior cruciate ligament
This is the most frequently reconstructed knee ligament. Failure rate occurs as frequently as in 10% of cases, with subsequent indication for MR imaging.

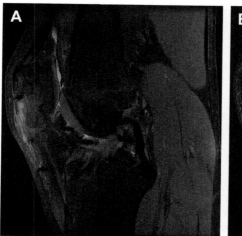
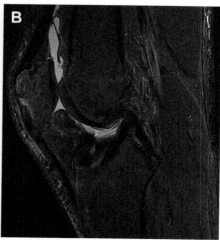

Fig. 20. The bone–patella–bone grafts are some of the most commonly used ones. (*A*) Sagittal PD fat sat 7 weeks after surgery demonstrates marked thickening and increased signal of the patellar tendon, as well as the inferior pole of the patella, where the bone–tendon has been harvested. Note the scattered punctate foci of magnetic susceptibility. Part of the tibial tunnel is visible, with the graft showing slight increase in signal. (*B*) Sagittal PD fat sat a year after surgery shows how the appearances of the patellar tendon have normalized and the ACL graft appears homogeneously low in signal.

Table 2
Normal appearances and pathologic findings in anterior cruciate ligament reconstruction

Expected Postsurgical Appearances	Pathologic Appearances
Position • The tibial tunnel should be at the back of the native ACL footprint to reproduce the function of the native ligament. If the tibial plateau is divided in four equal-length segments in the sagittal plane, numbered from anterior to posterior, the opening should be in segment 2. • The femoral tunnel courses oblique to the posterior cortex of the femur and the graft should be parallel to Blumensaat's line in the sagittal plane. If the roof of the intercondylar notch is divided in four equal-length segments in the sagittal plane, numbered from anterior to posterior, the opening should be located in segment 4 or posterior. In the axial plane, the opening should be in the 10–11 o'clock position (right) or 1–2 o'clock (left). • In the coronal plane, the graft should be angled about 15° Signal • Initially, a graft is of homogeneously low signal intensity. • After 2 months, the graft becomes higher in signal intensity during the vascularization phase. • From 6 months to 2 years, it again becomes of homogeneously low signal intensity. • Posterior to this, the graft should be a continuous low signal structure.	• If the tibial tunnel is too anterior, the graft will be too horizontal, with risk of impingement • If the femoral tunnel is too anterior, or the tibial too posterior, the graft will be too vertical, with instability. • During the revascularization stage, the graft is weak and susceptible to reinjury. • Degeneration (hyperintensity and thickening, with defined fibers) • Ganglion formation (in the spectrum of degeneration, similar appearances with sometimes discrete ganglion formation, extending into popliteal region). Ganglia may appear intratunnel and extend into the joint. • General complications such as infection may also occur. • Focal scar formation in the intercondylar notch: cyclops lesion This lesion may be related to inadequate removal of the native ACL or simply exuberant inflammatory response. Appears on MR imaging as low signal intensity tissue in the intercondylar notch. • Arthrofibrosis is due to extensive inflammatory response. Appears on MR imaging as low signal intensity tissue replacing the infrapatellar fat and extending from the femoral trochlea to the patella and patellar tendon.

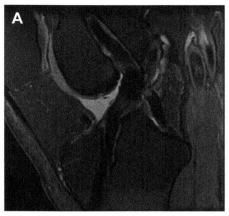
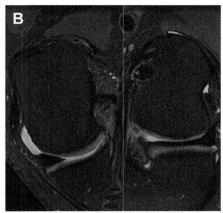

Fig. 21. ACL graft in an (A) oblique sagittal PD fat sat view and (B) coronal oblique PD fat sat view (different patients). These modified planes follow the course of the graft and allow seeing it in one plane, which is ideal to assess its signal and integrity. Approximately after 2 months of placement, the graft becomes higher in signal intensity during the vascularization phase (note how it appears slightly more hyperintense in B).

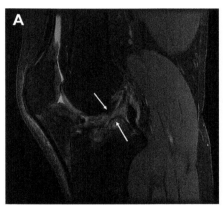
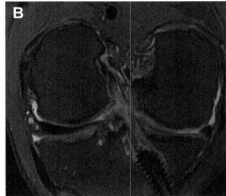

Fig. 22. Graft impingement. (A) Sagittal PD fat sat demonstrates increased signal intensity in the ACL graft (arrows), with adjacent bone marrow edema in the tibia, in the intercondylar ridge. If the tibial tunnel is too anterior, the graft will be too horizontal, with risk of impingement. (B) Oblique coronal PD fat sat better demonstrates increased signal and segmental thickening of the graft, in keeping with impingement.

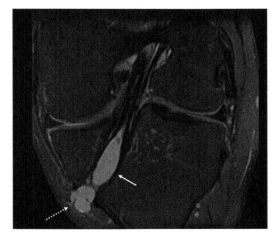

Fig. 23. Oblique coronal demonstrating an ACL graft ganglion, which in this case is mainly intra-tibial tunnel (bold arrow). This protrudes through the anterior opening of the tunnel (dotted arrow).

Artificial grafts and extra-articular techniques were used in the past, as well as different in situ grafts, with an autograft or allograft.

The most commonly used currently are either bone-patella-bone or hamstring auto or allografts (**Fig. 20**). Multiple fixation devices are used, the most common ones interference screws (these are from metal and therefore radiopaque or made from bioabsorbable polymers which are nonvisible on radiographs. Both have similar appearances on MR imaging), EndoButton devices (retain the graft outside of the bone preventing it from sliding into the tunnel) as well as horizontal femoral fixation devices and staples.

The hamstring tendon graft is usually folded on itself (up to four times), and sometimes the strands are sutured together (this may create artifact).

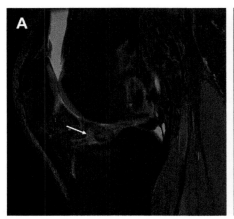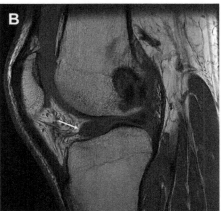

Fig. 24. Cyclops lesion. (*A*) Sagittal PD fat sat and (*B*) T1 demonstrating a nodular low-signal lesion anterior to the intercondylar notch, consistent with a cyclops lesion (*arrows*). This lesion may be related to inadequate removal of the native ACL or simply exuberant inflammatory response.

The graft is placed to have a linear, straight configuration on maximal flexion of the knee.

Adequate positioning of the graft is necessary to prevent complications such as impingement, knee instability, and laxity.

Most surgeons use one band of graft, reproducing the anteromedial bundle, but techniques using two bands to reproduce native appearances are also in use.[42,43] In these cases, two tunnels are needed.[44]

Ligament reconstructions go through a process of incorporation in which the graft initially serves as a stabilizer and then as a scaffold for a new fibrous support to form.

Nonanatomic techniques such as the over-the-top technique are useful to restore anterior and rotatory knee laxity in skeletally immature patients and in revision settings.[45]

Normal appearances and pathologic findings are summarized in **Table 2**[46,47] (**Figs. 21–24**).

Posterior cruciate ligament

Injuries to the PCL are less common than those of the ACL. They normally occur from a direct hit to the tibia with the knee in flexion (dashboard injury)

Table 3
Summary of appearances in collateral ligament repair

Ligament	Expected Postsurgical Appearances	Pathologic Appearances

MCL	• The healing MCL can be thick and exhibit high signal intensity on MR imaging.
	• A reconstructed ligament will have either interference screws or staples in the medial femoral condyle related to the surgery.
	• On MR imaging, the reconstructed ligament can be thick but should be low in signal and continuous.
	• On US, it should also be continuous and show homogeneous echogenicity.
		• Hardware failure (rare)
		• Reinjury: same appearances as a tear
		  – Thickening and hyperintensity
		  – Discontinuity
		• General complications: infection, inflammatory or granulomatous reaction to the graft or suture

Lateral Complex/ Posterolateral Corner	• Often combined with reconstruction of the ACL • Anchoring devices • Homogeneous low signal	• Hardware failure • Reinjury • General complications: infection, inflammatory or granulomatous reaction to the graft or suture

Abbreviations: US, ultrasound

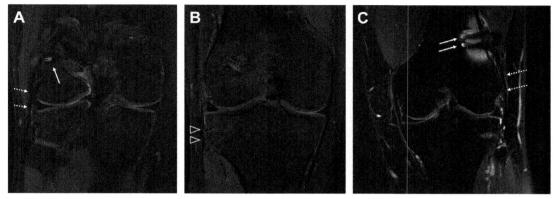

Fig. 25. Reinforcement of the lateral ligament complex. This is normally performed in combination with an ACL reconstruction. (*A*) Coronal PD fat sat in the posterior knee demonstrates the anchor of a modified Lemaire procedure in the lateral aspect of the lateral condyle (*bold arrow*). The transposed segment of iliotibial band (ITB) is signaled with dotted arrows. (*B*) Coronal fat sat in an anterior plane demonstrates tiny foci of susceptibility artifact where the origin of the segment of ITB has been dissected (*arrowheads*). (*C*) Modified Lemaire in a different patient, with double anchoring more proximal in the lateral aspect of the femur (*bold arrows*) and the transposed segment of ITB (*dotted arrows*).

or from hyperextension or complete knee dislocation.

The reconstruction is more commonly performed with two bundles.

The complications are similar to the complications described for the ACL: general (infection) related to position (instability or impingement) with the particularity that arthrofibrosis and cyclops lesions are less common.[47]

Collateral ligaments/lateral complexes

These are normally sports-related injuries and appear in association with tears of the ACL. The MCL usually heals without help, and treatment is conservative, but in some cases, surgery is

necessary. Reinforcement of the lateral ligament complex, with a modified Lemaire lateral extra-articular tenodesis, for example, is performed as an augmentation technique to reduce anterolateral rotatory laxity.

A summary of appearances is provided in **Table 3**[47,48] (**Figs. 25** and **26**).

Meniscal Interventions

Meniscal tears are very common, caused by degenerative and traumatic processes. The tears can cause pain, catching, and clicking. Displacement of portions of the torn meniscus may cause locking of the knee. There are multiple types of meniscal intervention.

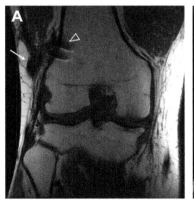
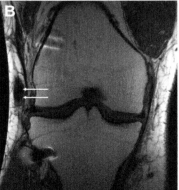
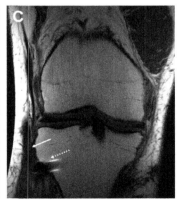

Fig. 26. Over-the-top ACL reconstruction technique. T1 coronal, three slices, from posterior to anterior (*A–C*). The tendon (hamstring in this case) passes through the tibial and femoral tunnels, to come out posterolaterally in the intercondylar notch and glide over the lateral condyle, where it is anchored (*arrowhead*), to then descend (*arrows* in *A*, *B*, and *C*) to be attached in the lateral tibial plateau (*dotted arrow*). This technique is used to restore anterior and rotatory knee instability in the immature skeleton or in the setting of revision.

Table 4
Summary of characteristics, indication, and expected and pathologic appearances in meniscal interventions

Technique	Characteristics / Indications	Expected Postsurgical Appearances	Pathologic Appearances
Meniscectomy	• Partial or total removal of the meniscus. Partial removal (the process of shaving an irregular edge) may simply be referred to as debridement. • Performed arthroscopically.	• Partial meniscectomy: the meniscus appears smaller, blunted. • Cases of large tear: smaller meniscus with persistent oblique increased signal intensity in the meniscal remnant (may persist for years after surgery) • If the meniscus is severely degenerated or so extensively torn that it cannot be salvaged, most of the meniscus will be removed.	• On MR imaging or MR arthrography, if there is a linear hyperintensity, unless the signal intensity is as high as that of fluid, or fluid is definitely in the prior defect, it is not sure there is a re-tear. • Parameniscal cysts are usually, but not always, drained at the time of meniscal surgery, so their presence does not indicate there is a re-tear. • Different types of tear to the original one • Appearance of a fragment • Dislocation
Meniscal Repair	• Preservation of meniscal tissue	• Appearances of a normal meniscus • Appearances of partial meniscectomy. • There may be some irregularity at the repair site, but there will be no contrast imbibition. • Foci of susceptibility artifact in meniscus (tack fixation has more artifact) and soft tissues, minimal scarring in soft tissues. • The site of a normal meniscal repair can have abnormal signal in the orientation of the original tear that represents fibrous tissue. • Persistent increased signal intensity is part of the normal healing process and can remain for up to 2 y after surgery. This intermediate signal, however, will not be as high as the signal intensity of joint fluid.	• On MR imaging or MR arthrography, if there is a linear hyperintensity, unless the signal intensity is as high as that of fluid, or fluid is definitely in the prior defect, it is not there is a re-tear. • Fluid can also dissect into the meniscus from the capsular side. This suggests that the meniscal repair is not healing well and that there is breakdown of the repair, but it this does not extend to an articular surface, is not considered a re-tear • Parameniscal cysts are usually, but not always, drained at the time of meniscal surgery, so their presence does not indicate there is a re-tear.

| Meniscal Transplant | • Cadaveric
• Potential way to prevent arthrosis in patients who have required meniscectomy (indication is patients without menisci who have not yet developed arthrosis).
• For the allograft to work, alignment and mechanics of the joint have to be normal. Sometimes concomitant osteotomy is necessary.
• The size that is requested for the meniscal allograft is determined by measurements made from preoperative radiographs. | • The meniscus should maintain normal signal and morphology: it should be of low signal intensity without tear (using the criteria for a native meniscus)
• The allograft is sutured to the native capsule circumferentially (there may be susceptibility artifact). This attachment can have high signal, but there should be no separation or fluid interposition. They usually heal to the capsule very well. The signal of the capsule varies from high to low on intermediate echo time, T2-weighted sequences.
• The plugs should be placed near to the native tibial attachments so that the meniscus can be anatomically located. Sometimes, it is hard to place the plugs exactly because many meniscal transplants have concomitant ACL grafts, and the space is limited.
• Evaluate chondral loss, status of the other meniscus, and ligaments. | • Re-tears of the meniscal allograft have the same appearance as that of the native meniscus
• Fluid signal indicates capsular detachment.
• Bone plugs or slots can fail to incorporate, yielding a persistent line of demarcation. This may occur when the bone becomes ischemic (persistent increased intermediate. T2-weighted signal) or necrotic (low signal on all sequences).
• The allograft may be too big or too small for the knee. Then, it appears as if the meniscus does not get to the edge of the joint (too small) or the opposite, it looks redundant. |

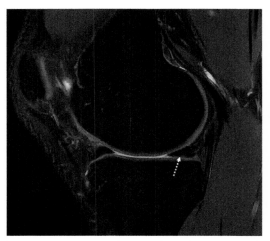

Fig. 27. Appearances of a partial meniscectomy in the context of a long horizontal tear. Sagittal PD fat sat demonstrates blunting of the meniscus, with mild inferior surface irregularity, residual from the tear (*dotted arrow*).

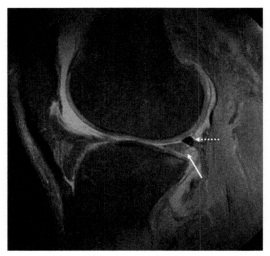

Fig. 29. Meniscal implant. Sagittal PD fat sat demonstrating the appearances of a meniscal implant (*bold arrow*). The meniscofemoral ligament is seen adjacent to it (*dotted arrows*).

The characteristics of meniscal repairs are summarized in **Table 4**[1,49–53] (**Figs. 27–29**).

Cartilage techniques

These consist of mosaicplasty/osteochondral autograft transfer system, autologous chondrocyte implantation, and osteochondral allograft, as summarized in **Table 5**[51,54–57] (**Fig. 30**).

Osteochondritis dissecans treatment

This consists of an osteochondral defect that occurs in characteristic locations. Etiology is likely posttraumatic. The fragment may become unstable and detach, leaving a defect.

Because of the potential consequences of development of osteoarthritis, repairing or replacing native bone is important. In younger patients especially, if a thin piece of bone, even if invisible

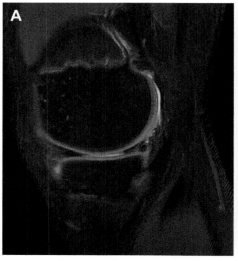

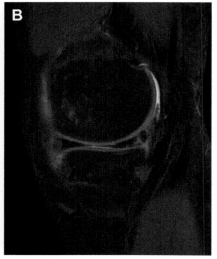

Fig. 28. Appearances of a sutured meniscus. (*A*) Sagittal PD fat sat demonstrates a posterior medial meniscal horn with an oblique linear band of increased signal intensity, in keeping with the line of suture. (*B*) Sagittal PD fat sat in a more medial location demonstrates higher inhomogeneity in signal. The patient underwent meniscal suture after a bucket handle tear of the medial meniscus. Past and surgical history is paramount to elucidate findings. These appearances may look indistinct from a tear.

Table 5
Summary of characteristics, indication, and expected appearances in cartilage techniques

Technique	Characteristics / Indications	Expected Postsurgical Appearances
Mosaicplasty/Osteochondral Autograft Transfer System Mosaicplasty and osteochondral autograft transfer system are essentially the same. They involve taking osteochondral plugs from one aspect of the joint to another part where there is a chondral defect, usually of the same joint. In the knee, donor sites tend to be at the peripheral trochlea where there is less stress on the cartilage. The region of chondral defect is prepared by having a hole drilled of the same size. The donor site fills in with bone and reparative fibrocartilage. Recently, resorbable scaffolds have been created to use in the donor sites to promote healing, or even as a treatment for a chondral injury. These scaffolds are resorbable.	• Mosaicplasty is usually used for lesions larger than microfracture or when microfracture has failed. • Lesions should be focal. • Multiple plugs may be needed to fill a defect. • Sometimes, because of the geometry of the defect, the plugs do not fill the entire defect, and there are some gaps. The hope is that cartilage spreads to fill the gaps.	Donor Site: if not filled with a scaffolding plug, looks initially like a hole and gradually, over a few months, fills in. The site is of high signal intensity on fat-suppressed images, with grafted sites being lower in signal intensity. The donor sites should fill in with time, with reparative fibrocartilage at the site of the original defect. Receiver Site: the bone and cartilage are both important. • The plug is initially of high signal intensity and becomes of lower signal intensity over time. • An interface between native and transferred bone (or adjacent plugs), at first, is sharp. Over time, the interface disappears as the bone becomes incorporated. • The cartilage should have the appearance of normal hyaline cartilage with a smooth interface with the surface of surrounding cartilage. The thickness of the cartilage may be different. This is normal. • In the cases in which scaffold plugs are used to fill the primary defect, they have a similar appearance to those used to fill donor sites. Some of the composite plugs look like autograft plugs on MR imaging.

(continued on next page)

Table 5
(continued)

Technique	Characteristics / Indications	Expected Postsurgical Appearances
Autologous Chondrocyte Implantation	Alternative to mosaicplasty for lesions that are too big for microfracture or in whom microfracture has failed.	• A periosteal flap may be visible, especially if thickened. • Underneath the flap, the cartilage should be similar in signal to normal hyaline cartilage but may vary. • Contours, although often a bit proud, should be smooth as should the interface with adjacent cartilage.
Osteochondral Allograft The allograft, which includes bone and overlying cartilage, is placed into an appropriately sized defect, in the area where the chondral defect is (usually on the femoral condyle). The allograft should heal to the native bone and restore the articular surface, blending the articular surfaces. Artificial scaffolds are being developed that will replace the need for allograft.	Osteochondral allografts are used on large but isolated chondral defects on one of the articular surfaces. They may be used after other techniques have failed.	• Initially, the allograft bone shows high signal with a sharp interface of native bone. • Over time, the interface becomes less sharp, gradually, the allograft and native bone fuse. • Ideally, the articular surfaces are smooth, and the geometry of the allograft is similar to the geometry of the native bone that it is replacing.

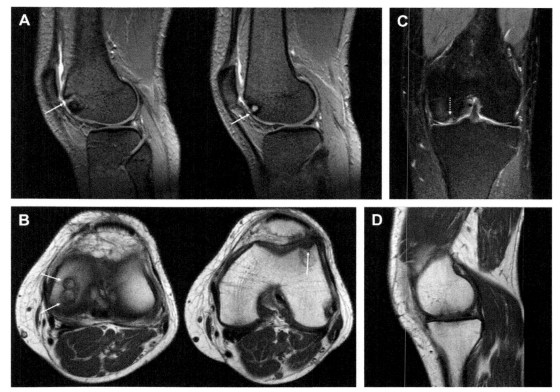

Fig. 30. Osteochondral allograft. (*A*) Sagittal T2* in consecutive slices demonstrates the osteochondral lesions in the peripheral lateral aspect of the trochlea, left by the harvesting of osteochondral allograft plugs (*bold arrows*). (*B*) Axial T1 images in two different planes demonstrate the location of the allograft plugs in the medial condyle (*left*) and one of the donor defects in the lateral aspect of the trochlea (*right*) (*bold arrows*). (*C*) Coronal PD fat sat demonstrates the region in the medial condyle where the allograft is incorporating, with continuity of the cartilage (*dotted arrow*). (*D*) Sagittal T1 demonstrates continuity of the subchondral bone, which appears homogeneous in this location.

on imaging, is present on a chondral surface, it can heal if reattached.[58]

For non-displaced fragments or fragments that have displaced but are viable, thin absorbable nails may be used. The nails used for fixation have a typical appearance on MR imaging as thin, straight, low signal intensity lines. They are radiolucent.

If the articular surface is intact, the lesion may be drilled from the nonarticular side to promote adherence of the fragment. This also appears as thin, low signal intensity lines on MR imaging.[58]

When the fragment is not viable, symptomatic patients may undergo the chondral repair techniques described previously.[59] The repaired fragment initially has high signal intensity and irregularity at the interface with underlying bone. Eventually, it fuses with the underlying bone.

If the overlying chondral surface deteriorates, or if the defect is left untreated, the subchondral bone, with time, becomes of normal signal intensity, but a defect remains in the overlying cartilage.

As a complication, the treatment may fail, and the piece may displace or collapse. The osteochondral fragment may not become incorporated; it may become a loose intra-articular body.

Arthroplasty

A summary of characteristics, indication, and expected and pathologic appearance is provided in **Table 6**[60,61] (**Fig. 31**).

Tendon repairs

The quadriceps and patellar tendons may be repaired or sutured. Depending on the quality of the stump, transpatellar tendon fixation is necessary.[62]

In the case of end-to-end sutures, postoperatively, the tendons should be continuous, with no discontinuity of gaps between ends.

Table 6
Summary of characteristics, indication, and expected and pathologic appearances in knee arthroplasty

Technique	Indications	Expected Postsurgical Appearances	Pathologic Appearances
Constrained Arthroplasty The patient's ligaments are not used to support the knee structure. A constrained arthroplasty has an additional metal piece between femoral and tibial components. Unconstrained Arthroplasty The patient's ligaments are used to stabilize the joint. Some are able to spare the native PCL.	Arthrosis (degenerative or inflammatory) A unicondylar arthroplasty (partial knee replacement) is used in patients with only medial or lateral compartment arthrosis as an alternative to osteotomy to relieve pain, improve alignment, and delay the need for a total arthroplasty.	• Joint alignment is normal. • The arthroplasty is radiopaque, and the space in between the femoral and tibial components is radiolucent (unconstrained), or has an additional metal piece (constrained) • Often, a layer of cement is used around the arthroplasty that is radiopaque • Generally, no more than 2 mm of lucency between the cement and bone or between the cement and component is present. • The patella should be aligned on the femoral component.	• An increase in the amount of lucency suggests that there is bone absorption (osteolysis), which often occurs from component wear and the body's reaction to the particles produced by that wear (particle disease). Smaller lucencies can be detected on computed tomography (CT) and MR imaging • Loosening • Adverse local tissue reaction • Infection is suggested on MR imaging when there is an abnormal increased signal extending into the soft tissues. Synovitis may also be found. Rapid osteolysis on radiographs or CT suggests infection. • Fracture • Recurrence of pathologic processes, such as tumor and synovitis. • Tendon and ligament injuries may also occur. • Problems with the components themselves (fractured polyethylene, incomplete seating of a prosthesis). • Recurrent synovitis may be apparent on MR imaging and is best seen on the axial images anteriorly around the patella. MR imaging may also show subtle abnormalities, such as synovial hypertrophy within the patellofemoral joint that can cause a click.

Abbreviations: CT, computed tomography

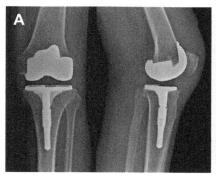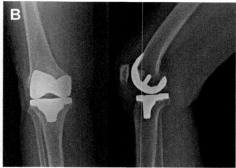

Fig. 31. Total knee unconstrained arthroplasty, two different types. (*A*) AP and lateral views demonstrate no lucency around the prosthetic components, which are correctly aligned and placed. The patella remains native. (*B*) AP and lateral radiographs demonstrate normal expected appearances. The tibial component has a shorter stem in the tibia, and the patella has been coated with a polyethylene cap.

Ultrasound is particularly useful for the evaluation of repaired tendons in early postsurgical status to demonstrate continuity.[48]

The tendons appear markedly thickened and hyperintense on MR imaging in early postsurgical status. Over time, appearances normalize.

Table 7
Summary of characteristics, indication, and expected and pathologic appearances in patellar realignment techniques

Technique	Characteristics / Indications	Expected Postsurgical Appearances	Pathologic Appearances
Proximal Realignment Release of the lateral retinaculum and patellofemoral ligament Medial retinaculum repair or tightening	• Abnormal patellar tracking. • Lateral dislocation • Generally performed arthroscopically	• Fascial defect just anterior to the iliotibial band on axial and coronal images at the level of the patella • Thicker medial retinaculum • Q angle should be normal	• Abnormal Q angle • Failure of medial retinaculum repair
Distal Realingment Distal realignments should not be performed in children because they interfere with the anterior growth plate and may lead to genu recurvatum	• Indicated when there is chondral loss to prevent further loss. • Indicated in cases of dysplasia that would not respond to noninvolved or less involved surgical methods. • Indicated when proximal realignments fail to solve the problem.	Radiographs • Fixation screws present (usually two) • The osteotomy site and bone block are also visible until they become incorporated, after which there is simply a prominent anterior tibial tubercle. • On patellar views, there should be a more normal Q angle. • Patella alta persists MR imaging • Only the remaining instrumentation and artifact persist. • Assessment of patellar cartilage.	• Failure of fixation, with the appearance of non-united osteotomy.

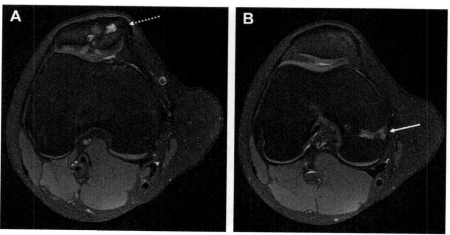

Fig. 32. Reconstruction of the medial patellar retinaculum. (*A*) Axial PD fat sat demonstrates anchors in the patella, with a small amount of fluid tracking within the anchor tunnel (*dotted arrow*). (*B*) Axial PD fat sat in a slightly more distal level demonstrates the anchor in the medial aspect of the medial condyle (*bold arrow*).

Table 8 Normal appearances and pathologic findings in fracture fixation	
Normal Expected Appearances	**Pathologic Appearances**
• There should be no radiographic spaces or step-offs. • Imaging appearances immediately after surgery should be identical on follow-up evaluations. • The screws should be continuous, and normal anatomy should be restored. • As long as a portion of the fracture is healing and creating a stable fixation, fracture lines may still be visible. • On MR imaging, acute or active healing fractures show high signal on fat-suppressed T2 or inversion recovery sequences.	• Fracture nonunion (fracture line still visible) • Loss of fixation (loosening of devices, rupture) • Infection (has the appearance of osteomyelitis) • Peroneal nerve palsy can occur. Proximal fibular fractures, because of the close proximity of the peroneal nerve to the fibula, can displace or injure the peroneal nerve.

The main possible complication is re-tear, quadriceps atrophy, and knee stiffness.[62]

Patellar realignments

A summary of characteristics, indication, and expected and pathologic appearance is provided in **Table 7**[63–65] (**Fig. 32**).

Fractures

Fixation of fractures is performed to restore anatomy (especially in articular surfaces) and facilitate healing. This prevents the development of early osteoarthritis.

Many groups use fixation when there is a step-off of more than 3 mm or angulation of more than 5°.

Fixations may be internal or external. The internal ones are performed with plate and screws and Kirschner wires, and the external ones usually seek to unload the joint and use intraosseous fixation points, connected externally.

Normal expected appearances and pathologic findings are summarized in **Table 8**[51,66]

SUMMARY

The knee is the largest, most stressed and therefore most frequently imaged joint in the body. The anatomy of the knee is complex. Knowledge of the anatomy helps to understand the mechanisms of injury and pathologic processes involving the knee. Familiarity with anatomic variants avoids misdiagnosis and potentially unnecessary intervention.

The correct understanding of the different types of surgical management approaches and the knowledge of the normal expected postsurgical appearances is extremely helpful in the assessment of potential postsurgical complications.

CLINICS CARE POINTS

- Knowledge of the complex anatomy and biomechanics of the knee, including its particularities and normal variation allows to understand the mechanisms of injury and provides a useful tool for accurate diagnosis and indications for treatment.
- Familiarity with the surgical procedures and normal postsurgical appearances and findings related to potential complications allows to provide relevant information to surgeons to favor a positive outcome for the patient.

DISCLOSURE

The authors have no funding information to disclose.

REFERENCES

1.. Bordalo-Rodrigues M, White LM. Knee. In: Hodler J, Kubik-Huch RA, von Schulthess GK, editors. Musculoskeletal diseases 2021-2024. IDKD springer series. Cham, Switzerland: Springer International Publishing; 2021. p. 83–106.

2. Raghavan S, Teo SH, Mohamed Al-Fayyadh MZ, et al. Variation in Kaplan fiber insertion to the distal femur and surgical implications: a cadaveric anatomical study comparing Asian and Caucasian knees. Knee 2022;38:56–61.

3. Lintin L, Chowdhury R, Yoong P, et al. The anterolateral ligament in acute knee trauma: patterns of injury on MR imaging. Skeletal Radiol 2020;49(11): 1765–72.

4. Campos JC, Chung CB, Lektrakul N, et al. Pathogenesis of the Segond fracture: anatomic and MR imaging evidence of an iliotibial tract or anterior oblique band avulsion. Radiology 2001;219(2):381–6.

5. Porrino J, Maloney E, Richardson M, et al. The anterolateral ligament of the knee: MRI appearance, association with the Segond fracture, and historical perspective. AJR Am J Roentgenol 2015;204(2): 367–73.

6. Getgood A, Brown C, Lording T, et al. The anterolateral complex of the knee: results from the International ALC Consensus Group Meeting. Knee Surg Sports Traumatol Arthrosc 2019;27(1):166–76.

7. Parsons EM, Gee AO, Spiekerman C, et al. The biomechanical function of the anterolateral ligament of the knee. Am J Sports Med 2015;43(3):669–74.

8. Rosas HG. Unraveling the posterolateral corner of the knee. RadioGraphics 2016;36(6):1776–91.

9. Perez Carro L, Sumillera Garcia M, Sunye Gracia C. Bifurcate popliteus tendon. Arthroscopy 1999;15(6): 638–9.

10. Doral MN, Atay AO, Bozkurt M, et al. Three-bundle popliteus tendon: a nonsymptomatic anatomical variation. Knee 2006;13(4):342–3.

11. Diamantopoulos A, Tokis A, Tzurbakis M, et al. The posterolateral corner of the knee: evaluation under microsurgical dissection. Arthroscopy 2005;21(7): 826–33.

12. Munshi M, Pretterklieber ML, Kwak S, et al. MR imaging, MR arthrography, and specimen correlation of the posterolateral corner of the knee: an anatomic study. AJR Am J Roentgenol 2003;180(4):1095–101.

13. Lundquist RB, Matcuk GR, Schein AJ, et al. Posteromedial corner of the knee: the neglected corner. RadioGraphics 2015;35(4):1123–37.

14. LaPrade RF, Morgan PM, Wentorf FA, et al. The anatomy of the posterior aspect of the knee. an anatomic study. J Bone Joint Surg Am 2007;89(4):758–64.

15. Saygi B, Yildirim Y, Berker N, et al. Evaluation of the neurosensory function of the medial meniscus in humans. Arthroscopy 2005;21(12):1468–72.

16. Hassebrock JD, Gulbrandsen MT, Asprey WL, et al. Knee ligament anatomy and biomechanics. Sports Med Arthrosc Rev 2020;28(3):80–6.

17. Mirai C, Otwock P, Bartoszewicz M. Dynamic ultrasonography in the diagnosis of acute anterior cruciate ligament injury – a case report. J Ultrason 2021; 21(85):e182–5.

18. Sonin AH, Fitzgerald SW, Hoff FL, et al. MR imaging of the posterior cruciate ligament: normal, abnormal, and associated injury patterns. RadioGraphics 1995;15(3):551–61.

19. Amis AA, Gupte CM, Bull AMJ, et al. Anatomy of the posterior cruciate ligament and the meniscofemoral ligaments. Knee Surg Sports Traumatol Arthrosc 2006;14(3):257–63.

20. Nacey NC, Geeslin MG, Miller GW, et al. Magnetic resonance imaging of the knee: an overview and update of conventional and state of the art imaging. J Magn Reson Imaging 2017;45(5): 1257–75.

21. Kang C, Wu L, Pu X, et al. Pseudotear Sign of the anterior horn of the meniscus. Arthrosc J Arthroscopic Relat Surg 2021;37(2):588–97.

22. Kumm J, Roemer FW, Guermazi A, et al. Natural history of intrameniscal signal intensity on knee MR images: six years of data from the osteoarthritis initiative. Radiology 2016;278(1):164–71.

23. Gaetke-Udager K, Yablon CM. Imaging of ligamentous structures within the knee includes

much more than the ACL. J Knee Surg 2018; 31(2):130–40.

24. Tubbs RS, Michelson J, Loukas M, et al. The transverse genicular ligament: anatomical study and review of the literature. Surg Radiol Anat 2008;30(1): 5–9.

25. Kim SH, Lipinski L, Pujol N. Meniscal allograft transplantation with soft-tissue fixation including the anterior intermeniscal ligament. Arthrosc Tech 2020;9(1): e137–42.

26. Deckey DG, Tummala S, Verhey JT, et al. Prevalence, biomechanics, and pathologies of the meniscofemoral ligaments: a systematic review. Arthrosc Sports Med Rehabil 2021;3(6):e2093–101.

27. Forkel P, Herbort M, Sprenker F, et al. The biomechanical effect of a lateral meniscus posterior root tear with and without damage to the meniscofemoral ligament: efficacy of different repair techniques. Arthroscopy 2014;30(7):833–40.

28. Pękala PA, Rosa MA, Łazarz DP, et al. Clinical Anatomy of the Anterior Meniscofemoral Ligament of humphrey: an original mri study, meta-analysis, and systematic review. Orthop J Sports Med 2021; 9(2). 2325967120973192.

29. Pękala PA, Łazarz DP, Rosa MA, et al. Clinical anatomy of the posterior meniscofemoral ligament of wrisberg: an original mri study, meta-analysis, and systematic review. Orthop J Sports Med 2021;9(2). 2325967120973195.

30. Savoye PY, Ravey JN, Dubois C, et al. Magnetic resonance diagnosis of posterior horn tears of the lateral meniscus using a thin axial plane: the zip sign–a preliminary study. Eur Radiol 2011;21(1): 151–9.

31. Mohankumar R, White LM, Naraghi A. Pitfalls and pearls in MRI of the knee. Am J Roentgenol 2014; 203(3):516–30.

32. Rohren EM, Kosarek FJ, Helms CA. Discoid lateral meniscus and the frequency of meniscal tears. Skeletal Radiol 2001;30(6):316–20.

33. Singh K, Helms CA, Jacobs MT, et al. MRI appearance of Wrisberg variant of discoid lateral meniscus. AJR Am J Roentgenol 2006;187(2): 384–7.

34. Moser MW, Dugas J, Hartzell J, et al. A hypermobile Wrisberg variant lateral discoid meniscus seen on MRI. Clin Orthop Relat Res 2007;456:264–7.

35. Collins MS, Tiegs-Heiden CA, Frick MA, et al. Medial patellofemoral ligament MRI abnormalities in the setting of MCL injuries: are they clinically relevant? Skeletal Radiol 2022;51(7):1381–9.

36. Krebs C, Tranovich M, Andrews K, et al. The medial patellofemoral ligament: Review of the literature. J Orthopaedics 2018;15(2):596–9.

37. Merican AM, Amis AA. Anatomy of the lateral retinaculum of the knee. J Bone Joint Surg Br 2008; 90(4):527–34.

38. García-Valtuille R, Abascal F, Cerezal L, et al. Anatomy and MR imaging appearances of synovial plicae of the knee. RadioGraphics 2002;22(4): 775–84.

39. Dupont JY. Synovial plicae of the knee. Controversies and review. Clin Sports Med 1997;16(1): 87–122.

40. Janzen DL, Peterfy CG, Forbes JR, et al. Cystic lesions around the knee joint: MR imaging findings. AJR Am J Roentgenol 1994;163(1):155–61.

41. Hirji Z, Hunjun JS, Choudur HN. Imaging of the bursae. J Clin Imaging Sci 2011;1:22.

42. Suomalainen P, Kannus P, Järvelä T. Double-bundle Anterior Cruciate Ligament reconstruction: a review of literature. Int Orthopaedics (Sicot) 2013;37(2): 227–32.

43. Zaffagnini S, Signorelli C, Lopomo N, et al. Anatomic double-bundle and over-the-top single-bundle with additional extra-articular tenodesis: an in vivo quantitative assessment of knee laxity in two different ACL reconstructions. Knee Surg Sports Traumatol Arthrosc 2012;20(1):153–9.

44. Casagranda BC, Maxwell NJ, Kavanagh EC, et al. Normal appearance and complications of double-bundle and selective-bundle anterior cruciate ligament reconstructions using optimal MRI techniques. Am J Roentgenology 2009;192(5): 1407–15.

45. Zaffagnini S, Marcheggiani Muccioli GM, Grassi A, et al. Over-the-top ACL reconstruction plus extra-articular lateral tenodesis with hamstring tendon grafts: prospective evaluation with 20-year minimum follow-up. Am J Sports Med 2017;45(14): 3233–42.

46. Wörtler K. MRT des Kniegelenks. Radiologe 2007; 47(12):1131–46.

47. Ilaslan H, Sundaram M, Miniaci A. Imaging evaluation of the postoperative knee ligaments. Eur J Radiol 2005;54(2):178–88.

48. Jacobson JA, Lax MJ. Musculoskeletal sonography of the postoperative orthopedic patient. Semin Musculoskelet Radiol 2002;6(1):67–77.

49. McCauley TR. MR imaging evaluation of the postoperative knee. Radiology 2005;234(1):53–61.

50. White LM, Kramer J, Recht MP. MR imaging evaluation of the postoperative knee: ligaments, menisci, and articular cartilage. Skeletal Radiol 2005;34(8): 431–52.

51. Frick MA, Collins MS, Adkins MC. Postoperative imaging of the knee. Radiol Clin North Am 2006;44(3): 367–89.

52. Gopez AG, Kavanagh EC. MR imaging of the postoperative meniscus: repair, resection, and

replacement. Semin Musculoskelet Radiol 2006; 10(3):229–40.

53. Grassi A, Zaffagnini S, Marcheggiani Muccioli GM, et al. Clinical outcomes and complications of a collagen meniscus implant: a systematic review. Int Orthop 2014;38(9):1945–53.

54. Hangody L, Füles P. Autologous osteochondral mosaicplasty for the treatment of full-thickness defects of weight-bearing joints: ten years of experimental and clinical experience. J Bone Joint Surg Am 2003;85(A Suppl 2):25–32.

55. Gross AE. Repair of cartilage defects in the knee. J Knee Surg 2002;15(3):167–9.

56. Choi YS, Potter HG, Chun TJ. MR imaging of cartilage repair in the knee and ankle. Radiographics 2008;28(4):1043–59.

57. Ho YY, Stanley AJ, Hui JHP, et al. Postoperative evaluation of the knee after autologous chondrocyte implantation: what radiologists need to know. Radiographics 2007;27(1):207–20. discussion 221-222.

58. Pascual-Garrido C, McNickle AG, Cole BJ. Surgical treatment options for osteochondritis dissecans of the knee. Sports Health 2009;1(4):326–34.

59. Filardo G, Kon E, Berruto M, et al. Arthroscopic second generation autologous chondrocytes implantation associated with bone grafting for the treatment of knee osteochondritis dissecans: Results at 6 years. Knee 2012;19(5):658–63.

60. Miller TT. Imaging of knee arthroplasty. Eur J Radiol 2005;54(2):164–77.

61. Fritz J, Lurie B, Potter HG. MR imaging of knee arthroplasty implants. Radiographics 2015;35(5):1483–501.

62. Lee D, Stinner D, Mir H. Quadriceps and patellar tendon ruptures. J Knee Surg 2013;26(5):301–8.

63. Jibri Z, Jamieson P, Rakhra KS, et al. Patellar maltracking: an update on the diagnosis and treatment strategies. Insights Imaging 2019; 10(1):65.

64. Zaffagnini S, Grassi A, Marcheggiani Muccioli GM, et al. Medial patellotibial ligament (MPTL) reconstruction for patellar instability. Knee Surg Sports Traumatol Arthrosc 2014;22(10):2491–8.

65. Zaffagnini S, Marcheggiani Muccioli GM, Grassi A, et al. Minimally invasive medial patellofemoral ligament reconstruction with fascia lata allograft: surgical technique. Knee Surg Sports Traumatol Arthrosc 2014;22(10):2426–30.

66. Mustonen AOT, Koivikko MP, Kiuru MJ, et al. Postoperative MDCT of tibial plateau fractures. Am J Roentgenology 2009;193(5):1354–60.

Overuse-Related Injuries of the Knee

Mohamed Jarraya, MD[a],*, Frank W. Roemer, MD[b,c], Daichi Hayashi, MD, PhD[d], Michel D. Crema, MD[e], Ali Guermazi, MD, PhD[b,f]

KEYWORDS

- Stress injuries • Knee • Overuse • Tendinopathy • Apophysitis • Bursitis • Friction • Impingement

KEY POINTS

- Overuse-related injuries often have nonspecific clinical presentations. Imaging helps guide the diagnosis and differentiate overuse-related injuries from other joint-related pathologic conditions.
- Bone stress injuries of the tibia plateau are rare and much less frequent that bone stress injuries of the tibial shaft. They are best depicted with MR imaging.
- In tendon overuse pathology and traction apophysitis, MR imaging can be helpful in severe cases, to rule out partial tears and avulsion injuries. Ultrasound may be helpful in characterizing chronicity.

INTRODUCTION

Overuse-related injuries of the knee joint and peri-articular tissues are a heterogenous group of sports-related and nonsports-related injuries, commonly seen in the adult and pediatric population. These injuries are common source of morbidity and often result in chronic functional impairment. Some of the described entities in this review may also be found with increased frequency in knee osteoarthritis, suggesting degenerative cause, as for knee bursitis and tendinopathy.

Although several imaging modalities can be helpful in making the diagnosis of overuse-related injuries, MR imaging is the most common and often the only modality performed. Other imaging modalities including conventional radiographs and ultrasound will be discussed, when relevant. Regardless, imaging examinations are an indispensable tool for diagnosing and sometimes managing these injuries.

In this review, we discuss imaging findings of overuse-related injuries around the knee, with particular focus on MR imaging. We limit our focus to entities that are either solely or mostly related to overuse.

SYNOVIAL IMPINGEMENT AND FRICTION SYNDROMES

Infrapatellar Fat Pad Impingement (Patellar Tendon-Lateral Femoral Condyle Friction Syndrome)

Infrapatellar fat pad impingement is also referred to as patellar tendon-lateral femoral condyle friction syndrome. Its main MR imaging hallmark is superolateral Hoffa fat pad (SHFP) edema.[1] SHFP edema is very common in routine knee MR imagings, especially in younger women with

[a] Department of Radiology, Massachusetts General Hospital, Harvard Medical School, 32 Fruit Street YAW 6044, Boston, MA 02114, USA; [b] Department of Radiology, Boston University School of Medicine, 820 Harrison Avenue, FGH Building 3rd Floor, Boston, MA 02118, USA; [c] Department of Radiology, Friedrich-Alexander University Erlangen-Nürnberg (FAU) and University Hospital Erlangen, Maximiliansplatz 391054 Erlangen, Germany; [d] Department of Radiology, Stony Brook University, 101 Nichols Road, HSc Level 4, Room 120, Dept of Radiology, Stony Brook, NY 11790, USA; [e] Institut d'Imagerie du Sport, Institut National du Sport, de l'Expertise et de la Performance (INSEP), 11 Avenue du Tremblay, 75012 Paris, France; [f] Department of Radiology, VA Boston Healthcare System, 1400 VFW Parkway, 1B105 West Roxbury, MA 02132, USA
* Corresponding author.
E-mail address: mjarraya@mgh.harvard.edu

or without anterior knee pain.[2] For instance, SHFP edema was reported in 1 in 2 female collegiate volleyball players[2] and was most frequent among Volleyball and Beach Volleyball Olympic athletes in the 2016 Olympic Games of Rio de Janeiro.[3] SHFP is thought to be secondary to impingement due to its association with high-riding patella, increased tibial tuberosity-trochlear groove (TT-TG) distance,[4] as well as other markers of patellofemoral maltracking.[5] SHFP edema was initially thought to be the imaging correlate of patellofemoral friction syndrome.[6] However, given it is high prevalence among asymptomatic young athletes, we hypothesize that isolated MR imaging-detected SHFP edema is the subclinical manifestation of infrapatellar tendon impingement. The frequent occurrence of SHFP edema among volleyball players suggest that it is secondary to overuse from repetitive jumping.

Increased TT-TG distance and high riding patella both result in exaggeration of valgus translational force during flexion and therefore result in a higher risk of friction of Hoffa fat pad between the lateral femoral condyle and the lateral aspect of the patellar tendon, as seen on MR imaging.[1] Of note, SHFP edema has also been linked to cartilage loss and osteoarthritis of the lateral patellofemoral compartment.[7]

Clinically, infrapatellar fat pad impingement is characterized by anterior knee pain and tenderness, typically at the lower pole of the patella. The pain is commonly exacerbated by hyperextension and physical examination can demonstrate focal point tenderness at the inferior pole of the patella.[1]

On MR imaging, sagittal and axial fluid-sensitive images such as short tau inversion recovery and T2-weighted fat-suppressed images reveal focal increased signal intensity in the superolateral portion of Hoffa fat pad, between the lateral femoral condyle and patellar tendon, described as edema, which may be enhancing after administration of contrast.[1] **Fig. 1** shows an example of classic SHFP edema. Focal proximal patellar tendinopathy apposing the lateral trochlea is another important MR imaging finding that was reported in association with patellar tendon-Lateral femoral condyle friction.[4] A short distance between the lateral femoral condyle and patellar ligament was also reported in association with the latter finding[4] (see **Fig. 1**).

The management of infrapatellar impingement is usually successfully managed with conservative therapy, including physical therapy targeted at restoring the biomechanics of patellar tracking, as well as taping to unload the inferior fat pad.[1]

Iliotibial Band Syndrome

Iliotibial band syndrome (ITBS) is the second leading cause of pain in runners. There are different hypotheses related to its cause, including anterior–posterior friction of the IT band on the lateral femoral condyle during knee flexion and extension activities, compression of a layer of fat near the IT band distal attachment, and inflammation of the IT band bursa.[8]

In a kinematic study of 9 runners with iliotibial friction syndrome, the impingement was found to occur near foot-strike, predominantly in the foot contact phase, between the posterior edge of the iliotibial band and the underlying lateral femoral epicondyle.[9] Downhill running is associated with reduced knee flexion angle at foot-strike, therefore predisposing to ITBS.[9] However, sprinting and faster running on the level ground were shown to be less likely to cause or aggravate ITBS symptoms because, at foot-strike, the knee is flexed beyond the angles at which friction occurs.[9]

A review exploring the biomechanical variables involved in the cause of ITBS in distance runners reported that although a clear biomechanical cause of ITBS is not known, a greater internal rotation at the knee joint and increased adduction angles of the hip may play a role in the cause of ITBS.[10]

On imaging, fluid-sensitive MR imaging sequences show an ill-defined area of increased signal in the soft tissues situated between the lateral femoral condyle and the IT band (**Fig. 2**). Note that imaging findings suggesting ITBS are often nonspecific and are also observed in asymptomatic individuals. Thickening and interstitial tear of the IT band can also be seen.[11] Osseous edema and underlying bone erosions have also been reported.[11] In chronic cases, an encapsulated cyst formation can be found between the IT tract and lateral femoral condyle.

Prepatellar Friction Syndrome

The prepatellar fascia, also referred to as the prepatellar quadriceps continuation, is formed by fibers from the rectus femoris tendon, connecting the quadriceps and patellar tendons.[12] It is a complex multilayer structure with a superficial layer comprising transverse fibers, an intermediate layer of obliquely oriented fibers, and a deep layer of longitudinally oriented fibers.[13]

Injuries to the prepatellar quadriceps continuation can occur in the setting of acute direct trauma or chronic overuse injuries and are commonly encountered among cyclists.[14] Of note, overuse injuries represent nearly two-thirds of all cycling-related injuries, and commonly involved the knee

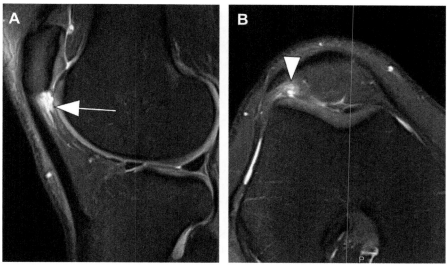

Fig. 1. Painful infrapatellar lateral inflammation of Hoffa's fat pad also known as infrapatellar fat pad impingement in a 34-year-old woman. (A) Sagittal proton density-weighted fat-suppressed MR imaging shows intense edematous changes in the superolateral aspect of Hoffa's fat pad (*arrow*) as a result of chronic friction due to maltracking. Note that the edema is located more laterally in comparison to classic tendinopathy of the patellar tendon (jumper's knee). (B) This is also well demonstrated on the corresponding axial proton density-weighted fat-suppressed MR imaging (*arrowhead*).

joint.[15] Prepatellar friction presents as anterior knee pain and is therefore in the differential of ITBS and patellofemoral degenerative disease. Although friction has been hypothetically used to define these injuries, other mechanisms could also explain it in athletes such as traction or overload directed to this part of the extensor mechanism.

MR imaging can show the normal or damaged trilaminar prepatellar structure, with possible edema along or within the prepatellar fascia (**Fig. 3**). Sometimes a defect along the fascia can

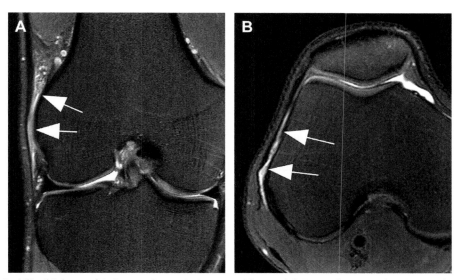

Fig. 2. Typical iliotibial tract friction syndrome in 27-year-old man. (A) Coronal proton density-weighted fat-suppressed MR imaging shows edematous changes between the iliotibial band and the lateral femoral condyle (*arrows*). (B) Such fibrovascular tissue between the iliotibial tract and the lateral femoral condyle is also well depicted on the corresponding axial proton density-weighted fat-suppressed MR imaging (*arrows*).

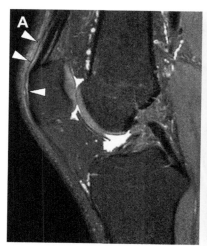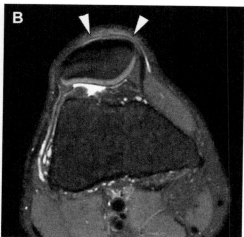

Fig. 3. Prepatellar fascia syndrome in a 30-year-old male elite triathlon athlete. (*A*) Sagittal proton density-weighted fat-suppressed MR imaging shows thickening and edema of the prepatellar and prequadriceps tendon soft tissue. In addition, the thickened prepatellar fascia is well depicted extending from the quadriceps tendon distally (*arrowheads*) with surrounding high-signal soft tissue changes. (*B*) Corresponding axial proton density-weighted fat-suppressed MR imaging shows predominantly medial involvement (*arrowheads*).

be seen.[14] Injury to the prepatellar fascia can also be associated with signal abnormality to the patellar or quadriceps tendon. High-frequency ultrasound was also reported to be highly effective for the localization of superficial pathologic condition in prepatellar friction injuries.

BURSITIS AROUND THE KNEE
Pes Anserine Bursitis

As for other bursitis, pes anserine bursitis can be secondary to different causes including overuse from sports activities such as running, mechanical derangement, direct trauma, and obesity.[16] Pes anserine symptoms may be related to either the tendons (sartorius, gracilis, and semitendinosus) or the associated brusa.[17] Medial compartment osteoarthritis is also commonly associated with pes anserine bursitis. Typically, pes anserine pain is located along the anteromedial tibia below the knee, whereas medial knee osteoarthritis pain lies along the medial joint line.

Although the bursa is typically described between the pes anserinus tendons and proximal tibia,[18] an ultrasound study in healthy asymptomatic volunteers showed variations that the pes anserine bursa can be identified between the pes anserinus and the medial collateral ligament (MCL) in 21%, or less commonly between the constituents of the pes anserinus (8%).[19] The distended bursa is usually noted distally and medially to the tibial tuberosity with possible invagination of fluid deep to the superficial MCL. The bursa can also extend above the joint line.[20]

A typical example of pes anserine bursitis on MR imaging is shown in **Fig. 4**.

Posteromedial Knee Friction and Pes Anserinus Snapping

Posteromedial knee friction is a cause of posteromedial pain in active patients. It occurs in the narrow space between the posteromedial femoral condyle and the sartorius and gracilis tendons. It is caused by friction between the tendons and the bone. MR imaging can show ill-defined edema between the gracilis and sartorius on one side and the medial femoral condyle on the other side.[21] Of note, edema in the same location can also be caused by acute meniscal tears, ligament injury, and leaking popliteal cysts.

Pes anserinus snapping occurs when the semitendinosus or gracilis snaps over the medial tibial condyle, or when the semimembranosus tendon snaps over the posteromedial aspect of the knee during the flexion-extension movements.[21,22] It is suggested that diminutive pes anserinus accessory fascial bands contribute to the snapping by allowing forward movements of the gracilis and semitendinosus over the posteromedial tibia.[16] Ultrasound is the preferred modality for the evaluation of posteromedial snapping considering its dynamic capability.[23]

BONE STRESS INJURIES

Bone stress injuries including stress fractures result from repetitive injury at areas of stress

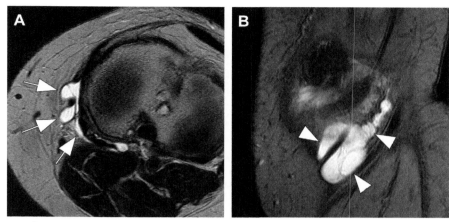

Fig. 4. Anserine bursitis with fluid between the pes anserine and the tibial plateau in a 45-year-old female patient. (*A*) Axial T2-weighted MR imaging shows irregular fluid collection adjacent to the medial tibial plateau surrounding the pes anserine attachment (*arrows*). (*B*) Fluid is also well depicted on the sagittal proton density-weighted fat-suppressed MR imaging (*arrowheads*).

concentration. These are very common among military recruit[24] as well as athletes.[25] The tibia is a commonly involved bone in stress injuries and fractures as demonstrated in prior reports from the Olympic Game of 2016[25] and 2020[26]; however, these injuries are most frequent at the diaphysis with the tibial plateau injury only found in 1 out of 6 cases of injuries involving the tibia in the Olympic games of Tokyo 2020.[26]

Although stress fractures of the tibial diaphysis are common among athletes, the proximal tibial metaphysis is an unusual location for such injuries. In addition, their proximity to the knee joint can obscure the diagnosis.

Imaging plays an important role in diagnosing tibial plateau stress injuries because they can be easily mistaken for intra-articular pathologic condition based on clinical presentation alone. **Fig. 5** gives an illustrative example of a typical epimetaphyseal stress reaction of the tibia due to overuse. Conventional radiographs can show linear or ill-defined sclerosis in the medial or lateral tibial plateau typically perpendicular to the cortex.[27] However, oftentimes the radiographs are negative at initial presentation and may only be positive at 4 weeks.[28] In some case, the radiograph never shows the bone stress fracture, which can only be detected on MR imaging.[27] Bone stress injuries are often bilateral.

MR imaging shows bone edema, with T1 hypo-intense and T2 hyperintense signal changes involving the medial or lateral tibial condyles away from the subchondral bone, either closely associated with epiphyseal plate scar,[27] or along it with some reports of stress fractures along persistent physis with biopsy evidence of cartilage at the fracture site.[29] T1-weighted imaging

superiorly depicts fracture lines, which can be obscured by bone marrow edema on fluid-sensitive fat-suppressed images (**Fig. 6**).

TENDINOPATHY AND TENDON OVERUSE-RELATED INJURIES

There is a common misconception that symptomatic tendon injuries are inflammatory; hence labeled as "tendonitis." In most cases, tendon-related symptoms are chronic suggesting a degenerative condition, related to overuse. The natural history is gradually increasing load-related localized pain coinciding with increased activity.[30] The most common overuse tendinopathies around the knee involve the extensor mechanism, as described below.

Patellar Tendinopathy and Overuse-Related Injuries

Overuse-related patellar tendon abnormalities include a spectrum of pathologic condition ranging from chronic degeneration to partial tearing. Patellar tendinopathy is classically seen in sports associated with jumping, hence often referred to as "Jumper's knee." Repetitive overload is the most commonly proposed theory in the pathogenesis of patellar tendinopathy with overload resulting in weakening of the tissues and eventually failure.[31,32] Patellofemoral morphology and alignment may also increase the risk of patellar tendinopathy.[33] The increased strain is located in the deep posterior portion of the tendon, closer to the center of rotation of the knee and the inferior pole of the patella, especially with increased knee flexion.[32] For this reason, lesions in patellar tendinopathy typically occur in

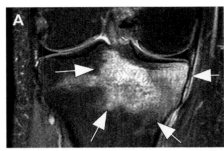
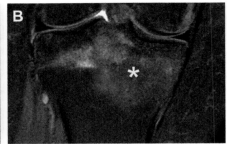

Fig. 5. Severe stress reaction in a 38-year-old woman, who had started a regime of intense running training 2 months earlier. (A) Coronal fat-suppressed proton density-weighted MR imaging shows marked epi-metaphyseal signal changes in the tibial plateau, reflecting a severe stress reaction (*arrows*). (B) A follow-up MR imaging 2 months later (not having exercised in the interval) shows only mild residual changes (*asterisk*).

the deep posterior portion of the proximal patellar tendon adjacent to the lower pole of the patella.[34] The mechanism of injury involves eccentric contraction of the quadriceps, usually with the foot planted and the knee flexed as the person falls.

Predisposing factors to tendon rupture include conditions associated with systemic inflammation such as diabetes, chronic renal failure, or systemic lupus erythematosus. In these cases, lower energy mechanisms can result in rupture.[35]

In the United States, the normal fibrillar pattern of the patellar tendon is altered with hypoechoic thickening of the tendon near its proximal insertion.[36] Increased Doppler flow can also be demonstrated indicating neovascularization, which can help localize the site of injury (Fig. 7). Because of its relatively higher resolution, ultrasound depicts better tendinous tears than MR imaging (usually anechoic in ultrasound). Moreover, tendinous calcifications are better depicted when performing ultrasound. Typical findings on MR imaging include

focal thickening of the proximal one-third of the patellar tendon with abnormal high-signal intensity on fluid-sensitive images.[37]

Ultimately chronic overuse injury of the patellar tendon may result in rupture, usually at the lower patellar pole (see Fig. 7). Rupture can be secondary to violent contraction of the quadriceps muscle against the fixed load of the patient's body weight with the knee in flexion, or can sometimes occur with less dramatic force. Conventional radiography shows a superiorly displaced patella with thickening of the infrapatellar silhouette. On MR imaging, the patellar tendon is ruptured from its patellar attachment with possible buckling.[38]

Quadriceps Tendon

Quadriceps tendinopathy usually occurs at the distal insertion of the quadriceps at the proximal patella and is often associated with underlying systemic disease and/or drug use such as steroid drug use.[39] However, repetitive microtrauma in

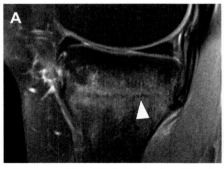
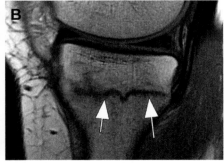

Fig. 6. Stress fracture of the tibial plateau in a 36-year-old female runner. (A) Sagittal proton density-weighted fat-suppressed MR imaging shows diffuse epiphyseal edema consistent with a stress reaction. In addition, there is a subtle fracture line (*arrowhead*) defining this injury as a stress fracture. (B) Corresponding sagittal T1-weighted MR imaging superiorly shows the fracture line (*arrows*) as surrounding edema is less conspicuous on the T1-weighted image.

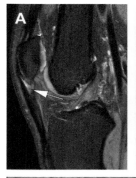
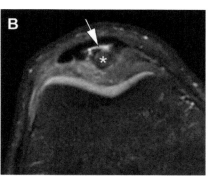
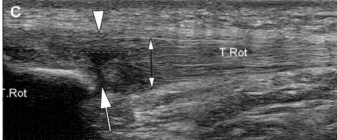
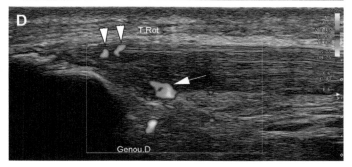

Fig. 7. Patellar tendinopathy. A 26-year-old male basketball player with a clinical diagnosis of jumpers' knee. (A) Sagittal proton density-weighted fat-suppressed MR imaging shows thickening of the proximal patellar tendon and a deep partial tendon disruption (arrow). (B) Corresponding axial proton density-weighted fat-suppressed MR imaging shows the central tendon rupture (arrow) and tendinopathic high signal changes of the deep portion of the tendon (asterisk). (C) Longitudinal corresponding ultrasound confirms partial rupture at the deep aspect of the tendon (arrow) while the superficial aspect of the tendon is still intact (arrowhead). The proximal patellar tendon is also thickened (two-sided arrow). (D) There is a moderate hypervascularity on Doppler mode of the deep (arrow) and superficial (arrowheads) portions of the patellar tendon.

athletes due to overloading from jumping and running activities[40–42] is also a contributing factor, especially in the pediatric population.[43] Patients often present with pain and tenderness at the superior pole of the patella, sometimes weakness on resisted quadriceps extension.[44]

Conventional radiography shows thickening of the quadriceps silhouette. The ultrasound features of quadriceps tendinopathy are quite similar to those described above for patellar tendinopathy. Attention to the trilaminar structure of the quadriceps tendon is useful as such pattern should be preserved on longitudinal and transverse ultrasound assessments.

MR imaging shows a thickened, abnormal tendon with increased intermediate signal in the tendon fibers.[45] When partial thickness tear occurs it usually extends from the superficial to the deep fibers, first involving the rectus femoris component. The vastus intermedius is usually involved last.

Other Tendinopathy: Semitendinosus, Semimembranosus, Biceps Femoris, and Gastrocnemius

Other overuse-related tendon injuries around the knee can mimic intra-articular joint pathologic condition and should, therefore, be recognized on imaging. Tendinopathy of the pes anserinus tendons can be associated with pes anserine bursitis, the semitendinosus tendon being more frequently affected in these cases. Tendinopathy at the distal insertion of the semimembranosus may also occur in athletes, isolated (Fig. 8) or associated with pes anserinus friction syndrome. Tendinopathy of the proximal medial gastrocnemius attachment along the posterior aspect of the medial femoral condyle can result in posterior knee pain and be mistaken for a popliteal cyst. Biceps tendinopathy can result in posterolateral knee pain. MR imaging and ultrasound features of tendinopathy

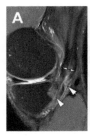
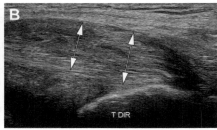
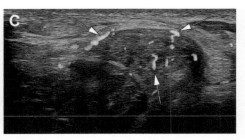

Fig. 8. A 36-year-old male soccer player with distal semimembranosus tendinopathy. (*A*) Sagittal intermediate-weighted fat suppressed MR imaging shows marked thickening (*two-sided arrow*) and longitudinal split of the distal semimembranosus tendon. In addition, there is a partial rupture of the posterior fibers (*arrow*) and marked signal change (*arrowhead*) near the attachment indicating tendinopathy. (*B*) Corresponding longitudinal ultrasound B-mode image shows diffuse thickening of the tendon (*two-sided arrows*). (*C*) Axial ultrasound mage with power Doppler shows neovascularization of the distal tendon (*arrows*).

affecting other tendons around the knee are quite similar to those described for the extensor mechanism above. For instance, MR imaging shows thinking and edema-like signal of the tendons, with possible partial tears in more severe cases.

Pediatric-Specific Overuse-Related Injuries: Traction Apophysitis

Young athletes with open growth plates are vulnerable to unique overuse injuries involving the apophyses, articular cartilage, and growth plate.[43] Traction apophysitis is referred to as Osgood-Schlatter when it involves the tibial tubercule apophysis and Sinding-Larsen-Johansson when it affects the inferior pole of the patella.

Osgood-Schlatter Syndrome

Osgood-Schlatter disease is more common in male adolescents between 11 and 13 years of age, with a higher incidence among athletes in comparison with nonathletes.[44]

Clinical examination shows anterior pain over the tibial tubercle, bilateral in up to 30% of the cases. Pain and discomfort are aggravated by sports involving jumping, squatting, and kneeling. Localized tenderness and sometimes swelling over the tibial tubercle are noted on examination. Conventional radiograph shows fragmentation of the tibial tubercle with soft tissue thickening.[46] MR imaging shows soft tissue edema on fluid-sensitive sequences with possible underlying bone edema (**Fig. 9**).

Sinding-Larsen-Johansson

This entity is secondary to repetitive traction at the inferior pole of the patella, resulting in tendonitis. In more severe cases, tendon avulsion with subsequent calcification can occur. It is often seen among adolescents between 10 and 13 years of age.[44]

This condition presents as intermittent anterior knee pain, related to activity, such as jumping and running. It is localized over the inferior pole of the patella and proximal attachment of the patellar tendon.[44]

Conventional radiographs show well-corticated mineralization and ossifications at the inferior pole of the patella. This should be differentiated

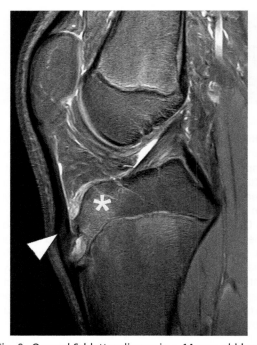

Fig. 9. Osgood-Schlatter disease in a 14-year-old boy. Sagittal proton density-weighted fat-suppressed MR imaging shows traction edema (*asterisk*) at the tibial tuberosity (=apophysitis) and edema at the deep infrapatellar bursa. Note, that the distal patellar tendon itself shows mildly increased signal as a sign of tendinopathy (*arrowhead*).

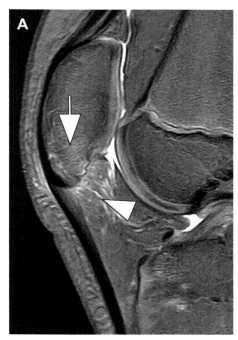
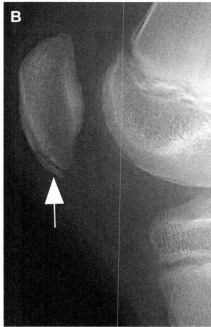

Fig. 10. Sinding-Larsen-Johansson syndrome in a 13-year-old boy. (*A*) Sagittal proton density-weighted fat-suppressed MR imaging shows traction edema at the inferior patellar pole (*arrow*) and edema in the superior aspect of Hoffa's fat pad (*arrowhead*). (*B*) Note that partial apophyseal avulsion is present and best seen on the corresponding lateral radiograph (*arrow*).

from a bipartite patella or a patellar sleeve fracture. MR imaging shows edema-like signal of the proximal patellar tendon and can help rule out patellar sleeve avulsion[44] (**Fig. 10**).

SUMMARY

Overuse-related injuries of the knee joint and the periarticular soft issues are a heterogenous group of pathologic conditions including friction and impingement syndromes, bursitis, tendon pathologic condition, bone stress–related injuries, and traction apophysitis in the pediatric population. MR imaging is the most common and often the only used imaging modality. Correlation to the clinical presentation is important because MR imaging findings consistent with impingement syndromes and bursitis can also be seen in asymptomatic individuals.

CLINICS CARE POINTS

- Bone stress innjuries are best depicted with MRI.2. Both MRI and ultrasound are helpful for overuse-related tendon injuries and bursits.

CONFLICT OF INTEREST

A. Guermazi: Consultant to Pfizer, Regeneron, MerckSerono, TissueGene, AstraZeneca and Novartis. Shareholder of Boston Imaging Core Lab (BICL), LLC. F.W. Roemer: Consultant to Calibr, Grünenthal (last 36 months). Shareholder of BICL, LLC. D. Hayashi: Publishing royalties from Wolters-Kluwer. M.D. Crema: Shareholder of BICL, LLC. M. Jarraya: None to declare.

REFERENCES

1. Jarraya M, Diaz LE, Roemer FW, et al. MRI Findings Consistent with Peripatellar Fat Pad Impingement: How Much Related to Patellofemoral Maltracking? Magn Reson Med Sci 2018;17(3):195–202.
2. Mehta K, Wissman R, England E, et al. Superolateral Hoffa's Fat Pad Edema in Collegiate Volleyball Players. J Comput Assist Tomogr 2015;39(6): 945–50.
3. Jarraya M, Roemer FW, Engebretsen L, et al. Association of markers of patellofemoral maltracking to cartilage damage and bone marrow lesions on MRI: Data from the 2016 Olympic Games of Rio De Janeiro. Eur J Radiol Open 2021;8:100381.
4. Campagna R, Pessis E, Biau DJ, et al. Is superolateral Hoffa fat pad edema a consequence of

impingement between lateral femoral condyle and patellar ligament? Radiology 2012;263(2):469–74.

5. Widjajahakim R, Roux M, Jarraya M, et al. Relationship of Trochlear Morphology and Patellofemoral Joint Alignment to Superolateral Hoffa Fat Pad Edema on MR Images in Individuals with or at Risk for Osteoarthritis of the Knee: The MOST Study. Radiology 2017;284(3):806–14.

6. Chung CB, Skaf A, Roger B, et al. Patellar tendon-lateral femoral condyle friction syndrome: MR imaging in 42 patients. Skeletal Radiol 2001;30(12):694–7.

7. Jarraya M, Guermazi A, Felson DT, et al. Is superolateral Hoffa's fat pad hyperintensity a marker of local patellofemoral joint disease? - The MOST study. Osteoarthritis Cartilage 2017;25(9):1459–67.

8. Charles D, Rodgers C. A literature review and clinical commentary on the development of iliotibial band syndrome in runners. Int J Sports Phys Ther 2020;15(3):460–70.

9. Orchard JW, Fricker PA, Abud AT, et al. Biomechanics of iliotibial band friction syndrome in runners. Am J Sports Med 1996;24(3):375–9.

10. Louw M, Deary C. The biomechanical variables involved in the aetiology of iliotibial band syndrome in distance runners - A systematic review of the literature. Phys Ther Sport Off J Assoc Chart Physiother Sports Med 2014;15(1):64–75.

11. Isusi M, Oleaga L, Campo M, et al. [MRI findings in iliotibial band friction syndrome: a report of two cases]. Radiologia 2007;49(6):433–5.

12. Wangwinyuvirat M, Dirim B, Pastore D, et al. Prepatellar quadriceps continuation: MRI of cadavers with gross anatomic and histologic correlation. AJR Am J Roentgenol 2009;192(3):W111–6.

13. Dye SF, Campagna-Pinto D, Dye CC, et al. Soft-tissue anatomy anterior to the human patella. J Bone Joint Surg Am 2003;85(6):1012–7.

14. Claes T, Claes S, De Roeck J, et al. Prepatellar Friction Syndrome: a common cause of knee pain in the elite cyclist. Acta Orthop Belg 2015;81(4):614–9.

15. De Bernardo N, Barrios C, Vera P, et al. Incidence and risk for traumatic and overuse injuries in top-level road cyclists. J Sports Sci 2012;30(10):1047–53.

16. Curtis BR, Huang BK, Pathria MN, et al. Pes Anserinus: Anatomy and Pathology of Native and Harvested Tendons. AJR Am J Roentgenol 2019;213(5):1107–16.

17. Sapp GH, Herman DC. Pay Attention to the Pes Anserine in Knee Osteoarthritis. Curr Sports Med Rep 2018;17(2):41.

18. Forbes JR, Helms CA, Janzen DL. Acute pes anserine bursitis: MR imaging. Radiology 1995;194(2):525–7.

19. Imani F, Rahimzadeh P, Abolhasan Gharehdag F, et al. Sonoanatomic variation of pes anserine bursa. Korean J Pain 2013;26(3):249–54.

20. Lee JH, Kim KJ, Jeong YG, et al. Pes anserinus and anserine bursa: anatomical study. Anat Cell Biol 2014;47(2):127–31.

21. Simeone FJ, Huang AJ, Chang CY, et al. Posteromedial knee friction syndrome: an entity with medial knee pain and edema between the femoral condyle, sartorius and gracilis. Skeletal Radiol 2015;44(4):557–63.

22. von Dercks N, Theopold JD, Marquass B, et al. Snapping knee syndrome caused by semitendinosus and semimembranosus tendons. A case report. The Knee 2016;23(6):1168–71.

23. Bollen SR, Arvinte D. Snapping pes syndrome: a report of four cases. J Bone Joint Surg Br 2008;90(3):334–5.

24. Jordaan G, Schwellnus MP. The incidence of overuse injuries in military recruits during basic military training. Mil Med 1994;159(6):421–6.

25. Hayashi D, Jarraya M, Engebretsen L, et al. Epidemiology of imaging-detected bone stress injuries in athletes participating in the Rio de Janeiro 2016 Summer Olympics. Br J Sports Med 2018;52(7):470–4.

26. Adachi T, Katagiri H, An JS, et al. Imaging-Detected Bone Stress Injuries at the Tokyo 2020 Summer Olympics: Epidemiology, Injury Onset, and Competition Withdrawal Rate. Review 2022. https://doi.org/10.21203/rs.3.rs-1463766/v1.

27. null Vossinakis, null Tasker. Stress fracture of the medial tibial condyle. The Knee 2000;7(3):187–90.

28. Engber WD. Stress fractures of the medial tibial plateau. J Bone Joint Surg Am 1977;59(6):767–9.

29. Carroll JJ, Kelly SP, Foster JN, et al. Bilateral Proximal Tibia Stress Fractures through Persistent Physes. Case Rep Orthop 2018;2018:8181547.

30. Wilson JJ, Best TM. Common overuse tendon problems: A review and recommendations for treatment. Am Fam Physician 2005;72(5):811–8.

31. Lavagnino M, Arnoczky SP, Elvin N, et al. Patellar tendon strain is increased at the site of the jumper's knee lesion during knee flexion and tendon loading: results and cadaveric testing of a computational model. Am J Sports Med 2008;36(11):2110–8.

32. Kannus P, Józsa L, Natri A, et al. Effects of training, immobilization and remobilization on tendons. Scand J Med Sci Sports 1997;7(2):67–71.

33. Crema MD, Cortinas LG, Lima GBP, et al. Magnetic resonance imaging-based morphological and alignment assessment of the patellofemoral joint and its relationship to proximal patellar tendinopathy. Skeletal Radiol 2018;47(3):341–9.

34. Tuong B, White J, Louis L, et al. Get a kick out of this: the spectrum of knee extensor mechanism injuries. Br J Sports Med 2011;45(2):140–6.

35. Dupuis CS, Westra SJ, Makris J, et al. Injuries and conditions of the extensor mechanism of the pediatric knee. Radiogr Rev Publ Radiol Soc N Am Inc 2009;29(3):877–86.

36. Khan KM, Bonar F, Desmond PM, et al. Patellar tendinosis (jumper's knee): findings at histopathologic examination, US, and MR imaging. Victorian Institute of Sport Tendon Study Group. Radiology 1996; 200(3):821–7.

37. Yu JS, Popp JE, Kaeding CC, et al. Correlation of MR imaging and pathologic findings in athletes undergoing surgery for chronic patellar tendinitis. AJR Am J Roentgenol 1995;165(1):115–8.

38. Matava null. Patellar Tendon Ruptures. J Am Acad Orthop Surg 1996;4(6):287–96.

39. Zaiter M, Ayoub A, Mohana A, et al. Beirut port explosion: unusual presentation of bilateral blast-related extensor mechanism rupture. Skeletal Radiol 2021;50(7):1479–83.

40. Zwerver J, Bredeweg SW, van den Akker-Scheek I. Prevalence of Jumper's knee among nonelite athletes from different sports: a cross-sectional survey. Am J Sports Med 2011;39(9):1984–8.

41. Lian OB, Engebretsen L, Bahr R. Prevalence of jumper's knee among elite athletes from different sports: a cross-sectional study. Am J Sports Med 2005;33(4):561–7.

42. King D, Yakubek G, Chughtai M, et al. Quadriceps tendinopathy: a review-part 1: epidemiology and diagnosis. Ann Transl Med 2019;7(4):71.

43. Seto CK, Statuta SM, Solari IL. Pediatric running injuries. Clin Sports Med 2010;29(3):499–511.

44. Patel DR, Villalobos A. Evaluation and management of knee pain in young athletes: overuse injuries of the knee. Transl Pediatr 2017;6(3):190–8.

45. Yablon CM, Pai D, Dong Q, et al. Magnetic resonance imaging of the extensor mechanism. Magn Reson Imaging Clin N Am 2014;22(4):601–20.

46. Vaishya R, Azizi AT, Agarwal AK, et al. Apophysitis of the Tibial Tuberosity (Osgood-Schlatter Disease): A Review. Cureus 2016;8(9):e780.

MR Imaging of Acute Knee Injuries
Systematic Evaluation and Reporting

Benjamin Fritz, MD[a,b], Jan Fritz, MD[c,*]

KEYWORDS

- MR imaging • Computed tomography • Imaging • knee • trauma • sports injury

KEY POINTS

- MR imaging is the most accurate imaging test for evaluating acute injuries of bone, articular cartilage, menisci, ligaments, tendons, nerves, and vessels.
- MR imaging interpretation and accurate reporting of acute knee injuries benefit from a systematic checklist.
- Several pulse sequence acquisition and postprocessing techniques are available for rapid 5-sequence 5-minute trauma knee MR imaging protocols in a clinical setting.
- Identifying contusive bone marrow edema lesions on MR imaging is a useful strategy to understand better the injury mechanism and predict internal derangement injuries.
- Acute traumatic osteochondral injuries represent a spectrum of bone contusions, condyle fractures, subchondral fractures, and osteochondral fractures.

INTRODUCTION

Acute knee injury ranges among the most common joint injuries in professional and recreational athletes, accounting for more than 500,000 visits to emergency departments annually in the United States.[1] Virtually any structure of the knee can be injured in acute knee trauma; however, the most important injuries are osteochondral injuries, cruciate ligament tears, meniscus tears and ramp lesions, anterolateral complex and collateral ligament injuries, patellofemoral translation, extensor mechanism tears, and nerve and vascular injuries. Accurate diagnosis of meniscus tears, tears of the cruciate and collateral ligaments, and chondral fractures is important for surgical decision-making. With history and clinical examination, imaging is employed in many knee injuries to confirm a clinically suspected diagnosis and evaluate for concomitant injuries.

According to American College of Radiology (ACR) guidelines, radiography is the appropriate first imaging test in adults and children 5 years of age and older.[2] Radiographs can detect joint effusion, fractures, deformities, and malalignment. Depending on the severity of the injury, clinical symptoms, and concordance of radiographic findings, computed tomography (CT) or MR imaging is indicated. CT visualizes osseous structures with the highest detail allowing for the detection of radiographically occult fractures and accurate characterization for surgical decision making and surgical planning. Dual energy-based monoenergetic extrapolation and iterative image reconstruction substantially reduce metal artifacts arising from orthopedic implants.[3–7] CT is readily available at many emergency departments worldwide; however, its drawback is radiation exposure, and, perhaps more importantly, limited soft tissue contrast, which typically does

a Department of Radiology, Balgrist University Hospital, Forchstrasse 340, Zürich, 8008, Switzerland; b Faculty of Medicine, University of Zurich, Zurich, Switzerland; c Department of Radiology, Division of Musculoskeletal Radiology, New York University Grossman School of Medicine, 660 1st Avenue, 3 Road Floor, Room 313, New York, NY 10016, USA
* Corresponding author.
E-mail address: jan.fritz@nyulangone.org
Twitter: JanFritzMSK (J.F.)

Radiol Clin N Am 61 (2023) 261–280
https://doi.org/10.1016/j.rcl.2022.10.005
0033-8389/23/© 2022 Elsevier Inc. All rights reserved.

not permit accurate detection and characterization of ligamentous, tendinous, meniscus, and cartilaginous injuries.

MR imaging is the most accurate test for evaluating bone marrow and cancellous bone, articular cartilage, menisci, ligaments, tendons, nerves, and vessels. The high soft tissue contrast of MR imaging augments the limitations of radiography and CT. Modern pulse sequences for creating MR imaging-based synthetic CT images can be included in trauma MR imaging protocols for improved characterization of osseous and mineralized structures.[8] In knee dislocation injuries, CT-, MR imaging-, or fluoroscopy-based angiography should be performed to detect and characterize vascular injury.[9,10]

This article reviews the MR imaging appearances of the core spectrum of traumatic knee injuries using a structured checklist approach for systematic MR imaging evaluation and reporting.

CHECKLIST

MR imaging interpretation and accurate reporting of acute knee injuries benefit from a systematic checklist of articular structures. We use a compartmentalized reporting template (**Table 1**).

MR IMAGING TECHNIQUE

Typical knee trauma MR imaging protocols include 4 to 5 turbo spin-echo pulse sequences in axial, sagittal, and coronal orientation. Nonfat-suppressed proton density-weighted turbo spin-echo pulse sequences are most versatile for morphologic evaluation, including articular cartilage, ligaments, menisci, and joint fluid, whereas fat-suppressed fluid-sensitive pulse sequences with echo times of 60 milliseconds are best for contrast evaluations, including joint fluid, bone marrow edema, and ligamentous and tendinous tears.[11] T1-weighted pulse sequences may be used to improve fracture visualization; however, the combination of proton density-weighted and fat-suppressed T2-weighted pulse sequences is often equally accurate. Spatial in-plane resolution of approximately 500 μm is typically sufficient for accurately evaluating anatomic knee structures.

Fast protocols are essential for patients to tolerate knee MR imaging examinations (**Table 2**). Several pulse sequence acquisition and postprocessing techniques are available to realize 5-sequence 5-minute knee MR imaging protocols[7] in a clinical setting. For 2-dimensional MR imaging, combined fourfold accelerated simultaneous multislice and parallel imaging acquisition and three-to-fourfold accelerated parallel imaging

with deep learning image reconstruction are recommended.[12–17] During the COVID-19 (coronavirus disease 2019) pandemic, 5-minute MR imaging protocols were also helpful for short patient dwell times in the radiology department and reduced contact times.[18]

Proton density-weighted Dixon turbo spin-echo pulse sequences with repetition times of 3500-4000 ms and echo times between 30-40ms produce proton density-like, fat-suppressed fluid sensitive-like, opposed phase, and T1-like fat-only images, which can increase the sensitivity for detecting osseous injuries. Isotropic 3-dimensional turbo spin-echo pulse sequences, such as fat-suppressed T2-weighted CAIPIRINHA SPACE[19] and compressed sensing SPACE,[20]

Table 1
MR imaging template for evaluation and reporting of acute knee injuries

MR Imaging Finding	Characteristics
Joint fluid	Volume (physiologic, small, moderate, large), consistency (simple, hemorrhagic, lipo hemorrhagic), presence of a popliteal cyst, joint bodies (chondral, osteochondral, chronic degenerative)
Medial knee	Medial meniscus, medial femoral and tibial articular cartilage, medial collateral ligament, posteromedial corner
Laterally	Lateral meniscus, lateral femoral and tibial articular cartilage, anterolateral complex, lateral collateral ligament complex, posterolateral corner, proximal tibiofibular joint
Anterior knee	Alignment, quadriceps tendon, patella tendon, patellofemoral articular cartilage, Hoffa fat pad
Intercondylar region	Anterior cruciate ligament, posterior cruciate ligament
Bones	Bone marrow and edema pattern, fractures, osteonecrosis, bone lesions, and geodes.
Nerves	Common peroneal and tibial nerve abnormalities
Vessels	Popliteal and geniculate artery injury and occlusion Venous injury and thrombosis

Table 2
Fast knee trauma 3.0 Tesla MR imaging protocol

Parameters	Axial PDFS	Sagittal PD	Sagittal T2FS	Coronal PDFS	Coronal T1
Repetition time (ms)	3600	3480	3700	3510	546
Echo time (ms)	32	23	56	35	7.1
Echo train length	11	11	11	11	4
Bandwidth (Hz/px)	296	354	299	301	355
Field-of-view (mm)	140 x 140	140 x 140	140 x 140	140 x 140	140 x 140
Matrix size	272 x 204	336 x 252	304 x 228	272 x 204	256 x 179
Slice thickness (mm)	3	3	3	3	3.5
Number of slices	38	38	38	36	28
Parallel imaging acceleration factor	2	2	2	2	2
Simultaneous multislice acceleration factor	2	2	2	2	2
Acquisition time (ms)	1:00	1:08	1:23	1:15	0:22

Abbreviations: FS, fat suppression; PD, proton density weighting.

may be obtained in 5 minutes.[21,22] The ability for multiplanar reformation and advanced postprocessing with cinematic rendering is available.[23,24] Two-dimensional and 3-dimensional MR imaging have similar accuracies for detecting articular cartilage, anterior cruciate ligament, and meniscus injuries.[25–27]

In patients with metallic orthopedic implants about the knee, including screws, plates, rods, and unicompartmental and total knee arthroplasty implants, basic and advanced metal artifact reduction techniques can be added (**Fig. 1**).[4,28] Basic techniques include high receiver bandwidth, view angle tilting, transmit and receiver radiofrequency bandwidth matching, and inversion recovery instead of chemical shift fat suppression. Advanced techniques include slice encoding for metal artifact correction (SEMAC) and multiacquisition variable-resonance image combination (MAVRIC).[29] Compressed sensing acceleration of SEMAC permits eightfold faster image acquisition, amounting to approximately 70% shorter acquisition times with minimal residual metal artifacts on the MR images.[30–32]

JOINT FLUID

Joint effusions, capsular edema, and periarticular soft tissue edema are almost always present in acute knee injuries and serve as an MR imaging indicator for acuteness. Traumatic joint effusion may be simple, hemorrhagic, or lipohemorrhagic. Hemorrhagic joint effusions are also referred to as hemarthrosis and may result in intra-articular clot formation, erythrocyte sedimentation, or reduced T2 brightness of joint fluid (T2 shortening/shading). Lipohemarthrosis is a specific hemarthrosis type characterized by the presence of intra-articular fat forming a fat-fluid level. Lipohemarthrosis is highly predictive of the presence of an intra-articular fracture. Joint bodies may be acute or chronic. Joint bodies following an acute injury are typically sharply-marginated crescentic-shaped osteochondral fragments with a distinct articular cartilage signature (**Fig. 2**), whereas degenerative joint bodies in degenerative arthrosis are usually popcorn-like in shape with variable signal intensities. MR imaging accurately identifies the donor site and potentially guides arthroscopic reattachment in sizable osteochondral fragments in acute osteochondral and chondral injuries.

BONE MARROW EDEMA

Common knee injury mechanisms often result in typical bone contusion patterns. Identifying contusive bone marrow edema lesions on MR imaging is a useful strategy to understand better the injury mechanism and predict internal derangement injuries. Pivot shift (**Fig. 3**), dashboard, hyperextension, clipping, and lateral patellar dislocation (**Fig. 2**) injuries result in typical bone contusion patterns (**Table 3**). Hyperflexion injuries with axial loading result in characteristic coup-contrecoup far posterior femoral condyle and posterior tibial plateau bone contusions with posterior corner injuries and optional posterior medial and lateral meniscus injuries.

ACUTE TRAUMATIC OSTEOCHONDRAL INJURY

Acute knee injuries are often associated with acute traumatic osteochondral injuries, representing a

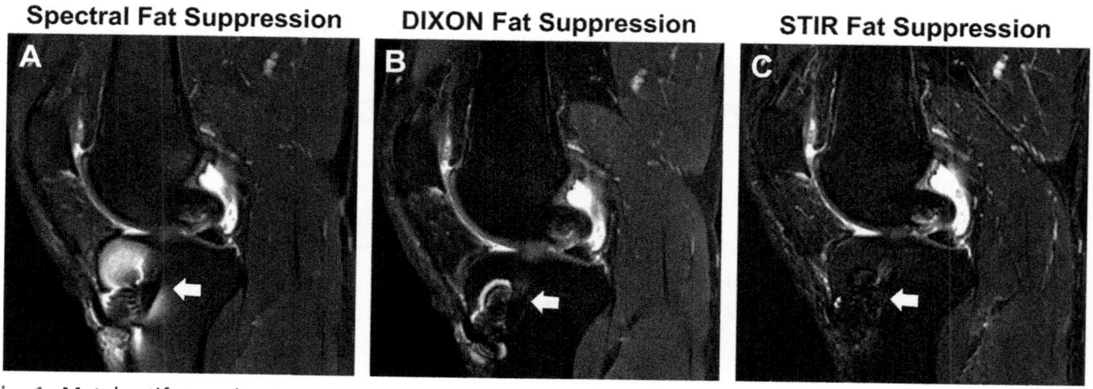

Spectral Fat Suppression   **DIXON Fat Suppression**   **STIR Fat Suppression**

Fig. 1. Metal artifact reduction MR imaging in the presence of orthopedic implants. 52-year-old man with an acute knee injury and previous anterior cruciate ligament reconstruction with tibial tunnel interference screw. Sagittal fat-suppressed T2-weighted MR images with spectral fat suppression (A), Dixon-based fat suppression (B), and Short-tau inversion recovery (STIR) fat suppression (C) show reducing metal artifacts and improving fat suppression (arrows) from left to right.

spectrum of bone contusions, condyle fractures, subchondral fractures (**Fig. 4**), osteochondral fractures, and chondral shear fractures (see **Fig. 2**).[33] As with the characteristic bone marrow edema patterns in the knee (**Table 4**), certain osteochondral injury sites are associated with specific mechanisms of injury. MR imaging is highly accurate in detecting and classifying acute traumatic osteochondral injuries. MR imaging reports should describe the anatomic location, involved osteochondral layers, 3-dimensional size, contour deformities, and degree of displacement. In the case of displaced chondral or osteochondral fragments, size and location should be reported for the displaced fragment and donor site.

The term "transchondral fracture" may be used for subchondral fractures with focally convex surface contour deformities of the condylopatellar sulcus after pivot-shift type tibial translation injuries with femorotibial shear and impaction. In acute transchondral fractures, MR imaging typically shows T2 signal hyperintensity of the overlying articular cartilage but no discrete chondral fractures or defects. However, at follow-up, articular cartilage defects often occur at this location, indicating initial morphologic underestimation of the microstructural damage on MRI in the acute setting.[34]

ANTERIOR CRUCIATE LIGAMENT INJURY

Anterior cruciate ligament (ACL) injuries are destabilizing knee injuries that often require surgery. Several mechanisms can result in ACL tears, including high-energy trauma with a direct blow to the knee joint and severe hyperextension. However, noncontact injuries during high-speed landing and cutting movements are the prevalent mechanisms of injury in team sport athletes, such as soccer, basketball, and European handball.[35] Female athletes are more at risk for noncontact ACL tears, with a 1:5 male-to-female ratio.[36]

The so-called pivot shift injury is the typical mechanism of noncontact ACL tears with a distinct bone marrow edema pattern on MR imaging (see **Fig. 3**) (see **Table 3**). The knee undergoes excessive valgus stress in combination with knee flexion and external rotation on the planted foot. Valgus overload and anterior translation caused by quadriceps traction result in ACL tearing. The lateral femoral condyle collides with the posterolateral tibial plateau during the transient rotatory posterolateral subluxation. Impact-related deepened deformity of the lateral femoral condyle at the condylopatellar sulcus or terminal sulcus describes the shallow anatomic concavity at the junction of the lateral trochlea facette and anterior femoral condyle that creates the deep sulcus sign or lateral femoral notch sign.[37] The deepened concave deformity may be occasionally diagnosed on radiographs; however, MR imaging is most accurate.

On MR imaging, the characteristic coup-contrecoup-type bone marrow edema pattern at the condylopatellar sulcus and lateral femoral condyle is diagnostic for a recent pivot shift-type knee translation injury. The deep sulcus contour deformity may or may not be present, which is the reason for the lower accuracies of radiographs. Nondisplaced and displaced osteochondral or chondral fractures occur with higher-grade femorotibial impact.

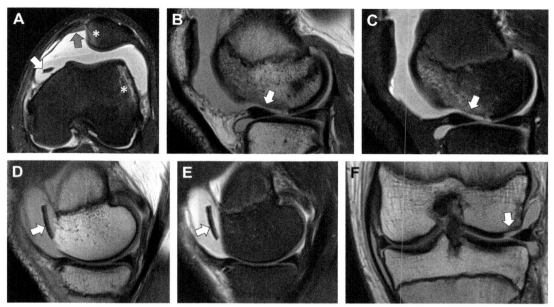

Fig. 2. 12-year-old boy with recent patellofemoral dislocation injury and displaced chondral fracture during skiing. Axial fat-suppressed proton density-weighted MR image (*A*) shows the characteristic contusion pattern (*asterisks*) of the inferomedial patella and lateral femoral condyle cortex, joint effusion with lipohemarthrosis fluid-fluid level (*gray arrow*), and floating chondral fragment (*white arrow*). Sagittal proton density-weighted (*B*), fat-suppressed T2-weighted (*C*), and coronal proton density-weighted (*F*) MR images show the donor site (*arrows*) of the chondral fragment at the lateral femoral condyle. Sagittal proton density-weighted (*D*) and fat-suppressed T2-weighted (*E*) MR images show the displaced chondral fragment (*arrows*) with characteristic cartilage signature.

ACL tears can be categorized into proximal third femoral attachment tears, midsubstance tears, and distal third tibial attachment tears. Midsubstance tears are most common, followed by proximal tears.[38] Distal third ACL tears are rare in adults.[38] MR imaging report should include a characterization of location, which has implications for surgical decision making. Primary ACL repair

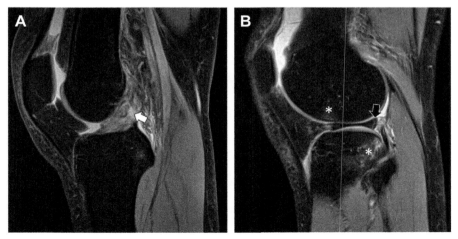

Fig. 3. 39-year-old woman with an acute knee injury during skiing. Sagittal fat-suppressed T2-weighted MR images demonstrate a proximal tear of the anterior cruciate ligament (*white arrow* in *A*), coup-contrecoup-type bone marrow edema pattern (*asterisks*) at the condylopatellar sulcus and lateral posterior tibia plateau indicating a recent pivot shift-type knee translation, and a longitudinal-vertical peripheral lateral meniscus tear (*black arrow* in *B*).

Table 3
Bone contusion pattern of common knee injuries

Injury Type	Bone Contusion Pattern	Injury Mechanism	Associated Injuries
Pivot shift injury	Condylopatella sulcus of the lateral femoral condyle, posterior lateral tibia plateau	Valgus stress and external rotation in flexion	Anterior cruciate ligament tear
Dashboard injury	Anterior tibia, sometimes posterior patella	Forceful posterior tibia translation in flexion	Posterior cruciate ligament tear
Hyperextension injury	Anterior femoral condyles, anterior tibia plateaus	Hyperextension and axial loading	Anterior cruciate ligament tear, posterior cruciate ligament tear, meniscus injuries, knee dislocation, posterolateral corner injury
Clipping injury	Lateral femoral condyle, lateral tibia plateau, medial femoral condyle	Valgus stress and flexion	Medial collateral ligament tear
Lateral patellar dislocation	Anterolateral cortex of the lateral femoral condyle, inferomedial patella	Rotation and flexion	Osteochondral injury of the patella, medial patellofemoral retinaculum tear

techniques benefit from proximal tear locations (see **Fig. 3**),[39] whereas distal tears may require ACL reconstruction surgery.[40]

Skilled clinical examination accurately detects ACL tears in most patients. The role of MR imaging includes confirming ACL tear in indeterminate cases, characterizing tears grade (interstitial tear, partial-thickness tear, full-thickness tear), location (proximal tear, midsubstance tear, distal tear), and diagnosing associated injuries. For the MR imaging diagnosis of the tear grade, the morphologic criterion of fiber continuity is more accurate than abnormal signal hyperintensity. Fiber disruption can be seen on any plane, but most readers prefer sagittal and coronal MR images. Fluid-sensitive intermediate- and T2-weighted MR images without or with fat suppression are most accurate, whereas T1-weighted images are inaccurate for detecting and characterizing ACL tears.

ACL thickening, defined as an increase in cross-sectional diameter, and higher than normal signal intensity have low accuracies for diagnosing ACL tears because of overlap with mucoid degeneration. Diagnosing partial-thickness ACL

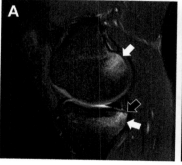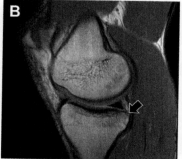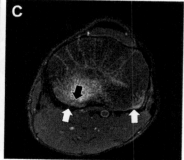

Fig. 4. 22-year-old man with an acute knee injury after squatting exercise accident with knee hyperflexion. Sagittal fat-suppressed T2-weighted (*A*), sagittal proton density-weighted (*B*), and axial fat-suppressed proton density-weighted (*C*) MR images demonstrate a characteristic coup-contrecoup bone marrow edema pattern (*white arrows*) of the far posterior femoral condyle and posterior tibial plateau with posterior corner fracture (*black arrows*).

Table 4 Types of acute traumatic osteochondral injury	
Type	MR Imaging Appearance
Bone contusion	Focal bone marrow edema pattern. Absent cortical contour deformity. Absent fracture lines. The overlying cartilage is structurally intact.
Subchondral fracture	Focal bone marrow edema pattern. Absent cortical contour deformity. Subcortically located fracture line that parallels the articular surface. The overlying cartilage is structurally intact.
Osteochondral fracture	Focal bone marrow edema pattern. Typically presents with contour deformities, articular surface step-off, or displaced fragment. Fracture line extends through bone and articular cartilage.
Chondral fracture	Focal bone marrow edema pattern. Presents with articular cartilage contour irregularities. The separation typically occurs at the calcified-noncalcified cartilage interface near the tidemark layer. Chondral fragments may remain in situ or float in the joint cavity.

tears requires the MR imaging visualization of fiber disruption, bundle attenuation, or both. However, the diagnosis of partial-thickness tears represents a spectrum from low-grade partial-thickness to high-grade partial-thickness tears, which scales with the percentage of fiber disruption. With a lower amount of torn fibers, the MR imaging accuracy decreases because of overlapping with natural variations in ACL volumes and obscuration by edema and joint fluid. Abnormal ACL orientation relative to Blumensaat line may help diagnose a partial ACL tear. Dedicated double-angulated 2- and 3-dimensional ACL profile views may also increase accuracy, especially in ACL grafts.[19,22,41]

A major role of MR imaging after ACL tear is the detection of associated knee injuries, including various types of meniscus injuries, collateral ligament injuries, and osteochondral fractures.

Acute knee injuries may be designated as multiligament knee injuries when there is tearing of 2 or more ligaments of the intercondylar notch (cruciate ligaments), posteromedial corner (including medial collateral ligament), and posterolateral corner (including lateral collateral ligament) (Fig. 5).[42] The recognition of multiligament knee injuries is important because of higher associations with knee dislocations, neurovascular injuries (up to 65% popliteal artery injuries), and disability. The number of torn ligaments scales with injury severity. High-energy trauma is associated with tearing 3 or more ligaments, whereas low-energy trauma is typically associated with tearing 1 cruciate and 1 collateral ligament.[43]

POSTERIOR CRUCIATE LIGAMENT INJURY

The posterior cruciate ligament (PCL) is the largest and strongest ligament in the knee. The PCL

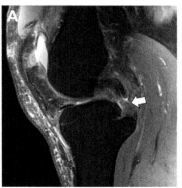 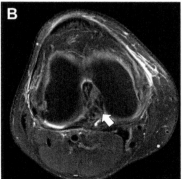 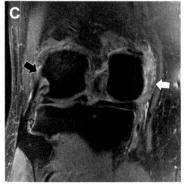

Fig. 5. 51-year-old man with multiligament knee injury. Sagittal (A) and axial (B) fat-suppressed T2-weighted MR images show a posterior cruciate ligament tear near the tibial attachment (white arrows). Coronal fat-suppressed proton density-weighted MR image (C) shows associated medial collateral ligament (*white arrow*) and lateral collateral ligament (*black arrow*) tears.

Table 5
Three-layer model of the medial knee stabilizers

Layer	Location	Structures
1	Superficial	Crural, sartorius, and vastus medialis fascia
2	Intermediate	Medial patellofemoral ligament and retinaculum, superficial medial collateral ligament (tibial collateral ligament), posterior oblique ligament, and semimembranosus muscle
3	Deep	Deep medial collateral ligament, coronary meniscofemoral and meniscotibial capsular ligaments, joint capsule

midsubstance is approximately 1.5 times thicker and twice as strong as the ACL.[44] Acute PCL tears most often occur during high-energy motor vehicle accidents, particularly motorcycle and dashboard injuries. In dashboard injuries, posterior tibia translation in knee flexion results in PCL rupture. In sports injuries, a common injury mechanism is falling on the flexed knee with a plantar flexed foot and subsequent knee joint hyperflexion.[45] The prevalence of PCL tears is approximately 3% in outpatient knee injuries and 38% in acute traumatic hemarthrosis.[46]

Almost all PCL tears occur in combination with other ligamentous injuries. On sagittal MR images, the intact PCL has a hooked appearance and shows hypointense signal on all sequences. The MR imaging signs of partial-thickness and full-thickness PCL tears are fiber disruption and abnormal signal hyperintensity on intermediate- and T2-weighted MR images (see **Fig. 7**). MR imaging has a diagnostic accuracy of almost 100% for detecting PCL tears.[47]

MEDIAL COLLATERAL LIGAMENT COMPLEX

The medial collateral ligament (MCL) complex includes the superficial medial collateral ligament (known as the tibial collateral ligament), deep medial collateral ligament including the coronary meniscofemoral and meniscotibial ligaments, posterior oblique ligament, and the medial patellofemoral ligament.[48] These structures have also been described in anatomic layers[49] (**Table 5**). The strong superficial MCL is the primary stabilizer of valgus loads and counters external tibia rotation and anterior tibial translation when the anterior cruciate ligament is torn. The deep MCL and posterior oblique ligament stabilize the medial knee joint line, menisci, and posteromedial corner.

In clinical practice, the most frequent acutely injured ligament is the MCL complex, with an annual incidence of 0.24 to 7.3 cases per 1000 individuals.[50] However, the number of MCL injuries on MR imaging is lower, as low-grade clinical MCL injuries do not require MR imaging. Forced valgus stress with knee flexion is the prototypical injury mechanism, occurring with or without opponent contact in athletes.

Clinical grading of MCL tears is based on laxity inferred by the degree of medial joint line opening and the presence or absence of valgus stress endpoints during physical examination (**Table 6**).[51] Clinical grade 1 or mild MCL injury is characterized by less than 5 mm medial joint line opening and solid valgus stress endpoint. Clinical grade 2 or moderate MCL injury is characterized by 5 to

Table 6
Clinical grading of medial collateral ligament tears and associated MR imaging findings

Clinical Grading	Medial Joint Line Opening with Valgus Stress	Endpoint with Valgus Stress	Ligamentous Integrity	MR Imaging Findings
Grade I	< 5 mm	Solid	Interstitial injury	Signal hyperintensity of the ligament without visualized fiber disruption
Grade II	5–9 mm	Soft or delayed	Partial-thickness tear	Disrupted and intact fibers
Grade III	≥ 10 mm	Absent	Full-thickness tear	All fibers disrupted optional fiber retraction and displacement

9 mm medial joint line opening and soft or late valgus stress endpoint. Clinical grade 3 or severe MCL injury is characterized by 10 mm and more medial joint line opening and absent valgus stress endpoint.

Attempts to equate the clinical MCL injury grades to specific MR imaging findings have repeatedly shown substantial inaccuracies in predicting the clinical degree of laxity.[52,53] Consequently, a grade 1 to 3 system should not be used in MR imaging reports to prevent the inadvertent equation with the clinical grades, which are based on functional testing. Instead, MR imaging reports should describe the injured medial collateral ligament complex portions, including the magnitude of fiber disruptions, detachments and degree of fiber retraction, displacement and interposition of torn ligaments, and associated injuries. Common associated injuries include anterior cruciate ligament tears, medial meniscus tears, and extensor mechanism tears. Clinical grade 1 medial collateral ligament injuries are often isolated, whereas 80% of clinical grade 3 injuries will have concomitant injuries.[51]

The location of superficial medial collateral ligament tears can be divided into proximal (femoral), midsubstance, and distal (tibial) tears. Osseous avulsion fractures at the medial femoral condyle are rare.[54] Proximal tears are the most common. Distal tears are rare but have a characteristic wavy MR imaging appearance of the torn distal tendon.[55] Coronal MR images should include the proximal and distal tibial collateral ligament attachments. Anatomic healing may fail in distal full-thickness tibial collateral ligament tears with a displacement of the torn tendon superficial to the adjacent pes anserine

tendons (**Fig. 6**).[56] Analogous to ulnar collateral ligament tears in the thump[57], such tears have been referred to as a Stener-like MCL lesions.[58] Soft tissue injuries of the posterior oblique ligament and the deep medial collateral ligaments have less specific injury patterns; however, a reversed Segond fracture describes an osseous avulsion fracture of the tibial attachment of the deep medial collateral ligament (**Fig. 7**).[59]

ANTEROLATERAL COMPLEX

Similar to the medial knee, the lateral knee stabilizers have been described with a 3-layer model (**Table 7**).[60] The term anterolateral complex encompasses the iliotibial band proper, iliotibial tract-associated deeper layers, and the joint capsule. The iliotibial band between the Kaplan fibers and Gerdy tubercle is the principal structure of the anterolateral complex. The iliotibial band anatomy is complex and comprises superficial, deep, and capsulosseous layers.[61]

The anterolateral structures are the joint capsule, quadriceps retinaculum extending from the lateral patella margin to the superficial iliotibial band, and superficial and deep iliotibial band, including the coronary meniscotibial and meniscofemoral ligaments. The anterolateral ligament has been described as a well-defined ligamentous structure spanning between lateral femoral epicondyle, lateral meniscus, and anterolateral tibial attachments between Gerdy tubercle and the tip of the fibular head.[62] The mid-third lateral capsular ligament, capsulo-osseous layer of the iliotibial band, and anterior oblique band of the fibular collateral ligament may describe the same anatomic structure. On MR imaging, this anatomic

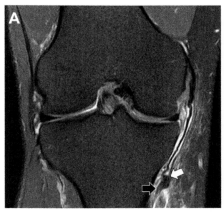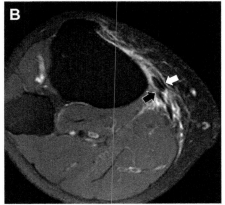

Fig. 6. 31-year-old man with Stener-type displaced medial collateral ligament tear after wrestling injury. Coronal (*A*) and axial (*B*) fat-suppressed proton density-weighted MR images demonstrate a distal medial collateral ligament tear (*white arrows*) with displacement of the torn ligament end superficially to the pes anserine tendons (*black arrows*).

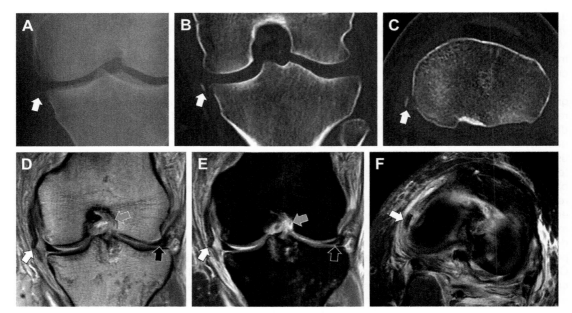

Fig. 7. 41-year-old woman with reverse Segond fracture after figure skating injury. Frontal radiograph (*A*), coronal CT image (*B*), axial CT image (*C*), coronal proton density-weighted MR image (*D*), coronal fat-suppressed T2-weighted MR image (*E*), and axial fat-suppressed T2-weighted MR image (*F*) show an osseous avulsion fracture (*white arrows*) of the tibial attachment of the deep medial collateral ligament (medial capsular sign). Additional injuries include an anterior cruciate ligament tear (*gray arrows* in *D* and *E*) and a lateral meniscus tear (*black arrows* in *D* and *E*).

region often appears as an anterolateral capsular thickening rather than a discrete ligamentous structure.[63] Functionally, the anterolateral ligament region appears to function synergically, rather than alone, within the anterolateral complex to control rotatory knee instability.

Table 7
Three-layer model of the lateral knee stabilizers

Layer	Location	Structures
1	Superficial	Iliotibial band with fascial expansions
2	Intermediate	patellar retinaculum, patellofemoral ligament, posterolateral capsule, and lateral gastrocnemius head
3	Deep	Joint capsule, lateral collateral ligament, fabellofibular ligament, coronary meniscofemoral and meniscotibial ligaments, and arcuate ligament

The tibial attachment site of the anterolateral ligament, mid-third lateral capsular ligament, capsuloosseous layer of the iliotibial band, and the anterior oblique band of the fibular collateral ligament coincide with the location of the Segond fracture (**Fig. 8**).[64] Internal knee rotation and varus stress comprise the principal mechanism of injury, resulting in anterolateral rotational instability. On MR imaging, acute Segond fractures are characterized by a small, mildly displaced cortical avulsion fracture of the anterolateral tibia (lateral capsular sign on radiographs) with associated bone marrow edema at the donor site. Acute Segond fractures, but especially subacute or chronic Segond fractures, can be notably subtle on MR imaging and often require correlation with radiographs and computed tomorgaphy to identify the thin cortical fragment. Associated injuries include anterior cruciate ligament tears, meniscus tears, and fibular attachment tears of the long head biceps femoris tendon and fibular collateral ligament.[65]

MENISCUS TEARS AND RAMP LESION

The medial meniscus and lateral meniscus distribute loads across the femoral and tibial articular surfaces, decreasing stress imparted during

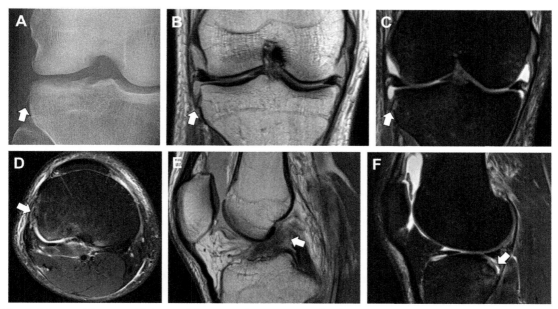

Fig. 8. 34-year-old man with Segond fracture after American football injury. Frontal radiograph (*A*), coronal proton-density-weighted MR image (*B*), coronal fat-suppressed proton density-weighted MR image (*C*), and axial fat-suppressed proton density-weighted MR image (*D*) show a mildly displaced cortical avulsion fracture (*arrows* in *A–D*) of the anterolateral tibia (lateral capsular sign). Sagittal proton density-weighted (*E*) and fat-suppressed T2-weighted MR images show an associated proximal anterior cruciate ligament tear (*arrow* in *E*) and posterior lateral tibial plateau osteochondral fracture (*arrow* in *F*).

weight bearing.[66] Intact menisci are hypointense on all MR images and have a triangular cross-sectional shape on sagittal and coronal MR images. Approximately 6% of acute knee injuries result in traumatic meniscus tears, of which 75% involve the medial meniscus.[67] In athletes with hemarthrosis, meniscus tears are present in 15% without ligamentous injuries.[68] The incidence of meniscus tears is higher with concomitant ligamentous injuries. In ACL tears, the overall incidence of a meniscus tear is 40% to 80%, with a slight preference for the lateral meniscus.[69] Traumatic meniscus tears, with or without associated ACL tears, carry a four- to sixfold increase in developing knee osteoarthritis.[70]

The role of MR imaging is to detect and characterize meniscus tears, including tear depth, concentric location, radial location, relationship to the popliteal hiatus, tear pattern, tissue quality, tear length, and location and volume of partial meniscectomy (**Table 8**).[71] Lateral meniscus tears at or extending to the popliteal hiatus are classified as central to the popliteal hiatus, where the lateral meniscus has no capsular attachment. Complex tears include more than 1 tear pattern. Degenerative tissue quality can be suggested when MR images show irregular and indistinct tear margins.

Table 8
MR imaging characteristics and descriptors of meniscus tears

Characteristics	Structures
Tear depth	Partial tear, complete tear
Concentric location	Outer zone 1 (<3 mm rim width), central zone 2 (3–5 mm rim width), inner zone 3 (>5 mm)
Radial location	Anterior segment, mid-body segment, posterior segment.
Central to popliteal hiatus	Yes or no
Tear pattern	Longitudinal-vertical (includes bucket-handle tears), horizontal, radial, vertical flap, horizontal flap, complex
Tissue quality	Nondegenerative, degenerative, indeterminate
Tear length	in mm
Partial meniscectomy location and volume	Location and percentage of absent meniscal tissue

In traumatic meniscus tears, longitudinal and complex tear patterns are most common (see **Fig. 3**),[72] whereas horizontal meniscus tears are typically associated with knee joint degeneration.[73] A retrospective study in patients undergoing arthroscopic knee surgery demonstrated that most lateral meniscus tears missed on MR imaging involved only one-third of the meniscus or were located in the posterior segment.[74]

Meniscal ramp injuries can destabilize the posteromedial corner and contribute to residual anterior-posterior instability after ACL reconstruction and failure of meniscus repair. Ramp lesions are difficult to diagnose on MR imaging and standard arthroscopy, requiring specialized techniques and portals.

The definitions of traumatic meniscal ramp lesions vary in anatomic location and involved structures. The original ramp lesion described a less than 2.5 cm longitudinal tear of the posterior medial meniscus segment at the meniscocapsular junction,[75] whereas later ramp lesions were described as injury of the meniscotibial attachment of the posterior medial meniscus segment.[76] Anatomic studies have suggested a conjoined meniscocapsular and meniscotibial ligament attachment at the posterior medial meniscus segment. Ramp lesions are present in up to 24% of acute knee injuries with ACL tears with a higher incidence in contact versus noncontact injuries.[77] The incidence of isolated ramp lesions is unknown, as they may be occult on MR imaging and may not undergo arthroscopic knee surgery. Applying the term ramp lesion has been suggested only in cases with concomitant ACL tears.[78] Two classifications have been described,[79,80] defining 5 tear types. Types 1 and 2 are stable on arthroscopic probing, whereas types 3 to 5 are unstable.

Published diagnostic accuracies of MR imaging vary, with sensitivities of 55% to 95% and specificities of 80% to 99%.[81–83] On MR imaging, meniscotibial and meniscocapsular attachment disruptions are the most specific sign of ramp lesions (**Fig. 9**). Sensitive but less specific signs include a thin layer of fluid and soft tissue edema between the posterior medial meniscus segment and the adjacent joint capsule, as well as bone marrow edema pattern of the posteromedial tibial plateau, particularly in ACL tears without medial meniscus tear.

LATERAL COLLATERAL LIGAMENT AND POSTEROLATERAL CORNER

The lateral collateral ligament (LCL), also known as the fibular collateral ligament, stabilizes the knee against varus stress and posterolateral rotation.

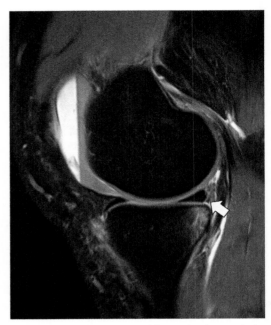

Fig. 9. 22-year-old woman with meniscal ramp lesion after a skiing accident. Sagittal fat-suppressed proton density-weighted MR image demonstrates a meniscus ramp lesion with tearing of the meniscocapsular and meniscotibial attachments of the posterior medial meniscus segment. Concomitant injuries included anterior cruciate ligament tear (not shown) and osteochondral fractures, with associated hemarthrosis (fluid-fluid level)

The femoral attachment locates slightly posteriorly at the lateral epicondyle, resulting in an oblique course to the distal fibular head.[84] Isolated LCL injuries are rare. Most LCL injuries occur with injuries to other posterolateral corner structures, cruciate ligaments, menisci, and medial collateral ligament complex.[85]

The LCL, popliteus tendon, and popliteofibular ligament are the 3 major structures of the posterolateral corner.[85] The popliteus muscle-tendon unit extends from the posterior medial tibia to the lateral femoral condyle (**Fig. 10**).[84] The popliteofibular ligament extends from the popliteus muscle attachment to the fibular head.[84]

Injury mechanisms of the posterolateral corner include direct posterolateral force to the tibia on the extended knee and external rotation and hyperextension without contact.[86] Missed posterolateral corner injuries can result in persisting knee instability and disability.[87] Posterolateral corner injuries are present in approximately 16% of knee injuries and 9% with hemarthrosis.[88] Ninety percent of posterolateral corner injuries are in combination with other knee ligament injuries (**Fig. 11**), whereas

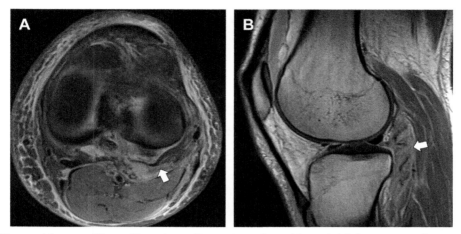

Fig. 10. 37-year-old man with popliteus tear after motorcycle accident. Axial fat-suppressed proton density-weighted (*A*) and sagittal proton density-weighted (*B*) MR images demonstrate a full-thickness tear of the popliteus muscle-tendon junction (*arrows*).

PCL tears are present in up to 62% of posterolateral corner injuries.[89]

Some studies suggest that the LCL may be the most important structure for posterolateral rotational stability.[89] The intact LCL is usually well depicted on MR imaging as a cord-like structure with hypointense signal on all pulse sequences. Acute LCL injury may present as low-grade interstitial injuries, partial-thickness tears, and full-thickness tears, which may occur at the femoral attachment, midsubstance, or distal attachment.

Less frequent findings are distal osseous avulsions of the lateral aspect of the fibular head.

Similarly, acute injuries of the popliteus tendon comprise the entire spectrum from low-grade interstitial to full-thickness tears, which may be located at the muscle-tendon junction or less frequently at the femoral attachment. Osseous femoral avulsions are rare. Concomitant knee injuries are frequent, most notably meniscus tears and PCL injuries.[90] On MR imaging, the popliteus tendon is prone to magic angle effect signal

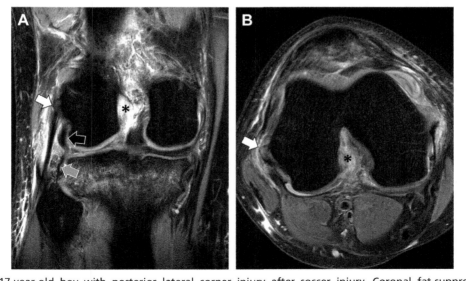

Fig. 11. 17-year-old boy with posterior lateral corner injury after soccer injury. Coronal fat-suppressed T2-weighted MR image (*A*) and axial fat-suppressed proton density-weighted (*B*) MR images demonstrate a partial-thickness lateral collateral ligament tear at the femoral attachment (*white arrows*), a partial-thickness tear of the popliteofibular ligament (*gray arrow*), a low-grade partial-thickness tear of the popliteus tendon (*black arrow*), and a tear of the anterior cruciate ligament (*asterisks*).

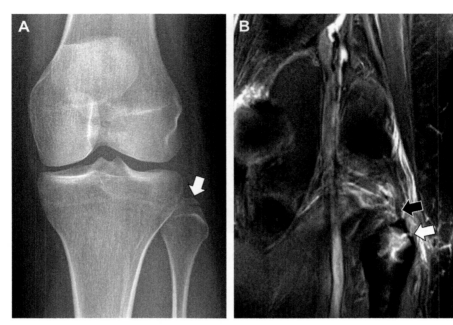

Fig. 12. 24-year-old woman with hyperextension knee injury. Anteroposterior radiograph (*A*) shows a small osseous avulsion fracture of the tip of the styloid process of the fibula ("arcuate sign"). Coronal STIR MR image (*B*) shows the osseous avulsion fracture with surrounding bone marrow edema pattern (*white arrow*) of the fibula and a partially torn popliteofibular ligament (*black arrow*).

alterations because of its curved course around the posterolateral corner. The popliteofibular ligament is often difficult to visualize on standard MR images because of its short length and oblique course. An acutely injured popliteofibular ligament can be recognized as a thickened structure with varying degrees of fiber disruption, often best visualized on coronal MR images. Surrounding edema often aids in unmasking the ligament (see **Fig. 12**).

Additional posterolateral corner structures are the distal biceps femoris tendon, the fabellofibular ligament, and the arcuate ligament.[85] The arcuate sign describes osseous avulsions of the arcuate, fabellofibular, and popliteofibular ligament attachments at the tip of the styloid process on MR images and radiographs (**Fig. 12**).[91] This injury often indicates a more severe posterolateral corner injury.

LATERAL PATELLOFEMORAL TRANSLATION

Acute traumatic patellofemoral subluxation and dislocation represent approximately 3% of all traumatic knee injuries. The most common mechanism of injury is noncontact twisting injuries in knee extension and external rotation. Direct impact collision injuries are less common. Noncontact twisting injuries are associated with osteochondral fractures upon the injury phase of patellar relocation. Predisposing factors include patella alta, trochlear dysplasia, hypoplastic lateral femoral condyle, high tibial tubercle trochlear groove distance and lateral patellar shift, vastus medialis obliquus dysfunction, increased Q angle, increased iliotibial tract and vastus lateralis tension, and ligament laxity caused by collagen vascular disease.

Medial stabilizers restrain lateral patellofemoral translation and include the medial patellar retinaculum (layer 2), medial patellofemoral ligament (layer 2), quadriceps muscle-tendon unit, patella tendon, and joint capsule (layer 3)[49] (see **Table 5**). The superiorly positioned medial patellofemoral ligament and the inferiorly positioned medial retinaculum extend from the medial patellar surface to the medial femoral condyle. On MR imaging, both structures often present as 1 complex. The superior margin of the medial patellofemoral ligament exchanges fibers with the vastus medialis obliquus portion of the vastus medials, providing an important additional element of stability. Additional differentiations include the patellomeniscal and patellotibial ligament portions. The medial patellofemoral ligament has an anterior fiber connection with the anterior margin of the superficial medial collateral ligament.

On MR imaging, after a patellofemoral translation, the patella is either relocated with or without residual lateral patellar shift or remains acutely or habitually dislocated laterally. The inferomedial patellar and anterolateral femoral condyle bone marrow edema pattern is pathognomonic (see **Fig. 2**) (see **Table 3**). Nondisplaced or displaced inferomedial patellar osteochondral fractures are common and typically accompanied by hemarthrosis or lipohemarthrosis. Fracture fragments may remain positioned in situ or float in the joint cavity.

Edema pattern and linear fluid are typically present along layer 2 structures, indicating a medial patellar stabilizer injury, which is almost always present after a first-time dislocation. Medial patellofemoral ligament and medial retinaculum tears may be classified by location into patellar attachment, midsubstance, and femoral attachment tears, and by depth into partial-thickness or full-thickness tears. Often, tears occur at multiple locations. Femoral attachment tears often extend into the anterior margin of the superficial medial collateral ligament and may present with edema of the adductor tubercle. Osseous avulsion and vastus medialis obliquus tears should be reported, as they may predict post-traumatic instability.[92]

EXTENSOR MECHANISM
Quadriceps Tendon

Quadriceps tendon tears are more common than patella tendon tears, are substantially more common in male than female patients, and occur predominantly in patients over 40 years of age. Predisposing risk factors include renal failure, diabetes, rheumatoid arthritis, hyperparathyroidism, connective tissue disorders, steroid use, and intra-articular injections. The typical mechanism of injury is eccentric loading with planted foot and mild knee flexion.

The distal quadriceps tendon is formed by tendinous contributions of the rectus femoris (superficial layer), vastus medialis and lateralis (intermediate layer), and vastus intermedius (deep layer). On sagittal MR imaging, individual patient variations result in the visibility of 4 (6%), 3 (56%), 2 (30%), or only 1 (8%) distal quadriceps tendon layer.[93] The patellar base attachment anatomy is variable, but typically, the rectus femoris forms the superficial fibers; the vastus medialis and lateralis form the central, medial and lateral fibers, and the vastus intermedius forms the articular-sided fibers.[94]

Quadriceps tendon tears may be classified into partial-thickness and full-thickness tears. Full-thickness tears are classically associated with patella baja and tendon retraction. Further differentiations include osseous and nonosseous patella attachment tears. Partial-thickness tears more often include the deep vastus intermedius

fibers, whereas tears of the rectus femoris, vastus medialis, and vastus lateralis tears are more commonly associated with full-thickness tears.[95] In full-thickness tears, the average tendon retraction is 2.5 cm. As such, sagittal images should extend at least 5 cm proximal to the anatomic location of the patella. Quadriceps tendon tears may extend into the patellar fascia lata attachments.

Patella Tendon

Patella tendon tears are uncommon, with an approximate annual incidence of 1:100,000, amounting to approximately half the incidence of quadriceps tendon tears. Patella tendon tears are more common in male than female patients and typically occur in the third and fourth decade of life. Risk factors include systemic metabolic diseases, patellofemoral joint degeneration, patella tendinopathy, and corticosteroid injections. The most common mechanism of injury is tensile overload caused by sudden quadriceps contraction in knee flexion.

On MR imaging, the normal patella tendon presents as a single-layer tendon in most cases. Tears may be classified by depth into partial-thickness and full-thickness tears and by location into proximal injuries at the inferior patellar pole (most common in traumatic knee injury), midsubstance injuries, and distal tibial tubercle attachment injuries. Full-thickness patella tendon tears typically result in patella alta. Associated injuries include patella fractures and retinacular tears. Complete patella tendon tears are typically surgical indications, whereas partial-thickness tears may be treated nonoperatively.

Anatomically, the patella tendon is the distal continuation of the quadriceps tendon. Acute patellar tendon tears should be differentiated from chronic tendinopathy, which typically presents with tendon expansion, increased intrasubstance signal, and partial articular surface fiber tears that are typically located in the proximal or midsubstance tendon. In adults, traumatic patella tendon tears may extend into the sleeve fibers surrounding the patella, whereas in children, patella sleeve fractures are the typical pattern where the cartilage sleeve layer separates from the ossified inferior patella.

NERVES

In acute knee injuries, the incidence and severity of common peroneal and tibial nerve injuries increase with the severity of the mechanisms of injury. Concomitant common peroneal nerve injuries are more frequent than tibial nerve injuries, likely

Table 9
MR imaging findings of common peroneal and tibial nerve injuries

	Neurapraxia	Axonotmesis	Neurotmesis
MR neurography	Abnormal T2 signal hyperintensity	Nerve enlargement and abnormal T2 signal hyperintensity distal to injury followed by normalization if nerve regeneration ensues	Nerve discontinuity with abnormal T2 signal hyperintensity distal to injury followed by delayed normalization
MR Imaging muscle denervation effects	None	Muscle edema pattern, followed by normalization if nerve regeneration ensues	Muscle edema pattern, followed by progressive atrophy and fatty infiltration

because of the relative anatomic fixation of the common peroneal nerve around the fibular head. Peroneal nerve injuries accompany up to 25% of multiligament knee injuries, whereas the incidence of tibial nerve injuries is reportedly less than 10%. Accompanying clinical symptoms include sensory deficits, motor deficits, or combinations thereof. A recent study found significant peripheral nerve abnormalities in 0.6% of all knee MR imaging examinations, of which the common peroneal nerve was more commonly abnormal than the tibial nerve, and 36% required surgical treatment.[96] The most common associated injuries were meniscus tears, followed by cruciate ligament tears.

The Seddon classification categorizes nerve injuries as neurapraxia, axonotmesis, and neurotmesis (**Table 9**). Neuropraxia is a nerve injury without axonal disruption and is typically clinically transient. On MR imaging, neuropraxia typically shows focal increased T2 hyperintensity at the side of nerve injury and no muscle denervation effects. Axonotmesis is a nerve injury with axonal disruption but preserved myelin sheath. Axonotmesis spans a spectrum of severity. It is typically accompanied by muscle denervation effects, motor deficit, abnormal T2 signal hyperintensity of a longer segment of the injured nerves, and nerve enlargement. In high-grade axonotmesis, muscle denervation may not recover, and internal nerve scarring may develop with fusiform nerve enlargement and effacement of the internal fascicular pattern.[97] Neurotmesis is nerve discontinuity with disruption of the surrounding myelin sheath and connective tissue.

VESSELS

Vascular injury is a feared complication with an incidence of up to 18% in multiligament and knee dislocation injuries. Vascular knee injuries are associated with lateral ligament injuries, posterior knee dislocation, and peroneal nerve injury. The popliteal artery is the most commonly injured vessel, with an incidence of 76% in a systematic review, of which 80% required vascular repair and 12% amputation because of failed repair.[98] Vascular stretch injuries and intimal tears are typically associated with anterior knee dislocation, whereas posterior knee dislocation is more commonly associated with dissection and transection. Geniculate artery injuries may also be seen with lower-grade knee injuries.

CLINICS CARE POINTS

- Acute knee injury ranges among the most common joint injuries in professional and recreational athletes, accounting for more than 500,000 visits to emergency departments annually in the United States.
- Pivot shift, dashboard, hyperextension, clipping, and lateral patellar dislocation injuries result in typical bone contusion patterns.
- Attempts to equate the clinical MCL injury grades to specific MR imaging findings have repeatedly shown substantial inaccuracies in predicting the clinical degree of laxity.
- The anterolateral ligament, mid-third lateral capsular ligament, capsulo-osseous layer of the iliotibial band, and anterior oblique band of the fibular collateral ligament may describe the same anatomic structure.
- Posterolateral corner injuries are present in approximately 16% of knee injuries and 9% with hemarthrosis.
- Peroneal nerve injuries accompany up to 25% of multiligament knee injuries, whereas the incidence of tibial nerve injuries is reportedly less than 10%.

DISCLOSURE

B. Fritz has nothing to disclose. J. Fritz received institutional research support from Siemens AG, BTG International Ltd., United Kingdom, Zimmer Biomed, DePuy Synthes, QED, and SyntheticMR; is a scientific advisor for Siemens AG, SyntheticMR, GE Healthcare, QED, BTG, ImageBiopsy Lab, Boston Scientific, and Mirata Pharma; and has shared patents with Siemens Healthcare, Johns Hopkins University, and New York University.

REFERENCES

1. Niska R, Bhuiya F, Xu J. National Hospital Ambulatory Medical Care Survey: 2007 emergency department summary. Natl Health Stat Rep 2010;26:1–31.
2. Expert Panel on Musculoskeletal I, Taljanovic MS, Chang EY, et al. ACR Appropriateness Criteria R acute trauma to the knee. J Am Coll Radiol 2020; 17(5S):S12–25.
3. Ghodasara N, Yi PH, Clark K, et al. Postoperative spinal CT: what the radiologist needs to know. Radiographics 2019;39(6):1840–61.
4. Khodarahmi I, Fishman EK, Fritz J. Dedicated CT and MRI techniques for the evaluation of the postoperative knee. Semin Musculoskelet Radiol 2018; 22(4):444–56.
5. Khodarahmi I, Haroun RR, Lee M, et al. Metal artifact reduction computed tomography of arthroplasty implants: effects of combined modeled iterative reconstruction and dual-energy virtual monoenergetic extrapolation at higher photon energies. Invest Radiol 2018;53(12):728–35.
6. Fritz J, Henes JC, Fuld MK, et al. Dual-energy computed tomography of the knee, ankle, and foot: noninvasive diagnosis of gout and quantification of monosodium urate in tendons and ligaments. Semin Musculoskelet Radiol 2016;20(1):130–6.
7. Fritz J, Fishman EK, Corl F, et al. Imaging of limb salvage surgery. AJR Am J Roentgenol 2012; 198(3):647–60.
8. Bharadwaj UU, Coy A, Motamedi D, et al. CT-like MRI: a qualitative assessment of ZTE sequences for knee osseous abnormalities. Skeletal Radiol 2022;51(8):1585–94.
9. Fritz J, Efron DT, Fishman EK. State-of-the-art 3DCT angiography assessment of lower extremity trauma: typical findings, pearls, and pitfalls. Emerg Radiol 2013;20(3):175–84.
10. Fritz J, Efron DT, Fishman EK. Multidetector CT and three-dimensional CT angiography of upper extremity arterial injury. Emerg Radiol 2015;22(3):269–82.
11. Del Grande F, Guggenberger R, Fritz J. Rapid musculoskeletal MRI in 2021: value and optimized use of widely accessible techniques. AJR Am J Roentgenol 2021;216(3):704–17.

12. Fritz J, Guggenberger R, Del Grande F. Rapid musculoskeletal MRI in 2021: clinical application of advanced accelerated techniques. AJR Am J Roentgenol 2021;216(3):718–33.
13. Fritz J, Fritz B, Zhang J, et al. Simultaneous multislice accelerated turbo spin echo magnetic resonance imaging: comparison and combination with in-plane parallel imaging acceleration for high-resolution magnetic resonance imaging of the knee. Invest Radiol 2017;52(9):529–37.
14. Khodarahmi I, Fritz J. The value of 3 tesla field strength for musculoskeletal magnetic resonance imaging. Invest Radiol 2021;56(11):749–63.
15. Lin D, Fritz J. AI-based fast and quality-augmented MSK MRI: from 2-fold parallel imaging to 10-fold combined simultaneous multislice-parallel imaging acceleration. Invest Radiol 2023;58(1): 28–42.
16. Khodarahmi I, Keerthivasan MB, Brinkmann IM, et al. Modern low-field MRI of the musculoskeletal system: practice considerations, opportunities, and challenges. Invest Radiol 2023;58(1):76–87.
17. Fritz J, Kijowski R, Recht MP. Artificial intelligence in musculoskeletal imaging: a perspective on value propositions, clinical use, and obstacles. Skeletal Radiol 2022;51(2):239–43.
18. Rashidi A, Fritz J. Sports imaging of COVID-19: a multi-organ system review of indications and imaging findings. Sports Health 2022;14(5):618–31, 19417381221106448.
19. Del Grande F, Delcogliano M, Guglielmi R, et al. Fully automated 10-minute 3D CAIPIRINHA SPACE TSE MRI of the knee in adults: a multicenter, multi-reader, multifield-strength validation study. Invest Radiol 2018;53(11):689–97.
20. Fritz J, Raithel E, Thawait GK, et al. Six-fold acceleration of high-spatial resolution 3D SPACE MRI of the knee through incoherent k-space undersampling and iterative reconstruction-first experience. Invest Radiol 2016;51(6):400–9.
21. Fritz J, Fritz B, Thawait GG, et al. Three-dimensional CAIPIRINHA SPACE TSE for 5-minute high-resolution MRI of the knee. Invest Radiol 2016; 51(10):609–17.
22. Fritz J, Ahlawat S, Fritz B, et al. 10-Min 3D turbo spin echo MRI of the knee in children: arthroscopy-validated accuracy for the diagnosis of internal derangement. J Magn Reson Imaging 2019;49(7): e139–51.
23. Fritz J, Ahlawat S. High-resolution three-dimensional and cinematic rendering MR neurography. Radiology 2018;288(1):25.
24. Rowe SP, Fritz J, Fishman EK. CT evaluation of musculoskeletal trauma: initial experience with cinematic rendering. Emerg Radiol 2018;25(1):93–101.
25. Shakoor D, Guermazi A, Kijowski R, et al. Diagnostic performance of three-dimensional MRI for depicting

cartilage defects in the knee: a meta-analysis. Radiology 2018;289(1):71–82.

26. Shakoor D, Guermazi A, Kijowski R, et al. Cruciate ligament injuries of the knee: a meta-analysis of the diagnostic performance of 3D MRI. J Magn Reson Imaging 2019;50(5):1545–60.

27. Shakoor D, Kijowski R, Guermazi A, et al. Diagnosis of knee meniscal injuries by using three-dimensional MRI: a systematic review and meta-analysis of diagnostic performance. Radiology 2019;290(2):435–45.

28. Khodarahmi I, Isaac A, Fishman EK, et al. Metal about the hip and artifact reduction techniques: from basic concepts to advanced imaging. Semin Musculoskelet Radiol 2019;23(3):e68–81.

29. Fritz J, Lurie B, Potter HG. MR imaging of knee arthroplasty implants. Radiographics 2015;35(5): 1483–501.

30. Fritz J, Ahlawat S, Demehri S, et al. Compressed sensing SEMAC: 8-fold accelerated high resolution metal artifact reduction MRI of cobalt-chromium knee arthroplasty implants. Invest Radiol 2016; 51(10):666–76.

31. Fritz J, Fritz B, Thawait GK, et al. Advanced metal artifact reduction MRI of metal-on-metal hip resurfacing arthroplasty implants: compressed sensing acceleration enables the time-neutral use of SEMAC. Skeletal Radiol 2016;45(10):1345–56.

32. Fritz J, Meshram P, Stern SE, et al. Diagnostic performance of advanced metal artifact reduction MRI for periprosthetic shoulder infection. J Bone Joint Surg Am 2022;104(15):1352–61.

33. Expert Panel on Musculoskeletal I, Fox MG, Chang EY, Amini B, et al. ACR Appropriateness Criteria R chronic knee pain. J Am Coll Radiol 2018;15(11S):S302–12.

34. Potter HG, Jain SK, Ma Y, et al. Cartilage injury after acute, isolated anterior cruciate ligament tear: immediate and longitudinal effect with clinical/MRI follow-up. Am J Sports Med 2012;40(2):276–85.

35. Fritz B, Parkar AP, Cerezal L, et al. Sports imaging of team handball injuries. Semin Musculoskelet Radiol 2020;24(3):227–45.

36. Renstrom P, Ljungqvist A, Arendt E, et al. Non-contact ACL injuries in female athletes: an International Olympic Committee current concepts statement. Br J Sports Med 2008;42(6):394–412.

37. Cobby MJ, Schweitzer ME, Resnick D. The deep lateral femoral notch: an indirect sign of a torn anterior cruciate ligament. Radiology 1992;184(3): 855–8.

38. van der List JP, Mintz DN, DiFelice GS. The location of anterior cruciate ligament tears: a prevalence study using magnetic resonance imaging. Orthop J Sports Med 2017;5(6). 2325967117709966.

39. DiFelice GS, Villegas C, Taylor S. Anterior cruciate ligament preservation: early results of a novel arthroscopic technique for suture anchor primary anterior

cruciate ligament repair. Arthroscopy 2015;31(11): 2162–71.

40. Daniels SP, van der List JP, Kazam JJ, et al. Arthroscopic primary repair of the anterior cruciate ligament: what the radiologist needs to know. Skeletal Radiol 2018;47(5):619–29.

41. Thakur U, Gulati V, Shah J, et al. Anterior cruciate ligament reconstruction related complications: 2D and 3D high-resolution magnetic resonance imaging evaluation. Skeletal Radiol 2022;51(7):1347–64.

42. Levy BA, Dajani KA, Whelan DB, et al. Decision making in the multiligament-injured knee: an evidence-based systematic review. Arthroscopy 2009;25(4):430–8.

43. Buyukdogan K, Laidlaw MS, Miller MD. Surgical management of the multiple-ligament knee injury. Arthrosc Tech 2018;7(2):e147–64.

44. Harner CD, Xerogeanes JW, Livesay GA, et al. The human posterior cruciate ligament complex: an interdisciplinary study. Ligament morphology and biomechanical evaluation. Am J Sports Med 1995; 23(6):736–45.

45. Pache S, Aman ZS, Kennedy M, et al. Posterior cruciate ligament: current concepts review. Arch Bone Jt Surg 2018;6(1):8–18.

46. Fanelli GC, Edson CJ. Posterior cruciate ligament injuries in trauma patients: Part II. Arthroscopy 1995; 11(5):526–9.

47. Heron CW, Calvert PT. Three-dimensional gradient-echo MR imaging of the knee: comparison with arthroscopy in 100 patients. Radiology 1992; 183(3):839–44.

48. LaPrade RF, Engebretsen AH, Ly TV, et al. The anatomy of the medial part of the knee. J Bone Joint Surg Am 2007;89(9):2000–10.

49. Warren LF, Marshall JL. The supporting structures and layers on the medial side of the knee: an anatomical analysis. J Bone Joint Surg Am 1979; 61(1):56–62.

50. Roach CJ, Haley CA, Cameron KL, et al. The epidemiology of medial collateral ligament sprains in young athletes. Am J Sports Med 2014;42(5):1103–9.

51. Fetto JF, Marshall JL. Medial collateral ligament injuries of the knee: a rationale for treatment. Clin Orthop Relat Res 1978;132:206–18.

52. Schweitzer ME, Tran D, Deely DM, et al. Medial collateral ligament injuries: evaluation of multiple signs, prevalence and location of associated bone bruises, and assessment with MR imaging. Radiology 1995;194(3):825–9.

53. Watura C, Morgan C, Flaherty D, et al. Medial collateral ligament injury of the knee: correlations between MRI features and clinical gradings. Skeletal Radiol 2022;51(6):1225–33.

54. Albtoush OM, Horger M, Springer F, et al. Avulsion fracture of the medial collateral ligament association with Segond fracture. Clin Imaging 2019;53:32–4.

55. Taketomi S, Uchiyama E, Nakagawa T, et al. Clinical features and injury patterns of medial collateral ligament tibial side avulsions: "wave sign" on magnetic resonance imaging is essential for diagnosis. Knee 2014;21(6):1151–5.

56. Marchant MH Jr, Tibor LM, Sekiya JK, et al. Management of medial-sided knee injuries, part 1: medial collateral ligament. Am J Sports Med 2011;39(5): 1102–13.

57. Rashidi A, Haj-Mirzaian A, Dalili D, et al. Evidence-based use of clinical examination, ultrasonography, and MRI for diagnosing ulnar collateral ligament tears of the metacarpophalangeal joint of the thumb: systematic review and meta-analysis. Eur Radiol 2021;31(8):5699–712.

58. Alaia EF, Rosenberg ZS, Alaia MJ. Stener-like lesions of the superficial medial collateral ligament of the knee: mri features. AJR Am J Roentgenol 2019; 213(6):W272–6.

59. Escobedo EM, Mills WJ, Hunter JC. The reverse Segond fracture: association with a tear of the posterior cruciate ligament and medial meniscus. AJR Am J Roentgenol 2002;178(4):979–83.

60. Seebacher JR, Inglis AE, Marshall JL, et al. The structure of the posterolateral aspect of the knee. J Bone Joint Surg Am 1982;64(4):536–41.

61. Kowalczuk M, Herbst E, Burnham JM, et al. A layered anatomic description of the anterolateral complex of the knee. Clin Sports Med 2018;37(1): 1–8.

62. Claes S, Vereecke E, Maes M, et al. Anatomy of the anterolateral ligament of the knee. J Anat 2013; 223(4):321–8.

63. Dombrowski ME, Costello JM, Ohashi B, et al. Macroscopic anatomical, histological and magnetic resonance imaging correlation of the lateral capsule of the knee. Knee Surg Sports Traumatol Arthrosc 2016;24(9):2854–60.

64. Campos JC, Chung CB, Lektrakul N, et al. Pathogenesis of the Segond fracture: anatomic and MR imaging evidence of an iliotibial tract or anterior oblique band avulsion. Radiology 2001;219(2):381–6.

65. Gottsegen CJ, Eyer BA, White EA, et al. Avulsion fractures of the knee: imaging findings and clinical significance. Radiographics 2008;28(6):1755–70.

66. Walker PS, Erkman MJ. The role of the menisci in force transmission across the knee. Clin Orthop Relat Res 1975;109:184–92.

67. Nielsen AB, Yde J. Epidemiology of acute knee injuries: a prospective hospital investigation. J Trauma 1991;31(12):1644–8.

68. DeHaven KE. Diagnosis of acute knee injuries with hemarthrosis. Am J Sports Med 1980;8(1):9–14.

69. Bellabarba C, Bush-Joseph CA, Bach BR Jr. Patterns of meniscal injury in the anterior cruciate-deficient knee: a review of the literature. Am J Orthop (Belle Mead Nj) 1997;26(1):18–23.

70. Poulsen E, Goncalves GH, Bricca A, et al. Knee osteoarthritis risk is increased 4-6 fold after knee injury - a systematic review and meta-analysis. Br J Sports Med 2019;53(23):1454–63.

71. Wadhwa V, Omar H, Coyner K, et al. ISAKOS classification of meniscal tears-illustration on 2D and 3D isotropic spin echo MR imaging. Eur J Radiol 2016;85(1):15–24.

72. Fetzer GB, Spindler KP, Amendola A, et al. Potential market for new meniscus repair strategies: evaluation of the MOON cohort. J Knee Surg 2009;22(3): 180–6.

73. Kopf S, Beaufils P, Hirschmann MT, et al. Management of traumatic meniscus tears: the 2019 ESSKA meniscus consensus. Knee Surg Sports Traumatol Arthrosc 2020;28(4):1177–94.

74. De Smet AA, Mukherjee R. Clinical, MRI, and arthroscopic findings associated with failure to diagnose a lateral meniscal tear on knee MRI. AJR Am J Roentgenol 2008;190(1):22–6.

75. Liu X, Feng H, Zhang H, et al. Arthroscopic prevalence of ramp lesion in 868 patients with anterior cruciate ligament injury. Am J Sports Med 2011;39(4): 832–7.

76. Sonnery-Cottet B, Conteduca J, Thaunat M, et al. Hidden lesions of the posterior horn of the medial meniscus: a systematic arthroscopic exploration of the concealed portion of the knee. Am J Sports Med 2014;42(4):921–6.

77. DePhillipo NN, Cinque ME, Chahla J, et al. Incidence and detection of meniscal ramp lesions on magnetic resonance imaging in patients with anterior cruciate ligament reconstruction. Am J Sports Med 2017;45(10):2233–7.

78. Hetsroni I, Lillemoe K, Marx RG. Small medial meniscocapsular separations: a potential cause of chronic medial-side knee pain. Arthroscopy 2011;27(11): 1536–42.

79. Greif DN, Baraga MG, Rizzo MG, et al. MRI appearance of the different meniscal ramp lesion types, with clinical and arthroscopic correlation. Skeletal Radiol 2020;49(5):677–89.

80. Thaunat M, Fayard JM, Guimaraes TM, et al. Classification and surgical repair of ramp lesions of the medial meniscus. Arthrosc Tech 2016;5(4): e871–5.

81. Arner JW, Herbst E, Burnham JM, et al. MRI can accurately detect meniscal ramp lesions of the knee. Knee Surg Sports Traumatol Arthrosc 2017; 25(12):3955–60.

82. Yeo Y, Ahn JM, Kim H, et al. MR evaluation of the meniscal ramp lesion in patients with anterior cruciate ligament tear. Skeletal Radiol 2018;47(12): 1683–9.

83. Laurens M, Cavaignac E, Fayolle H, et al. The accuracy of MRI for the diagnosis of ramp lesions. Skeletal Radiol 2022;51(3):525–33.

84. LaPrade RF, Ly TV, Wentorf FA, et al. The posterolateral attachments of the knee: a qualitative and quantitative morphologic analysis of the fibular collateral ligament, popliteus tendon, popliteofibular ligament, and lateral gastrocnemius tendon. Am J Sports Med 2003;31(6):854–60.

85. Rosas HG. Unraveling the Posterolateral Corner of the Knee. Radiographics 2016;36(6):1776–91.

86. DeLee JC, Riley MB, Rockwood CA Jr. Acute posterolateral rotatory instability of the knee. Am J Sports Med 1983;11(4):199–207.

87. Yaras RJ, O'Neill N, Yaish AM. Lateral collateral ligament knee injuries. Treasure Island (FL): StatPearls; 2022.

88. LaPrade RF, Wentorf FA, Fritts H, et al. A prospective magnetic resonance imaging study of the incidence of posterolateral and multiple ligament injuries in acute knee injuries presenting with a hemarthrosis. Arthroscopy 2007;23(12):1341–7.

89. LaPrade RF, Terry GC. Injuries to the posterolateral aspect of the knee. Association of anatomic injury patterns with clinical instability. Am J Sports Med 1997;25(4):433–8.

90. Brown TR, Quinn SF, Wensel JP, et al. Diagnosis of popliteus injuries with MR imaging. Skeletal Radiol 1995;24(7):511–4.

91. Fanelli GC. Posterior cruciate ligament injuries in trauma patients. Arthroscopy 1993;9(3):291–4.

92. Sillanpaa PJ, Peltola E, Mattila VM, et al. Femoral avulsion of the medial patellofemoral ligament after primary traumatic patellar dislocation predicts subsequent instability in men: a mean 7-year nonoperative follow-up study. Am J Sports Med 2009;37(8):1513–21.

93. Zeiss J, Saddemi SR, Ebraheim NA. MR imaging of the quadriceps tendon: normal layered configuration and its importance in cases of tendon rupture. AJR Am J Roentgenol 1992;159(5):1031–4.

94. Waligora AC, Johanson NA, Hirsch BE. Clinical anatomy of the quadriceps femoris and extensor apparatus of the knee. Clin Orthop Relat Res 2009;467(12):3297–306.

95. Falkowski AL, Jacobson JA, Hirschmann MT, et al. MR imaging of the quadriceps femoris tendon: distal tear characterization and clinical significance of rupture types. Eur Radiol 2021;31(10):7674–83.

96. Dalili D, Isaac A, Fayad LM, et al. Routine knee MRI: how common are peripheral nerve abnormalities, and why does it matter? Skeletal Radiol 2021;50(2):321–32.

97. Chhabra A, Ahlawat S, Belzberg A, et al. Peripheral nerve injury grading simplified on MR neurography: as referenced to Seddon and Sunderland classifications. Indian J Radiol Imaging 2014;24(3):217–24.

98. Medina O, Arom GA, Yeranosian MG, et al. Vascular and nerve injury after knee dislocation: a systematic review. Clin Orthop Relat Res 2014;472(9):2621–9.

Particularities on Anatomy and Normal Postsurgical Appearances of the Ankle and Foot

Maria Pilar Aparisi Gómez, MBChB, FRANZCR[a,b,]*, Francisco Aparisi, MD, PhD[c], Giuseppe Guglielmi, MD[d,e], Alberto Bazzocchi, MD, PhD[f]

KEYWORDS

• Ankle • Foot • Anatomy • Postoperative period • Radiology • MR imaging

KEY POINTS

- The ankle and foot are anatomically complex. A sound knowledge of the anatomy and biomechanics helps to understand the mechanisms of injury and provides a useful tool for accurate diagnosis, with a positive impact on management and prognosis.
- A good understanding of the different surgical procedures used to treat pathology helps in providing as much information as possible to guarantee a favorable outcome, improving levels of care and prognosis.
- Familiarity with the expected postsurgical appearances is mandatory, to be able to discern these from complications.

INTRODUCTION

The ankle and foot are very complex anatomic regions. The function of walking involves the coordination of many different joints.

Detailed knowledge of anatomy is necessary to understand the pathology.

In this article, we will focus on reviewing the components of the anatomy of the ankle and foot, with special attention to those concepts that have been the object of recent study or anatomic features that have a clear association with the development of symptoms or are a frequent location for injury, elucidating why this is the case.

Frequently encountered anatomic variants and other common findings in asymptomatic patients are also described.

Finally, we will highlight what are the commonly expected postsurgical appearances and the most common postsurgical complications.

ANATOMY
Talocrural Joint

This consists of the tibia, fibula, and talus.

The distal tibia is covered by hyaline cartilage and articulates with the dorsal surface of the talus, in a trochlear joint. The dorsal surface of the talus has a concave configuration, from anterior to posterior, and the tibia is convex. From medial to

The authors have no funding information to disclose.

[a] Department of Radiology, Auckland City Hospital, 2 Park Road, Grafton, Auckland 1023, New Zealand; [b] Department of Radiology, IMSKE, Calle Suiza, 11, Valencia 46024, Spain; [c] Department of Radiology, Hospital Vithas Nueve de Octubre, Calle Valle de la Ballestera, 59, Valencia 46015, Spain; [d] Department of Radiology, Hospital San Giovanni Rotondo, Italy; [e] Department of Radiology, University of Foggia, Viale Luigi Pinto 1, Foggia 71100, Italy; [f] Diagnostic and Interventional Radiology, IRCCS Istituto Ortopedico Rizzoli, Via G. C. Pupilli 1, Bologna 40136, Italy
* Corresponding author. Auckland City Hospital, 2 Park Road, Grafton, Auckland 1023, New Zealand.
E-mail addresses: pilara@adhb.govt.nz; pilucaparisi193@gmail.com; pilara@adhb.govt.nz

lateral, the talus is mildly convex, and the tibia is mildly concave.

In the medial aspect, the lateral surface of the medial malleolus articulates with the medial articular facet of the talus. It is formed by the anterior and posterior colliculus and the intercollicular groove to which the deltoid ligament attaches. The medial ankle mortise is fairly rigid and strong.

In the lateral aspect, in opposition, the mortise tends to be flexible. The medial facet of the lateral malleolus and the lateral aspect of the talus configure a small triangular articulation. The lateral surface of the distal tibia has the shape of a convex triangular notch, with which the distal fibular shaft articulates. This joint is stabilized by the syndesmotic ligament, the interosseous ligament, and membrane.[1]

The fibrous capsule attaches to the inferior ridge of the distal tibia and medial and lateral malleoli. It follows the trochlear margins, except for the anterior aspect, where it leaves a bit of extra room attaching to the talar neck. The anterior and posterior aspects of the capsule are relatively weak, and covered by the synovial layer.

The Syndesmotic Ligament Complex

The ligaments of the complex are the anteroinferior and the posteroinferior (Fig. 1).

The anteroinferior tibiofibular ligament has multiple small fascicles in a flat, fibrous laminar band-like configuration. Its origin is the anteromedial tubercle of the distal fibula. It inserts on the anterolateral tubercle of the distal tibia (Fig. 2).

There is a common anatomic variant, which consists of an accessory anteroinferior tibiofibular ligament (Also known as Bassett's ligament).[2] This is a distal separate fascicle that is located parallel and distal to the anteroinferior tibiofibular ligament (Fig. 3).

Variations in the width, length (wider and longer fascicles), and course (distal fibular attachment) of the Bassett's ligament may increase the risk of pathology. Pathologic thickening of the Bassett's ligament (in the setting of an inversion injury, for example) can cause anterior impingement.

The presence of anterior, anterolateral, and superolateral talar dome chondral abrasion is associated with pathologic accessory anteroinferior tibiofibular ligament.[3]

The posteroinferior tibiofibular ligament is made up of a deep transverse component, and a superficial component. The deep transverse component is a very strong, thick fibrous band. Its origin is in the posterior fibular tubercle. It attaches across the whole posterior tibial plafond to the medial border of the malleolus. It courses inferiorly to the tibial plafond, and in this way deepens the articular surface of the tibia, with the same function that a labrum would have. The triangular fibular origin forms an articular surface for the talar facet[4] (Fig. 4).

The superficial syndesmotic ligament is broad and has the shape of a fan. Its origin is in the posterior crest of the fibula. It extends above and below the posterior fibular tubercle and has two attachments. The first attachment is to the posterolateral tibial tubercle, and the second is a broad attachment across the tibial plafond to the border of the tibialis posterior tendon groove (Fig. 5).

The interosseous ligament is a short, dense band that extends from the medial surface of the fibula to the lateral surface of the tibia.[5]

The posterosuperior tibiofibular recess may contain a synovial fold extending from the talocrural joint, and is located below the syndesmotic ligament.

The Medial Collateral Ligament Complex

The medial collateral ligament complex is also known as the deltoid ligament.

Based on MR appearances, the description consists of a deep and a superficial ligament.[5]

The deep deltoid ligament (posterior and anterior tibiotalar fibers) (Fig. 6) is broad, with a shape that resembles a fan. It originates from the intercollicular groove and adjacent surfaces of the anterior and posterior colliculus. It is lined by synovium, intraarticular.

The superficial deltoid ligament (posterior and anterior tibiotalar, tibionavicular, and tibiocalcaneal fibers) (Fig. 7) is also broad, flat, with a triangular shape. It originates from the anteromedial

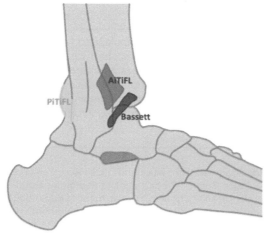

Fig. 1. Syndesmotic complex. AiTiFL, anteroinferior tibiofibular ligament; PiTiFL, posteroinferior tibiofibular ligament; Bassett ligament (accessory anteroinferior tibiofibular).

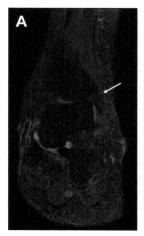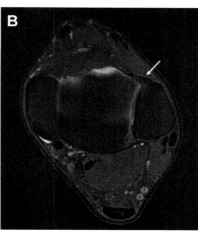

Fig. 2. Anteroinferior tibiofibular ligament (*arrow*) in the (*A*) coronal and (*B*) axial plane (PD fat sat images).

surface of the anterior colliculus and medial subcutaneous surface of the malleolus. The distal fibers merge with the superomedial fibers of the calcaneonavicular ligament in the tibiospring ligament[6] (**Fig. 8**).

The Lateral Collateral Ligament Complex

The lateral collateral ligament complex is formed by the anterior talofibular ligament (ATFL), calcaneofibular ligament (CFL), and posterior talofibular ligament (PTFL) (**Fig. 9**).

The ATFL is composed of various flat, thick, fibrous bands. The cranial band is thicker and stronger and originates from the anteromedial distal fibula and attaches to the lateral neck of the talus.[7] There may be up to three fiber bundles (Type I, II, and III depending on the number).[8] In a

cadaveric study, type II (two bundles) was found to be the most common.[9]

The CFL is a fibrous band that originates from the deep posterior lateral malleolar fossa and courses inferiorly and posteriorly to the lateral surface of the calcaneus. The medial aspect of the peroneal tendon sheath is attached to the CFL in the inframalleolar course.

There are variations in the number of ATFL and CFL, and variations in fiber connections between them.[8,10]

The PTFL is a broad, flat, triangular ligament interspersed with fatty fibers.[11] The widest portion of the ligament originates from the deep posterior lateral malleolar fossa and attaches to the lateral tubercle of the talus (**Fig. 10**).

A recent cadaveric study by Kobayashi and colleagues[9] found that the ATFL, CFL, and PTFL

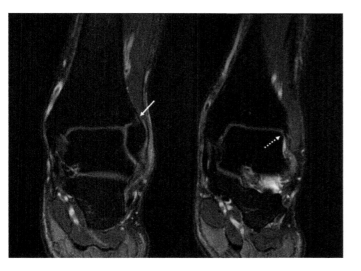

Fig. 3. Consecutive coronal PD fat sat, from posterior to anterior show the anteroinferior tibiofibular ligament (*bold arrow*) and slightly more anterior and inferior, the accessory anteroinferior tibiofibular ligament (Bassett's ligament) (*dotted arrow*).

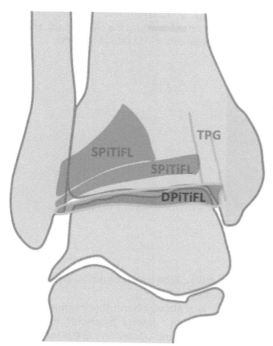

Fig. 4. Posteroinferior tibiofibular ligament. SPiTiFL, superficial component. The superficial syndesmotic ligament is broad and has the shape of a fan. It has two attachments, to the posterolateral tibial tubercle and across the tibial plafond to the border of the tibialis posterior tendon groove (TPG). DPiTiFL, deep component, a strong thick fibrous band that courses inferiorly to the tibial plafond, and deepens the articular surface of the tibia, with the same function that a labrum.

connect at the anterior/inferior tip of the lateral malleolus, suggesting that stabilization of the lateral ankle is reinforced by ligament connections. This could also suggest that injuries involving the tip of the fibula may have a different pattern to the typically seen ones, with the instability of several ligaments.

The tibial slip or posterior intermalleolar ligament is an anatomic variant. The ligament originates from the fibers of the PTFL and inserts onto the posteromedial malleolus. It may cause crowding of the posterior joint and contribute to posterior impingement.[12]

Talocalcaneal joint

The talocalcaneal joint is composed of two independent synovial articulations: the anterior (talocalcaneonavicular) and the posterior (talocalcaneal) subtalar joints.

The Anterior Subtalar Joint
The anterior subtalar joint is formed by the head of the talus, which has an oval convex shape, and is

medially rotated, and the proximal concave facet of the navicular.

The plantar surface of the head of the talus articulates anterolaterally with the superior surface of the calcaneus and posteriorly with the sustentaculum tali of the calcaneus. The plantar and medial articulation is supported by the deltoid ligament and the calcaneonavicular ligament (spring ligament complex).

The Posterior Subtalar Joint
The posterior calcaneal facet of the talus articulates with the posterior talar facet of the calcaneus. The posterior subtalar joint communicates with the talocrural joint in up to 20% of cases.

The Spring Ligament Complex
This ligament complex supports the head of the talus at the anterior and middle facets of the calcaneus. The complex is the primary static stabilizer of the medial arch of the foot. In combination with the tibialis posterior tendon, they maintain normal hindfoot relations. The ligament complex has three bands.[13]

The superomedial band originates from the medial anterior surface of the sustentaculum tali, and merges with inferior fibers of the tibiospring ligament (superficial deltoid ligament), attaching to the superior and peripheral border of the navicular tuberosity (wide insertion). It forms a sling that suspends the head of the talus. This is the strongest and most important longitudinal arch stabilizer, and the most frequently injured.

The medioplantar oblique band (lateral calcaneonavicular) originates from the medial margin of the coronoid fossa and attaches to the caudal surface of the navicular tuberosity.

The inferoplantar ligament (intermedial calcaneonavicular) originates from the coronoid fossa of the calcaneus and inserts on the navicular beak. It has a minor role in stabilizing the hindfoot and longitudinal arch.

The failure of the tibialis posterior and spring ligament complex leads to hindfoot valgus and pes planovalgus[13] **(Fig. 11)**.

The Sinus Tarsi
The sinus tarsi is a canal that has a conical configuration. The apex is medial, called the tarsal canal, and the outlet is lateral. It separates the anterior and medial talar facets from the posterior talar facet. The sinus tarsi contains fat and branches of the posterior tibial artery and nerve, peroneal artery and nerve, and supporting ligaments.[14]

These supporting ligaments are the medial, intermediate, and lateral roots of the inferior extensor retinaculum (fibers anchored to the talus and calcaneus), the lateral cervical

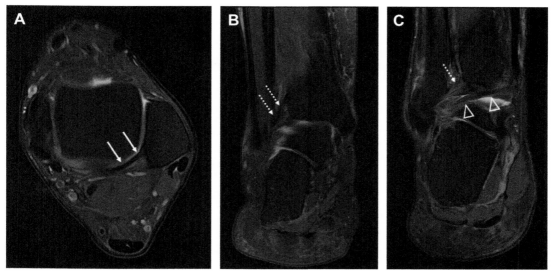

Fig. 5. Posteroinferior tibiofibular ligament. (*A*) Axial PD fat sat shows the deep transverse component (*bold arrows*). This is very strong, a thick fibrous band that courses inferiorly to the tibial plafond, and in this way deepens the articular surface of the tibia, with the same function that a labrum would have. The triangular fibular origin forms an articular surface for the talar facet. The superficial syndesmotic ligament is broad and has the shape of a fan. Its origin is in the posterior crest of the fibula. It extends above and below the posterior fibular tubercle and has two attachments. (*B*) Coronal PD fats sat shows the first attachment, to the posterolateral tibial tubercle (*dotted arrows*). (*C*) Coronal PD fat sat in a different patient shows the second attachment, across the tibial plafond to the border of the posterior tibial tendon groove (*arrowheads*). Note the first attachment is also visible (*dotted arrow*).

ligament, and the medial talocalcaneal interosseous ligament.

The Talocalcaneonavicular Ligament Complex
The ligament complex supports the subtalar joint and comprises the extensor retinaculum, the lateral cervical ligament, and the medial talocalcaneal interosseous ligament.

Other minor supporting ligaments are also present, but normally not identifiable with MR imaging. There are multiple variations of the anatomy.[14]

The cervical ligament originates from the anteromedial floor of the sinus tarsi (cervical tubercle) and courses anteromedially and upward to attach to the neck of the talus. This is the strongest ligament of the sinus tarsi.

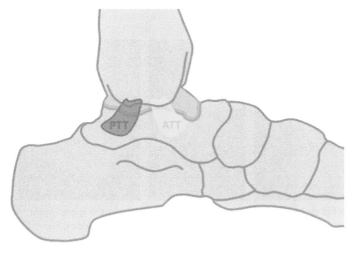

Fig. 6. Deep deltoid ligament components. ATT, anterior tibiotalar; PTT, posterior tibiotalar.

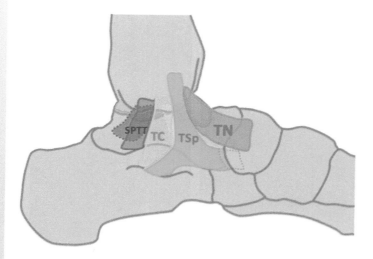

Fig. 7. Superficial deltoid ligament components. SPTT, superficial posterior tibio talar; TC, tibiocalcaneal; TSp, tibiospring fibers, which are tibiocalcaneal fibers that merge with the superomedial fibers of the calcaneonavicular ligament; TN, tibionavicular.

The posterior and medial reflections of the inferior extensor retinaculum course parallelly to the cervical ligament in the lateral aspect and form a strong support for the lateral sinus tarsi.

The interosseous talocalcaneal ligament (ligament of the sinus tarsi or fundiform ligament)[15] is a broad, flat, oblique band that is medially oriented. Its origin is in the sulcus of the calcaneus at the anterior border of the posterior talocalcaneal joint. It inserts into the medial undersurface of the sustentaculum tali. It has a lateral and a medial band.[15] The interosseous talocalcaneal and the medial component of the extensor retinaculum root form a "V" shape in the tarsal sinus[16] (Fig. 12).

The interosseous talocalcaneal maintains apposition of the talus and calcaneus in eversion—inversion movements. The cervical ligament limits the inversion of the hindfoot, assisted by the inferior extensor retinaculum (limits inversion of the subtalar joint). When there is a dorsal extension of the toes (phase of movement), the sinus tarsi complex forms a control mechanism for the longitudinal arch of the foot.

The lateral talocalcaneal ligament is parallel to the CFL, and is difficult to differentiate from it. Its origin is in the inferior surface of the lateral talar process. It inserts onto the lateral and posterior surfaces of the calcaneus. Normally it is located anterior and medial to the insertion of the CFL.[17]

The posterior talocalcaneal ligament is flat and short. Its origin is in the lateral surface of the talar tubercle. It inserts on the superior and medial aspect of the calcaneus. Fibers may merge with the PTFL. If there is an os trigonum, the ligament may have its origin in it, and form a trigonocalcaneal ligament.[18,19]

The medial talocalcaneal ligament has its origin in the posteromedial border of the talar tubercle

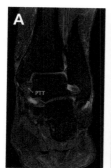
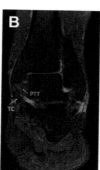
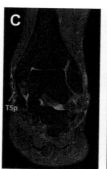
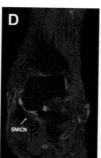
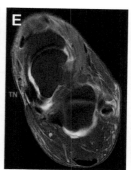

Fig. 8. Deltoid ligament. (A–D) Consecutive PD fat sat images, from posterior to anterior show the components of the deltoid ligament. PTT, posterior tibio talar (includes deep and superficial fibers); TC, tibiocalcaneal; TSp, tibiospring fibers, which are tibiocalcaneal fibers that merge distally with the superomedial fibers of the calcaneonavicular ligament (SMCN). (E) Axial PD fat sat shows the tibionavicular. TN, tibionavicular.

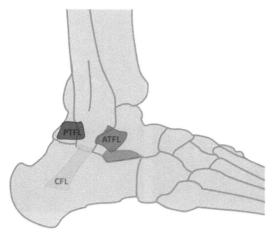

Fig. 9. Lateral complex. ATFL, anterior talofibular ligament; CFL, calcaneofibular ligament; PTFL, posterior talofibular ligament.

and its insertion in the posterior border of the sustentaculum tali.[17]

The talonavicular ligament has both a superficial and a deep component and crosses both dorsal and plantar to the superomedial calcaneonavicular ligament. The dorsal fibers merge with the ligament. They originate from the dorsal surface of the talar neck and insert on the dorsum of the navicular.[17]

The Calcaneocuboid Joint

The calcaneal and cuboid articular surface is rectangular. The joint is supported by a capsule, besides the long plantar ligament, and the bifurcate, dorsolateral, and plantar calcaneocuboid ligaments (short plantar ligament). The calcaneocuboid joint is part of the Chopart joint.

The bifurcate ligament arises from the anterior process of the calcaneus and has two components, with a "Y" shape. The calcaneonavicular component (lateral calcaneonavicular) extends medially and inserts onto the dorsolateral part of the navicular. The calcaneocuboid component (medial calcaneocuboid) extends laterally and inserts onto the dorsomedial part of the cuboid[20] (Fig. 13).

The long plantar ligament has the shape of an hourglass. Its origin is in the plantar aspect of the calcaneus, proximal to the origin of the short plantar ligament (plantar calcaneocuboid). It inserts onto the cuboid and the bases of the second to fourth metatarsals (fan-shaped insertion), covering the peroneus longus (PL) tunnel.[21]

There is anatomic variation, with the insertion sometimes reaching the fifth metatarsal base or involving the PL sheath.[21,22]

Chopart Joint

The Chopart joint (transverse tarsal joint) is a biomechanically intricate unit made up of the anterior subtalar joint (talocalcaneonavicular joint) and the calcaneocuboid joint and cubonavicular joint. The joints act in unison to coordinate the transmission of forces from hindfoot to forefoot and provide transverse arch support. There is a dorsal, plantar, and interosseous cubonavicular ligament.

Intertarsal Joints

These consist of the joints between navicular and proximal medial, intermediate, and lateral cuneiform. They are all reinforced by a single joint capsule. The cuboid and lateral cuneiform and the cuboid and navicular joints comprise two additional intertarsal joints. They conform to a

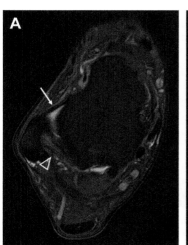

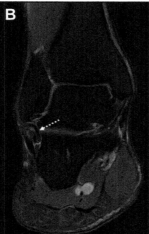

Fig. 10. Lateral complex. (A) Axial PD fat sat shows the anterior talofibular ligament (*bold arrow*) and the posterior talofibular ligament (*arrowhead*). (B) Coronal PD fat sat better shows the course of the calcaneofibular ligament (*dotted arrow*).

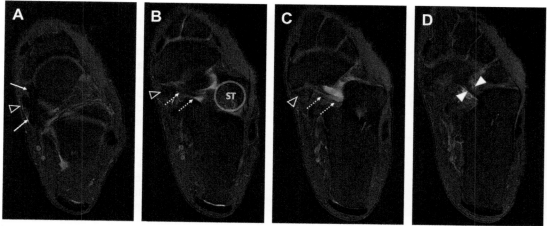

Fig. 11. Spring ligament complex. Consecutive axial PD fat sat images, from superior to inferior. (*A*) shows the superomedial band (*bold arrows*) that merges with inferior fibers of the tibiospring ligament superiorly. This forms a sling that suspends the head of the talus and is the strongest and most most frequently injured band. The tibialis posterior runs in close vicinity (*hollow arrowhead*). (*B, C*) At a more inferior level the medioplantar oblique band (lateral calcaneonavicular) is visible (*dotted arrows*). The tibialis posterior is also visible (*hollow arrowhead*). This is the level of the sinus tarsi (*ST, encircled*) (*D*) The inferoplantar ligament (intermedial calcaneonavicular) is visible more inferiorly (*solid arrowheads*).

functional unit. Each joint has a dorsal, plantar, and interosseous ligament named for the bone origin and bone insertion.

The Tarsometatarsal Joints (Lisfranc Joint)

There is a medial, intermediate, and lateral tarsometatarsal joint, with individual capsules. The medial tarsometatarsal joint is formed by the medial cuneiform and the first metatarsal. The intermediate tarsometatarsal joint is formed by the intermediate and lateral cuneiform articulation with the base of the second and third metatarsals. The lateral tarsometatarsal joint is formed by the cuboid and fourth and fifth metatarsal bases. The joint spaces extend to include the articulation between the metatarsal bases.

There are dorsal and plantar ligaments supporting each tarsometatarsal joint.

The dorsal ligaments are seven, with the first being the strongest. The plantar ligaments vary between five and seven. Medial plantar ligaments are generally present; lateral ligaments are variably present. The intermetatarsal bases of the second through fifth digits are supported by dorsal, plantar, and interosseous transverse metatarsal base ligaments.[23]

Lisfranc Ligament

The strongest interosseous cuneometatarsal ligament is the first ligament (Lisfranc ligament). This is an important stabilizer of the midfoot, connecting the medial cuneiform to the base of the second metatarsal. This creates a keystone configuration in the "arch" between the medial and lateral cuneiforms. The ligament has its origin in the lateral distal surface of the medial cuneiform and extends obliquely to insert onto the medial aspect of the base of the second metatarsal.

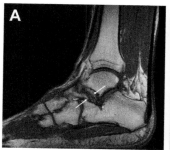
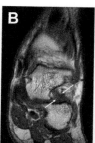
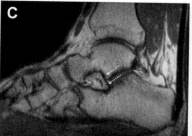
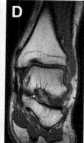

Fig. 12. Subtalar joint. (*A*) Sagittal T1 shows de cervical ligament (*arrows*), seen in coronal T1 as well (*B*). (*C*) Sagittal reconstruction from axial PD cube sequence shows the interosseus talocalcaneal (*dotted arrows*), also seen in coronal T1 (*D*).

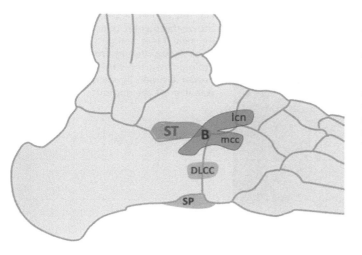

Fig. 13. Calcaneocuboid joint. The bifurcate ligament (B) arises from the anterior process of the calcaneus and has two components, with a "Y" shape, a calcaneonavicular component (lateral calcaneonavicular, lcn) and the calcaneocuboid component (medial calcaneocuboid, mcc). DLCC, dorsolateral calcaneocuboid; SP, short plantar ligament (plantar calcaneocuboid). ST, sinus tarsi.

The configuration of the ligament is variable.[24] There is a dorsal band, which is the weakest, an interosseous ligament (the Lisfranc proper ligament), and a plantar ligament that sends bundles to the second and third metatarsal bases.[25]

In 22% of the population, there are only two bands (**Fig. 14**).

A second ligament bridges the medial and intermediate cuneiforms in a direct transverse orientation.

The second and third interosseous cuneometatarsal ligaments have variable morphology but, in general, form attachments between the second and third metatarsal bases and the intermediate and lateral cuneiforms.

The ligament may have a homogeneous low signal or a striated appearance with low to intermediate signal on MR. The oblique coronal plane is the best one to assess the transverse arch of the foot and the cross-section of the Lisfranc ligament.[25]

Metatarsophalangeal Joints

The metatarsophalangeal joints (MTPJ) are condyloid synovial joints that allow flexion, extension, and limited adduction and abduction.

The first metatarsophalangeal joint is stabilized by a capsuloligamentous complex and multiple tendons. The capsuloligamentous complex components are the fibrous capsule, the collateral ligament complex, the sesamoid-phalangeal ligaments, and intersesamoid ligament, the plantar plate and the extensor hood. The tendons crossing the joint, from the flexor hallucis brevis and longus (FHL), abductor and adductor hallucis, and extensor hallucis longus (EHL) and brevis provide additional stability. Anatomic variability in the

configuration of the sesamoids has been described.[26]

The second to fifth metatarsophalangeal joints are stabilized by the plantar plate, which consists of a 20-mm long and 2-mm thick rectangular fibrocartilaginous ridge that arises from the plantar aspect of the metatarsal head fascial band and inserts on the plantar base of the phalanx. It is supported by the accessory collateral (suspensory glenoid ligaments or plantar plate ligaments) to either side, the medial and lateral collateral ligaments, and the deep transverse intermetatarsal ligaments[27,28] (**Fig. 15**).

The accessory collateral originates posteriorly and inferiorly to the lateral tubercle of the metatarsal head and is fan-shaped and broad distally where it inserts on the posterolateral and anterolateral surfaces of the plantar plate. The fibers are in continuity with the dependent border of the collateral ligaments.

The lateral collateral ligament tends to be thicker and stronger than the medial collateral ligament. Both originate from the metatarsal head lateral tubercle and are directed distally and anteriorly to the lateral tubercle of the phalanx base (**Fig. 16**).

The deep transverse metatarsal ligament attaches to the dorsal surface of the sides of the plantar plates at the junction of the interosseous muscle insertion.[27,28]

Tendons Crossing the Ankle

Anterior aspect

The tendons in the anterior aspect are the tibialis anterior, the EHL, the extensor digitorum longus (EDL), and the peroneus tertius, which is not always present but has a very high prevalence.[29]

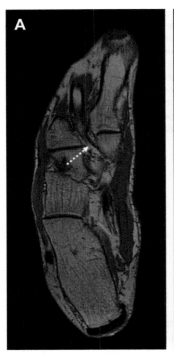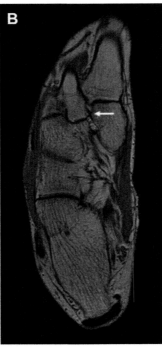

Fig. 14. Lisfranc ligament. (*A*) Axial T1 shows the plantar band (*dotted arrow*). (*B*) axial T1 at a slightly more superior level shows the interosseous ligament (*bold arrow*), the strongest one and the proper Lisfranc ligament, an important stabilizer of the midfoot.

Within the anterior aspect runs the tibial artery and vein and the deep peroneal nerve. These structures are supported by the superior and inferior extensor retinacula.

The superior extensor retinaculum attaches just medial to the tibialis anterior tendon at the medial margin of the distal tibia, extends across the extensor tendons and the anterior compartment, and attaches to the medial margin of the distal fibula.

The inferior extensor retinaculum has a "Y" shape and has its origin in the medial malleolus and the plantar fascia and inserts onto the anterior and lateral surface of the calcaneus.

Possible anatomic variation is the existence of accessory muscle tendons, such as the extensor hallucis capsularis tendon (up to 14% prevalence).

Other accessory muscles such as the anterior fibulocalcaneus, accessory extensor digiti secundus, and the tibioastragalus anticus of Gruber are very rare.[29]

Medial aspect

The medial group contains the tibialis posterior (the last 2 cm are not covered by tenosynovium), flexor digitorum longus (FDL), and flexor hallucis longus (FHL).

The tarsal tunnel is a fibro-osseous canal in the medial aspect of the ankle. The roof of this canal is the flexor retinaculum (spans from the medial malleolus to the medial calcaneal process and plantar aponeurosis) and the floor is the bony surfaces of the tibia, talus, and calcaneus. It contains, from anterior to posterior, the tendons of the tibialis posterior, FDL, the posterior tibial

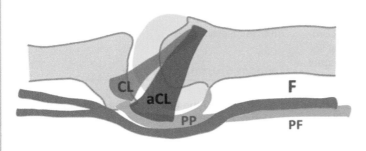

Fig. 15. The plantar plate complex. aCL, accessory collateral ligament; CL, proper collateral ligament; F, flexors; PF, plantar fascia; PP, plantar plate.

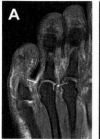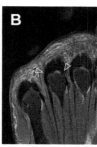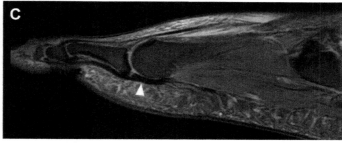

Fig. 16. Plantar plate complex. (A) axial PD fat sat shows in detail the proper collateral ligaments, lateral (*arrow*) and medial (*dotted arrow*). The lateral collateral ligament tends to be thicker and stronger than the medial collateral ligament. (B) axial PS fat sat at a more inferior level shows the attachment of the accessory ligaments to the plantar plate (*arrowheads*). (C) Sagittal PD fat sat shows the fibrocartilaginous plantar plate (*bold arrowhead*).

neurovascular bundle, and the FHL tendon. There are fibrous septae that extend from the retinaculum to the calcaneus, compartmentalizing each one of these structures. The tibial nerve divides into the medial and lateral branches at the tunnel, but there is anatomic variation, and the division may be proximal or distal. The tibialis posterior artery also has a variable level of bifurcation.[6]

Distally in the midfoot, at the level of the navicular, the master knot of Henry is the superficial crossing of the FDL tendon over the FHL tendon. Distally to this point, there are multiple connections between the two tendons. This is a location for FHL tenosynovitis and for an intersection syndrome[30] (**Fig. 17**).

Possible anatomic variations are tendons from accessory muscles such as the flexor digitorum accessorius longus (6%–8% prevalence), or much rarer the peroneocalcaneus internus or tibiocalcaneus internus.[29]

Lateral aspect

The lateral aspect contains the PL and brevis (PB) tendons. These are supported by the superior and inferior peroneal retinacula. A triangular component of the retinacula, called the fibrocartilaginous ridge, inserts onto the posterolateral tip of the fibula and supports the peroneal tendons in the lateral retromalleolar groove. The superior peroneal retinaculum has been seen to have connections with the ATFL, inferior extensor retinaculum, and peroneal tendon sheath, reinforcing these structures.[31]

Possible anatomic variation is the presence of a peroneus quartus, which may have different configurations, and for which a prevalence of up to 16% has been described.[29]

Posterior aspect

The posterior aspect contains the Achilles tendon and plantaris tendon.

The Achilles tendon is the confluence of the medial and lateral heads of the gastrocnemius and soleus muscles. The distal 2 cm of the tendon is not encased by tenosynovium. It is separated from the posterior ankle joint by the pre-Achilles fat or Kager's fat pad. Proximally, the tendon is flat and concave, and distally, it is more rounded cross-sectionally. Anteriorly, it is concave at its distal insertion on to the calcaneum.[32]

An anatomic variant that may mimic the existence of a solid mass is the presence of an accessory soleus[29] (**Fig. 18**).

Muscles

The muscle layers in the foot and their functions are summarized in **Table 1**.

The Plantar Aponeurosis

The plantar aponeurosis is a strong longitudinal fibrous band that supports the plantar aspect of the heel, arch, and foot. It has three components, a central, medial, and lateral band, originating from the medial process of the tuberosity of the calcaneus.

The central band is the thickest at the calcaneal tuberosity attachment.

Distally, the aponeurosis becomes thin and broad and then divides, just proximal to the heads of the metatarsals into five separate bundles that extend to attach to the distal toes. The superficial fibers insert onto the dermis, via the retinacula cutis (skin ligaments). The deep layers of each digit become septa that separate the digital flexor tendons from the lumbricals and the digital neurovascular bundles.

In the medial aspect, the fascia merges with the flexor retinaculum and dorsalis paedis fascia.[33]

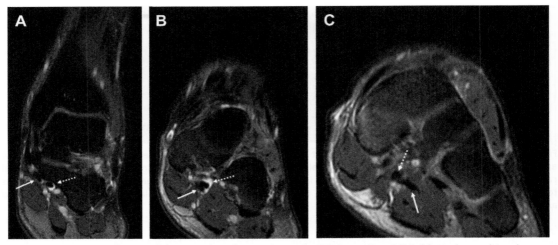

Fig. 17. Master Knot of Henry. (*A*) Coronal PD fat sat shows de FDL (*arrow*) and FHL (*dotted arrow*) tendons underneath the sustentaculum tali (there is a small amount of fluid in the FHL sheath). (*B*) Coronal PD fat sat slightly more anterior shows the crossing of the tendons (master knot of Henry). The FDL crosses plantar to the FHL. (*C*) More distal coronal PD fat sat images shows the tendons distally to the crossing.

POSTSURGICAL APPEARANCES

Multiple types of surgery can be performed in the ankle and foot. We will review the most common types.

Osteosynthesis Techniques

The most commonly performed surgeries in the ankle and foot are fracture fixation, osteotomy, and arthrodesis.

The goal is always to restore anatomy as precisely as possible. This can be done through open or close reductions, then using different procedures to maintain alignment of fragments until healing establishes.

A summary of the techniques, indications, and contraindications is provided in **Table 2**[34,35], and a summary of the expected postsurgical appearances and pathologic appearances is provided in **Table 3**[34,36,37] (**Figs. 19 and 20**).

The amount of bone fusion necessary has not been accurately established. Clinical success consists of lack of pain, absence of motion between bones or fragments under stress, and ability to function.

Arthroplasty

An alternative to ankle arthrodesis for the treatment of refractory pain, especially in the context

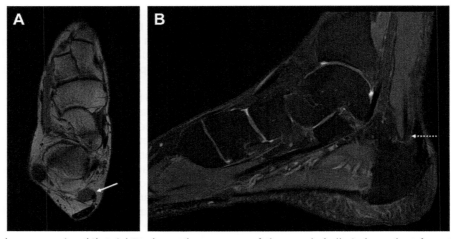

Fig. 18. Soleus accesorius. (*A*) Axial T1 shows the presence of the muscle belly independent from the Achilles tendon (*arrow*). (*B*) Sagittal PD fat sat shows the independent attachment of the tendon (*dotted arrow*), anterior to the Achilles. This may mimic the existence of a solid mass clinically and on radiographs.

Table 1
Muscles of the foot

Layer	Muscle	Origin	Insertion	Function	Innervation
First	Abductor Hallucis	Calcaneal tuberosity Flexor retinaculum Plantar aponeurosis	Base proximal phalanx great toe	Abduction and flexion of the great toe (MTPJ). Support the plantar aspect of the longitudinal arch	Medial plantar nerve
	Flexor digitorum brevis	Medial calcaneal tuberosity Plantar aponeurosis Intermuscular septum	Middle phalanges, second to fifth toes	Toe flexion (second to fifth) (MTPJ) Support the plantar aspect of the longitudinal arch	Medial plantar nerve
	Abductor digit minimi	Calcaneal tuberosity Plantar aponeurosis	Metatarsal, base proximal phalanx fifth	Abduction and flexion of the fifth toe (MTPJ). Support the plantar aspect of the longitudinal arch	Lateral plantar nerve
Second	Quadratus plantae	Lateral process calcaneal tuberosity Medial surface calcaneus	Tendon of the flexor digitorum longus	Toe flexion (second to fifth) (MTPJ)	Lateral plantar nerve
	Lumbrical muscles	Tendon of the flexor digitorum longus	Medial bases of the proximal phalanges and extensor expansion (second to fifth)	MTPJ flexion and adduction, second to fifth toes IPJ extension, second to fifth toes	First lumbrical: Medial plantar nerve Second to fourth lumbricals: Lateral plantar nerve
Third	Flexor hallucis brevis	Tendon of the tibialis posterior, medial, and lateral cuneiform, cuboid.	Lateral and medial aspects at base of the proximal phalanx great toe	MTPJ flexion Support longitudinal arch foot	Medial plantar nerve
	Adductor hallucis	Oblique head—bases second to fourth Metatarsals, cuboid, lateral cuneiform, peroneus longus tendon	Lateral aspect base of the proximal phalanx great toe	MTPJ adduction and flexion, great toe. Support longitudinal arch foot	Lateral plantar nerve

(continued on next page)

Table 1
(continued)

Layer	Muscle	Origin	Insertion	Function	Innervation
		Transverse head—plantar MTP ligaments toes third to fifth, deep transverse metatarsal ligaments toes third to fifth			
	Flexor digiti minimi brevis	Base fifth metatarsal Long plantar ligament	Base of proximal phalanx fifth toe	MTPJ flexion fifth toe	Lateral plantar nerve
Fourth	Interosseous muscles (plantar and dorsal)	Medial aspects of third to fifth metatarsals	Medial bases of proximal phalanges and extensor expansions of third to fifth toes	MTPJ flexion and adduction, third to fifth toes IPJ extension third to fifth toes	Lateral plantar nerve
	Extensor digitorum brevis	Superolateral surface of calcaneus bone, interosseous talocalcaneal ligament; stem of inferior extensor retinaculum	Extensor digitorum longus tendons second to fourth	DIPJ extension, second to fourth toes	Deep fibular/peroneal nerve

of end-stage arthritis, is the placement of a total ankle replacement.

These consist of a two- or three-component prosthesis. Prosthetic replacement preserves mobility, and prevents hindfoot osteoarthritis.

Total ankle replacement is a technique to consider in patients with relatively low functional demands. Obese patients, patients that are more active or younger have worse outcomes with this technique, and better outcomes with arthrodesis.[35] Indications and contraindications are summarized in **Table 4**.[35]

In the two-component type, a polyethylene liner is attached to the tibial component. In the three-component type, the liner is mobile. Sometimes, extra stabilization of the distal tibia and fibula is required, with syndesmotic arthrodesis. Sometimes, prophylactic screw fixation of the malleoli is performed, to avoid fracture. In some cases, to correct alignment abnormalities distal fibular osteotomy is performed[38] **(Fig. 21)**.

A summary of the expected postsurgical appearances and pathologic appearances is provided in **Table 5**[39–41]

Instability Treatment

Ankle sprains are one of the most common musculoskeletal injuries.

They generally heal with conservative treatment. In a small amount of patients, as a result of a major injury or repetitive ligament damage, chronic instability develops.

Instability of the syndesmosis is normally treated by arthrodesis.

The deltoid complex ligaments and sinus tarsi ligaments rarely require surgery.

Chronic lateral ankle instability still presents challenges for diagnosis.

A recent systematic review and meta-analysis[42] found a pooled sensitivity of MR imaging for the diagnosis of chronic injury of the ATFL of 0.83 and for the CFL of 0.56, whereas US had a pooled sensitivity of 0.90 for both ligaments. However, MR imaging is effective for the diagnosis of intraarticular lesion (osteochondral, cartilage lesions) syndesmotic injuries, and impingement syndromes, and therefore invaluable for surgical planning.

Surgery for the management of chronic lateral instability is indicated when conservative

Table 2
Osteosynthesis techniques, indications, and contraindications

Technique			Indication		Contraindication
Fracture fixation	Casting Non-weight-bearing Internal fixation		• Stable fractures		• Unstable fracture
			• Unstable fractures		• Ongoing infection
			• Intraarticular fractures		• Severe comminution
			• Non-unions		• Deficient soft tissue coverage
					• Acute phase of neuropathic disease.
	External fixation		• Contraindications for internal fixation		
Osteotomy Performed to correct malalignments Generally with fixation ± bone grafting May be associated with soft tissue procedures		Hindfoot Midfoot	Pes cavus Pes planus Pes equinus (varus) Pes valgus Pes adductus Pes abductus Neuromuscular Traumatic Degenerative Arthritis Complex malalignments due to congenital conditions		• Ongoing infection • Severe comminution • Deficient soft tissue coverage • Acute phase of neuropathic disease.
		Forefoot	Hallux valgus Metatarsus primum varus Quintus varus Finger deformities		
Arthrodesis Generally with fixation ± bone grafting May be associated with soft tissue procedures			• Posttraumatic osteoarthritis • Rheumatoid arthritis • Restore and maintain plantigrade alignment in congenital and acquired conditions (hidfoot triple arthrodesis—subtalar, talonavicular, and calcaneocuboid joints in severe planovalgus from end-stage posterior tibial tendon dysfunction)		• Ongoing infection • Severe comminution • Deficient soft tissue coverage • Acute phase of neuropathic disease.

treatment fails. If instability becomes interfering with every day activity, reconstruction is indicated.

More than 50 surgical procedures have been proposed in adults. Repairs are divided into primary anatomic, which may be non-augmented repairs (an example is the Broström procedure) or anatomic reconstructions (using grafts such as hamstring, fascia lata, etc.) and secondary extrinsic (augmented, such as the Evans, Watson-Jones and Chrisman and Snook).[43]

Anatomic repairs are the preferred type of repairs in patients who need full anatomic motion of the ankle—mechanics are preserved, in range of movement and gait, including subtalar motion. Repair techniques can be attempted when there is enough viable tissue left. These consist of end-to-end suture using suture anchors to reattach to bone (Broström technique), sometimes reinforced by regional periosteal flaps or the inferior retinaculum (Modified Broström) (**Fig. 22**).

Reconstruction with secondary tendon augmentation is the preferred method in cases where there is ligamentous laxity, ligamentous insufficiency and chronic ankle sprains, as well as cases in which anatomic repair has failed.[44–47] In general, these techniques use split peroneus brevis tendon to reinforce the ATFL and CFL. The tendon is passed through an antero-posterior tunnel drilled in the distal fibula, and then either resutured to itself or the PL or anchored

Table 3
Osteosynthesis techniques, expected postsurgical, and pathologic appearances

Expected Postsurgical Appearances	Pathologic Appearances
Radiographs	Radiographs/CT
• Progressive blurring and narrowing of the interface between opposing bone surfaces	• Nonunion
• Obliteration of the space between the bones by itself does not indicate fusion (with fixation, the bone surfaces will often be in full contact after procedure)	• Displacement or motion between the bones or fragments in interval assessment.
	• Loose or fractured implants
	• Progressive resorption of bone graft
• Sequential examination is required to fully document full osseous incorporation and healing.	• Persistent gap between bone surfaces
	• Lack of osseous bridging
• When evaluating alignment standing radiographs are needed.	• Neocortex formation along the bone ends is diagnostic.
CT	• Infection (appearances of osteomyelitis)
• Callus and bone graft between the bones will progressively increase in amount and attenuation before bridging the gap.	General intraoperative or postsurgical: traumatic neuroma wound infection dehiscence
• Bridging of trabeculae and or cortex	
MR imaging	
• In healing phase, marrow edema will be present in the bones adjacent to the operation site (mechanical trauma from the procedure and granulation tissue)	
Continuity of mature bone (continuity of the marrow fat) indicates fusion.	
• Mild surrounding marrow edema may persist even atter fusion occurs because of bone remodeling.	

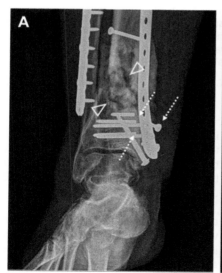
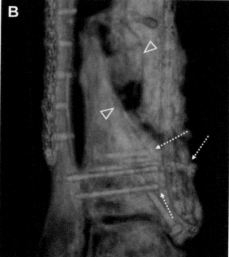

Fig. 19. Osteosynthesis failure. (*A*) Oblique ankle radiograph shows hardware material in distal tibia and fibula (plates and screws). Note several of the distal screws are broken (*dotted arrows*), which results in defective fixation of fragments. The fracture line is still visible (*arrowheads*) and there is hypertrophic bonne formation around it, in keeping with a pseudoarthrosis. (*B*) 3D reconstruction with metal hardware algorithm better shows the broken screws (*dotted arrows*) and the separation of the fragments (*arrowheads*).

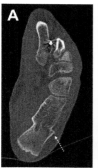 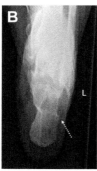 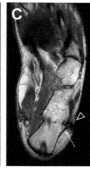 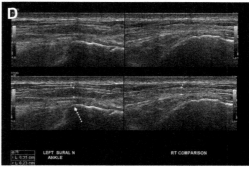

Fig. 20. Sural nerve neuroma as post osteotomy complication. Post-calcaneal osteotomy appearances on axial CT (*A*), calcaneal projection radiograph (*B*) and on axial PD (*C*). Note the residual step on the lateral aspect (*dotted arrow*). There is thickening with low signal in the adjacent subcutaneous fatty tissue, with thickening of the skin and punctate foci of metal susceptibility artifact (*arrowhead*). On ultrasound (*D*) the sural nerve appears thickened and hypoechoic at this level, in comparison with the contralateral side. The step in the calcaneus is obvious (*dotted arrow*).

to the talus (**Fig. 23**). In some cases the tendon may be tunneled under the talus or calcaneus. The use of a transferred extensor digitorum brevis or plantaris tendon has also been described.

Detailed expected postsurgical appearances and pathologic findings post lateral instability treatment are summarized in **Table 6**.[48,49]

The limitation of these procedures is the decrease in subtalar and talocrural motion and potential risk of adjacent cutaneous nerve injury. Besides, most of these procedures use a portion of the peroneus brevis, potentially modifying the dynamic stability of the ankle.

More recently, anatomic reconstruction has been developed, to allow tendon grafts to recreate anatomy, and thus preserve joint biomechanics.[50]

The postsurgical assessment in these patients heavily relies on clinical examinations, symptomatology and ability to return to activities.

Instability of the midfoot (Lisfranc injuries) is treated with open reduction and internal fixation if acute, and arthrodesis if chronic.

In the foot, instability caused by collateral ligament or plantar plate injuries is treated with osteotomy, fusion or tendon transfers if conservative.[35,49]

Surgical Procedures Involving the Tendons

Tendon disorders are a frequent problem in the hindfoot and ankle. The tendons most frequently affected by pathology are the Achilles, tibialis posterior, tibialis anterior, FHL, and peroneal tendons. Most tendon disorders result from chronic overuse, incomplete healing and degeneration. Surgery has a role when symptoms are refractory to conservative treatment or in cases when outcome studies show a clear advantage to surgical over conservative management.[51]

Tendonitis is normally treated conservatively. For tendinopathy refractory to conservative treatment, the indicated surgical procedures if there is no tear are tenosynovectomy, brisement (high pressure injection of fluid in the tendon sheath to break adhesions), and/or tendon débridement. If the tendon is torn, repair and potentially augmentation with adjacent tissue (neighboring tendons) is added to these techniques.

Lacerations and acute tendon tears in general are treated with repair procedures that consist on the suture of the tendon using a technique that minimizes scarring and preserves normal smooth movement. Longitudinal tears (typical of the tibialis posterior and the peroneus brevis) can

Table 4 Arthroplasty, indications, and contraindications	
Indications	**Contraindications**
End-stage ankle osteo-arthritis Traumatic Infectious Inflammatory Degenerative Congenital	• Active infection • Neuropathy • Talar osteonecrosis, • Deficient soft tissue coverage • Severe peripheral vascular disease • Poor bone stock • Coronal or sagittal plane deformity of the ankle exceeding 15° requires additional procedures to ensure good implant position

A   B

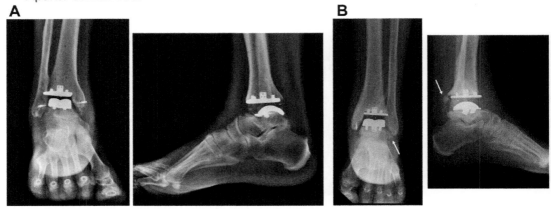

Fig. 21. Total ankle arthroplasty in two different patients. (*A*) AP and lateral demonstrating the correct alignment of the two components, A small radiolucent dot signals the location of the polyethylene lines (in the posterior midline). Note the anchors for combined ligament fixation in the malleoli. (*B*) AP and lateral. Note the anchor for deltoid repair in the medial malleolus. Heterotopic ossification (*bold arrow*) and an effusion are evident.

Table 5 Arthroplasty, expected postsurgical, and pathologic appearances	
Expected Postsurgical Appearances	**Pathologic Appearances**
Radiographs (Weight-bearing) • The tibial component should be positioned perpendicularly to the long axis of the tibia, and the articular surfaces of the talar and tibial components should be parallel. • The tibial tray (optimal size) extends from the anterior to the posterior cortical margin of the plafond. • Linear radiodense markers indicate the location of the polyethylene liner • Comparison of serial radiographs CT • Detailed information on the status of the subchondral bone • Direct visualization of the polyethylene liner	• Edge loading: leads to asymmetric polyethylene liner wear. Nonuniform narrowing of the medial of lateral joint space • Osteolysis: scalloped erosions • Implant loosening: migration on serial radiographs, bone resorption around the implant • Fracture or migration of the polyethylene bearing (three component type) • Lateral malposition: talofibular abutment • Heterotopic ossification, medial or lateral spur formation • Infection (appearances of osteomyelitis) • Periprosthetic fracture General intraoperative or postsurgical: Neurovascular injury (superficial peroneal nerve) Malleolar fracture.

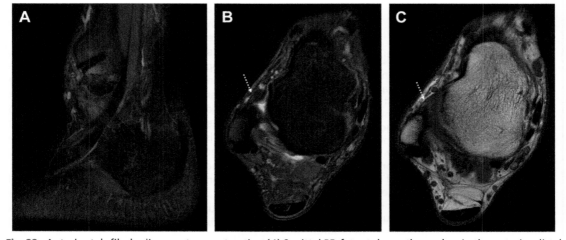

Fig. 22. Anterior talofibular ligament reconstruction (*A*) Sagittal PD fat sat shows the anchor in the anterior distal fibula. (*B*) Axial PD fat sat shows the reconstructed ligament as thick and slightly heterogeneous. (*B*) Axial PD fat sat and (*C*) axial T1 show the appearances of the reconstructed ligament (*dotted arrows*).

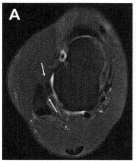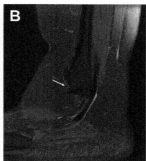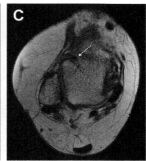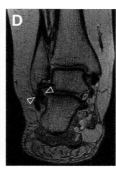

Fig. 23. Reconstruction with secondary tendon augmentation. In this case, the peroneus brevis tendon has been used to reinforce the anterior talofibular ligament. The tendon is passed through an antero-posterior tunnel drilled in the distal fibula (*bold arrows*), seen in (*A*) axial PD fat sat and (*B*) sagittal PD fat sat. This is anchored to the talus (*C*, axial T1, *dotted arrow*). (*D*) coronal T2 shows a calcaneofibular ligament repair—reinforcement suturing. The ligament appears thick and mildly heterogeneous as a result (*arrowheads*).

also be sutured (**Fig. 24**). Patients with Achilles tendon rupture which are not surgical candidates may be managed nonoperatively with casting of the ankle in plantar flexion.[52]

When there is a considerable gap between the ends of a completely torn tendon, there is muscle contracture that prevents tendon end approaching, or when a tendon has been stretched beyond its viscoelastic limits, repair is not possible and

Table 6
Instability treatment techniques, expected postsurgical, and pathologic appearances

Technique	Expected Postsurgical Appearances	Pathologic Appearances
Chronic Lateral Instability Treatment	Ligament Repair • Radiography may be normal, or there may be suture anchors visible in the talus, fibular tip, or calcaneus Ligament Reconstruction • Fibular tunnel/tunnels (peroneus brevis tendon transfer) MR imaging • Low signal intensity scar tissue in the incision and operative bed are typically visible. • Fibular tunnel/tunnels • Ligament or tendon thickening and ferromagnetic artifact from sutures or anchors • The course of the peroneus brevis tendon should be traced and correlated with the operation notes. • Tendon should be seen both entering and exiting the fibular tunnel/tunnels. Metal artifact from drilling may preclude visualization of the tendon within the bone. • Normal structures may no longer be found in their anatomic positions.	• Failure more likely if there is osteoarthritis in the hindfoot or hindfoot varus. • Clinical impression important because failure may be due to laxity, difficult to show on imaging • Discontinuity of the repaired tissue or rerouted peroneus brevis is relatively unusual • Peroneal tendon abnormalities visible in postsurgical context need to be carefully correlated with operation notes.

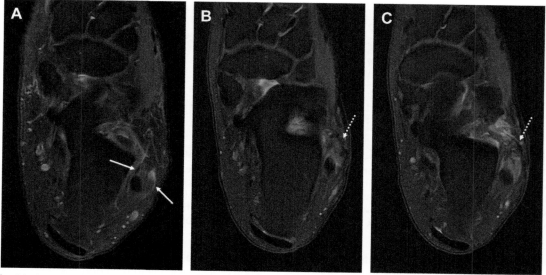

Fig. 24. Peroneus brevis repair. (*A*) axial PD fat sat shows a longitudinal tear of the peroneus brevis tendon (two separate fiber bundles marked with *bold arrows*). (*B*) and (*C*) axial PD fat sat at two consecutive levels after surgical repair shows the tendon is thickened, with increased signal intensity (*dotted arrows*). Repaired tendons often remain thicker than the native tendon for years.

tendon transfer or graft becomes necessary. Autologous sources of tendon grafts include the plantaris, palmaris, peroneus tertius, extensor digitorum, tibialis anterior, FDL, and FHL tendons. Cadaveric and synthetic grafts are also available. Tendon transfers are also performed to correct alignment deformity, create or support motor function, and generate tenodesis.[53]

In cases where advanced tendon dysfunction results in a fixed hindfoot malalignment or osteoarthritis, triple arthrodesis as a salvage procedure is

indicated. Corrective osteotomies combined with tendon transfer procedures can avoid the need for joint fusion in cases of flexible malalignment.

Malalignments or anatomic features that predispose to tendon injury may be addressed early if only tendinopathy is present, or at the time of tendon repair or transfer. Tendon débridement and/or re anchoring may accompany the osseous operation.[54] Tendon lengthening, especially for the Achilles, is an additional procedure used to redistribute forces on the foot in patients with

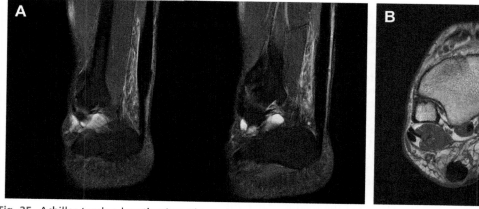

Fig. 25. Achilles tendon lengthening. This technique is used to redistribute forces on the foot in patients with conditions ranging from midfoot neuropathy to calcaneal equinus to plantar fasciitis. (*A*) Sagittal PD fat sat, in two consecutive images shows fusiform diffuse thickening of the tendon, with some posterior punctate foci of metal susceptibility artifact, where sutures are placed, and edema in Kager's fat pad and the paratenon. There is no loss of continuity of the fibers. (*B*) Axial T1 shows mildly heterogeneous signal within the thickened tendon.

Table 7
Tendon techniques, expected postsurgical, and pathologic appearances

Technique	Expected Postsurgical Appearances		Pathologic Appearances
	MR imaging • Information on bone, joint, and soft tissues.	US • Real-time, dynamic assessment, • If there is extensive metallic instrumentation • Allows guided intervention	
Tendon Repair	• Successfully repaired tendons are initially markedly thickened, with maximum thickness peaking approximately 3 mo after surgery. • Repaired tendons often remain thicker than the native tendon for years. • Regions of heterogeneous fiber orientation and mixed signal intensity on T1- and T2-weighted MR images within the tendon are common and do not correlate with clinical parameters.	• Tendon thickening, heterogeneous echo-texture with sutures visible as echogenic foci. Sometimes tiny foci of calcification • In some cases, impaired tendon movement on real-time evaluation.	• Typically, a normally healed tendon will not return to its normal pre-injury baseline appearance • Signal on MR imaging and sonographic echotexture changes and altered tendon morphology are insufficient to diagnose pathology • Tendon fiber discontinuity is the most reliable sign of a failed repair or failed tendon transfer • Postoperative scarring of the repaired tendon may limit mobility and can be diagnosed on MR or ultrasound by the presence of scar tissue tethering the tendon to adjacent tissues. • If infection is suspected, the use of contrast MR may be useful to show rim-enhancing collections or sinus tracts
Tendon Transfer/ Augmentation	• Tracing the course of the other tendons may be an important clue that a tendon transfer or augmentation has been performed. • Transferred tendons also feature alterations in morphology as well as MR signal and sonographic echotexture, but intact transfers display fiber continuity throughout the tendon.	• Transferred tendons feature alterations in morphology as well as sonographic echotexture, but intact transfers display fiber continuity throughout the tendon.	
Tendon lengthening	• Focal thickening, susceptibility artifact	• Focal thickening and sutures visible	

conditions ranging from midfoot neuropathy to calcaneal equinus to plantar fasciitis (**Fig. 25**).

A summary of the expected postsurgical appearances and pathologic findings after tendon repair is presented in **Table 7**.[34,54,55]

Plantar Fasciotomy

Plantar fasciotomy is indicates in cases or plantar fasciitis refractory to conservative/orthotic treatment.

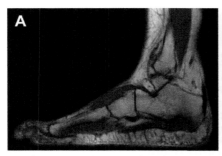
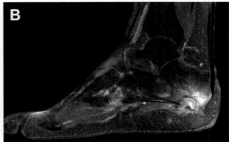

Fig. 26. Plantar fasciotomy. (*A*) sagittal T1 shows residually thickened fascia, and a defect in the inferior calcaneus where a calcaneal spur has been removed. (*B*) sagittal T1 fat sat after gadolinium administration shows intense enhancement of the bone and granulation tissue in the bony defect. There is only minimal edema in the plantar subcutaneous fat.

The fascia normally appears thickened with poorly defined margins. If treatment is successful, the surrounding heel fat should not show increased signal. If a segment has been resected, a gap may or not be present[56] (**Fig. 26**).

Recurrent fasciitis shows perifascial edema on water sensitive sequences.

Development of flatfoot is a potential complication, which may lead to failure of the PT and the peroneus brevis.

Section of the lateral plantar branch may lead to numbness and subsequent insensitive injury. Recurrent plantar fibromatosis after resection may be difficult to distinguish from postoperative scarring on cross-sectional imaging studies. Enhancement in the operative bed with associated mass effect favors recurrence.[57,58]

Nerve Decompression

Tarsal tunnel decompression

The presence of masses, such as ganglia, nerve sheath tumors, or muscle anomalies, can compress the posterior tibial nerve. Sometimes, similar to the carpal tunnel syndrome in the wrist, there may be idiopathic increased pressure within the tunnel.

Surgical treatment consists of decompression of the space around the nerve, with excision of the cause for compression.[59]

Decompression consists of the section of the flexor retinaculum, division of deep fascia of the abductor hallucis, and neurolysis.

The expected postsurgical appearances and pathologic findings after surgical decompression of the tarsal tunnel are summarized in **Table 8**[53]

Table 8
Tarsal tunnel decompression, expected postsurgical, and pathologic appearances

Technique	Expected Postsurgical Appearances	Pathologic Appearances

Tarsal Tunnel Decompression	• Low-signal intensity scar tissue is present in the surrounding subcutaneous fat on MR images
	• The sectioned retinaculum is visible
	• Denervation changes in the muscles supplied by the posterior tibial nerve may persist (if fatty infiltration) medial branch
	  ○ Abductor hallucis
	  ○ Flexor digitorum brevis lateral branch
	  ○ Quadratus plantae
	  ○ Abductor digiti minimi
	• Tarsal tunnel syndrome may coexist with other hindfoot conditions (plantar fasciitis, tibialis posterior tendon dysfunction)
		• Unresolved or recurrent symptoms may be due to incomplete sectioning of the retinaculum or abductor hallucis fascia, scar tissue entrapping the nerve roots or reestablishing the flexor retinaculum, or a persistent or recurrent mass.
		• Low signal intensity scar completely encircling a nerve branch suggests entrapment (more conspicuous after contrast administration)
		General intraoperative or postsurgical:
		• Wound infection
		• Iatrogenic injury to the posterior tibial artery
		• Sectioning of the posterior tibial nerve.

Repeated decompression does not have good outcomes in general.[60]

Morton Neuroma

Morton neuroma or interdigital neuritis results from irritation of a plantar interdigital nerve, attributed to nerve compression by the metatarsal heads and the transverse metatarsal ligament.

Traditional surgical treatment consists of neurolysis or nerve excision, often with release of the transverse metatarsal ligament.[51,61] Percutaneous techniques tend to be favored and surgery used when these fail.

Recurrent pain is a problem after Morton's neuroma surgery, happening in up to one-third of the patients. MR imaging is useful to rule out potential causes for pain, which may be due to scar tissue, recurrence of the neuroma, intermetatarsal bursitis and other like stress fracture.

In postoperative MR imaging, it is common to see neuroma-like masses in 50% of symptomatic spaces, but also, 26% of asymptomatic web spaces show similar findings.[62] The presence of a hour-glass or comma-shaped mass deep to the transverse ligament which is isointense on T1 and isointense or slightly hyperintense on fat suppressed images suggests recurrence. Contrast enhancement may be useful to better demarcate lesions.[62]

CLINICS CARE POINTS

- Knowledge of the complex anatomy and biomechanics of the ankle and foot, including its particularities, and normal variation allows to understand the mechanisms of injury and provides a useful tool for accurate diagnosis and indications for treatment.

- Familiarity with the surgical procedures and normal postsurgical appearances and findings related to potential complications allows to provide relevant information to surgeons to favor a positive outcome for the patient.

REFERENCES

1. Kirsch MD, Erickson SJ. Normal magnetic resonance imaging anatomy of the ankle and foot. Magn Reson Imaging Clin N Am 1994;2(1):1–21.

2. Bassett FH, Gates HS, Billys JB, et al. Talar impingement by the anteroinferior tibiofibular ligament. A cause of chronic pain in the ankle after inversion sprain. J Bone Joint Surg Am 1990;72(1):55–9.

3. van den Bekerom MPJ, Raven EEJ. The distal fascicle of the anterior inferior tibiofibular ligament as a cause of tibiotalar impingement syndrome: a current concepts review. Knee Surg Sports Traumatol Arthrosc 2007;15(4):465–71.

4. Hermans JJ, Beumer A, De Jong TAW, et al. Anatomy of the distal tibiofibular syndesmosis in adults: a pictorial essay with a multimodality approach: Anatomy of the distal tibiofibular syndesmosis. J Anat 2010;217(6):633–45.

5. Golanó P, Vega J, de Leeuw PAJ, et al. Anatomy of the ankle ligaments: a pictorial essay. Knee Surg Sports Traumatol Arthrosc 2016;24(4):944–56.

6. Rosenberg ZS, Beltran J, Bencardino JT. From the RSNA Refresher Courses. Radiological Society of North America. MR imaging of the ankle and foot. Radiographics 2000. 20 Spec No:S153-S179.

7. Gimber LH, Daniel Latt L, Caruso C, et al. Ultrasound shear wave elastography of the anterior talofibular and calcaneofibular ligaments in healthy subjects. J Ultrason 2021;21(85):e86–94.

8. Edama M, Kageyama I, Kikumoto T, et al. Morphological features of the anterior talofibular ligament by the number of fiber bundles. Ann Anat 2018; 216:69–74.

9. Kobayashi T, Suzuki D, Kondo Y, et al. Morphological characteristics of the lateral ankle ligament complex. Surg Radiol Anat 2020;42(10):1153–9.

10. Vega J, Malagelada F, Manzanares Céspedes MC, et al. The lateral fibulotalocalcaneal ligament complex: an ankle stabilizing isometric structure. Knee Surg Sports Traumatol Arthrosc 2020;28(1):8–17.

11. Poboży T, Konarski W. Ultrasound imaging of the posterior talofibular ligament. J Ultrason 2021;21(84):82–3.

12. Oh CS, Won HS, Hur MS, et al. Anatomic Variations and MRI of the Intermalleolar Ligament. Am J Roentgenology 2006;186(4):943–7.

13. Omar H, Saini V, Wadhwa V, et al. Spring ligament complex: Illustrated normal anatomy and spectrum of pathologies on 3T MR imaging. Eur J Radiol 2016;85(11):2133–43.

14. Lektrakul N, Chung CB, null Lai Ym, et al. Tarsal sinus: arthrographic, MR imaging, MR arthrographic, and pathologic findings in cadavers and retrospective study data in patients with sinus tarsi syndrome. Radiology 2001;219(3):802–10.

15. Herrmann M, Pieper KS. [Sinus tarsi syndrome: what hurts?]. Unfallchirurg 2008;111(2):132–6.

16. Mittlmeier T, Rammelt S. Update on Subtalar Joint Instability. Foot Ankle Clin 2018;23(3):397–413.

17. Michels F, Matricali G, Vereecke E, et al. The intrinsic subtalar ligaments have a consistent presence, location and morphology. Foot Ankle Surg 2021; 27(1):101–9.

18. Iovane A, Palma A, Messina G, et al. The posterior talocalcaneal ligament: an MRI evaluation. Surg Radiol Anat 2020;42(10):1167–74.

19. Szaro P, Ghali Gataa K, Polaczek M. Ligaments of the os trigonum: an anatomical study. Surg Radiol Anat 2021;43(7):1083–90.

20. Walter WR, Hirschmann A, Alaia EF, et al. Normal Anatomy and Traumatic Injury of the Midtarsal (Chopart) Joint Complex: An Imaging Primer. RadioGraphics 2019;39(1):136–52.

21. Melão L, Canella C, Weber M, et al. Ligaments of the Transverse Tarsal Joint Complex: MRI–Anatomic Correlation in Cadavers. Am J Roentgenology 2009;193(3):662–71.

22. Walter WR, Goldman LH, Rosenberg ZS. Pitfalls in MRI of the Developing Pediatric Ankle. RadioGraphics 2021;41(1):210–23.

23. Arastu MH, Buckley RE. Tarsometatarsal joint complex and midtarsal injuries. Acta Chir Orthop Traumatol Cech 2012;79(1):21–30.

24. Sripanich Y, Steadman J, Krähenbühl N, et al. Anatomy and biomechanics of the Lisfranc ligamentous complex: A systematic literature review. J Biomech 2021;119:110287.

25. Siddiqui NA, Galizia MS, Almusa E, et al. Evaluation of the Tarsometatarsal Joint Using Conventional Radiography, CT, and MR Imaging. RadioGraphics 2014;34(2):514–31.

26. Aparisi Gómez MP, Aparisi F, Bartoloni A, et al. Anatomical variation in the ankle and foot: from incidental finding to inductor of pathology. Part II: midfooot and forefoot. Insights Imaging 2019;10(1):69.

27. Gregg J, Silberstein M, Schneider T, et al. Sonographic and MRI evaluation of the plantar plate: a prospective study. Eur Radiol 2006;16(12):2661–9.

28. Gregg JM, Silberstein M, Schneider T, et al. Sonography of Plantar Plates in Cadavers: Correlation with MRI and Histology. Am J Roentgenology 2006; 186(4):948–55.

29. Aparisi Gómez MP, Aparisi F, Bartoloni A, et al. Anatomical variation in the ankle and foot: from incidental finding to inductor of pathology. Part I: ankle and hindfoot. Insights Imaging 2019;10(1):74.

30. Rajakulasingam R, Murphy J, Panchal H, et al. Master knot of Henry revisited: a radiologist's perspective on MRI. Clin Radiol 2019;74(12):972.e1–8.

31. Drakonaki EE, Gataa KG, Solidakis N, et al. Anatomical variations and interconnections of the superior peroneal retinaculum to adjacent lateral ankle structures: a preliminary imaging anatomy study. J Ultrason 2021;21(84):12–21.

32. Ciszkowska-Łysoń B, Zdanowicz U, Śmigielski R. The ultrasonographic dynamic heel-rise test of the Achilles tendon. J Ultrason 2021;21(86):e260–6.

33. Draghi F, Gitto S, Bortolotto C, et al. Imaging of plantar fascia disorders: findings on plain radiography, ultrasound and magnetic resonance imaging. Insights Imaging 2017;8(1):69–78.

34. Bergin D, Kearns S, Cullen E. Postoperative imaging of the ankle and foot. Semin Musculoskelet Radiol 2011;15(4):408–24.

35. Coughlin MJ, Saltzman CL, Anderson RB, et al, editors. Mann's surgery of the foot and ankle. Saunders Elsevier; 2014.

36. Linklater J. Imaging of the Postoperative Ankle and Foot. Semin Musculoskelet Radiol 2012;16(03): 175–6.

37. Sofka CM. Postoperative magnetic resonance imaging of the foot and ankle. J Magn Reson Imaging 2013;37(3):556–65.

38. Kim DR, Choi YS, Potter HG, et al. Total Ankle Arthroplasty: An Imaging Overview. Korean J Radiol 2016; 17(3):413.

39. Lee AY, Ha AS, Petscavage JM, et al. Total ankle arthroplasty: a radiographic outcome study. AJR Am J Roentgenol 2013;200(6):1310–6.

40. Spirt AA, Assal M, Hansen ST. Complications and failure after total ankle arthroplasty. J Bone Joint Surg Am 2004;86(6):1172–8.

41. Bestic JM, Peterson JJ, DeOrio JK, et al. Postoperative evaluation of the total ankle arthroplasty. AJR Am J Roentgenol 2008;190(4):1112–23.

42. Cao S, Wang C, Ma X, et al. Imaging diagnosis for chronic lateral ankle ligament injury: a systemic review with meta-analysis. J Orthop Surg Res 2018; 13(1):122.

43. Letts M, Davidson D, Mukhtar I. Surgical management of chronic lateral ankle instability in adolescents. J Pediatr Orthop 2003;23(3):392–7.

44. Barnum MJ, Ehrlich MG, Zaleske DJ. Long-term patient-oriented outcome study of a modified Evans procedure. J Pediatr Orthop 1998;18(6):783–8.

45. Marsh JS, Daigneault JP, Polzhofer GK. Treatment of ankle instability in children and adolescents with a modified Chrisman-Snook repair: a clinical and patient-based outcome study. J Pediatr Orthop 2006;26(1):94–9.

46. Yang J, Morscher MA, Weiner DS. Modified Chrisman–Snook repair for the treatment of chronic ankle ligamentous instability in children and adolescents. J Children's Orthopaedics 2010;4(6):561–70.

47. Snook GA, Chrisman OD, Wilson TC. Long-term results of the Chrisman-Snook operation for reconstruction of the lateral ligaments of the ankle. J Bone Joint Surg Am 1985;67(1):1–7.

48. Chien AJ, Jacobson JA, Jamadar DA, et al. Imaging appearances of lateral ankle ligament reconstruction. Radiographics 2004;24(4):999–1008.

49. Tourné Y, Mabit C. Lateral ligament reconstruction procedures for the ankle. Orthop Traumatol Surg Res 2017;103(1S):S171–81.

50. Jung HG, Kim TH, Park JY, et al. Anatomic reconstruction of the anterior talofibular and calcaneofibular ligaments using a semitendinosus tendon

allograft and interference screws. Knee Surg Sports Traumatol Arthrosc 2012;20(8):1432–7.

51. Sconfienza LM, Adriaensen M, Albano D, et al. Clinical indications for image-guided interventional procedures in the musculoskeletal system: a Delphi-based consensus paper from the European Society of Musculoskeletal Radiology (ESSR)-part VI, foot and ankle. Eur Radiol 2022;32(2):1384–94.

52. Soroceanu A, Sidhwa F, Aarabi S, et al. Surgical versus nonsurgical treatment of acute Achilles tendon rupture: a meta-analysis of randomized trials. J Bone Joint Surg Am 2012;94(23):2136–43.

53. LiMarzi GM, Scherer KF, Richardson ML, et al. CT and MR Imaging of the Postoperative Ankle and Foot. Radiographics 2016;36(6):1828–48.

54. Jesse MK, Hunt KJ, Strickland C. Postoperative Imaging of the Ankle. AJR Am J Roentgenol 2018; 211(3):496–505.

55. Chianca V, Zappia M, Oliva F, et al. Post-operative MRI and US appearance of the Achilles tendons. J Ultrasound 2020;23(3):387–95.

56. Yu JS, Smith G, Ashman C, et al. The plantar fasciotomy: MR imaging findings in asymptomatic volunteers. Skeletal Radiol 1999;28(8):447–52.

57. Yu JS, Spigos D, Tomczak R. Foot pain after a plantar fasciotomy: an MR analysis to determine potential causes. J Comput Assist Tomogr 1999;23(5): 707–12.

58. Woelffer KE, Figura MA, Sandberg NS, et al. Five-year follow-up results of instep plantar fasciotomy for chronic heel pain. J Foot Ankle Surg 2000; 39(4):218–23.

59. Khodatars D, Gupta A, Welck M, et al. An update on imaging of tarsal tunnel syndrome. Skeletal Radiol 2022. https://doi.org/10.1007/s00256-022-04072-y.

60. Sammarco GJ, Chang L. Outcome of surgical treatment of tarsal tunnel syndrome. Foot Ankle Int 2003; 24(2):125–31.

61. Zanetti M, Saupe N, Espinosa N. Postoperative MR imaging of the foot and ankle: tendon repair, ligament repair, and Morton's neuroma resection. Semin Musculoskelet Radiol 2010;14(3):357–64.

62. Espinosa N, Schmitt JW, Saupe N, et al. Morton neuroma: MR imaging after resection–postoperative MR and histologic findings in asymptomatic and symptomatic intermetatarsal spaces. Radiology 2010; 255(3):850–6.

Imaging of Overuse Injuries of the Ankle and Foot in Sport and Work

Kerensa M. Beekman, MD, PhD[a],*, P. Paul F.M. Kuijer, PhD[b],
Mario Maas, MD, PhD[a,c,d]

KEYWORDS

- Imaging • Overuse injuries • Ankle • Foot • MR imaging • Athletes

KEY POINTS

- Overuse injuries of the ankle and foot are common injuries in athletes but also in the working population.
- When imaging of suspected overuse injuries of the ankle and foot is necessary, different modalities can be used, starting with radiography mainly followed by MR imaging; however, new techniques such as dual energy computed tomography (CT) and weight-bearing CT can be of help, when available.
- Structured reporting is key to minimize errors, increase consistency in reporting, improve quality, facilitate efficient data mining and big data research, and helps the clinician to extract the most important information more easily from the report.
- We would like to advocate the use of structured reporting from a clinical perspective because patients present with pain lateral, medial, anterior, posterior, deep, midfoot, lateral, or medial side of the forefoot. Structuring the report according to these departments could help the clinician extract the most important information more easily.
- Radiology never stands alone, especially because imaging findings of overuse injuries of the ankle and foot can be subtle and/or nonspecific, the clinical epidemiological context is important for the interpretation of the imaging findings.

INTRODUCTION/BACKGROUND

Overuse injuries of the ankle and foot are common in both sports and work-related context. They account for lengthy sick leave and delayed return to play.[1–4] Early diagnosis and treatment can shorten sick leave and return to play. Imaging can detect overuse injuries in an early stage and therefore is key to increase at an early diagnosis and treatment plan.

Overuse injuries in general are defined as "repetitive application of submaximal stress to otherwise normal tissues, overwhelming the normal repair process."[5] In sports, overuse injuries are common, about 30% to 50% of the sport-related injuries are related to overuse,[6] and can restrain the subject from sport participation.[7,8] Incidences of overuse injuries of the ankle and foot vary widely, as studies on the incidence of overuse injuries in sports have heterogeneous methods and populations. Most studied sports are soccer, running, and gymnastics, and the most frequently studied injuries are tendinopathy, stress fractures,

[a] Department of Radiology and Nuclear Medicine, Amsterdam Movement Sciences, Amsterdam UMC, Location AMC, University of Amsterdam, Meibergdreef 9, 1105 AZ Amsterdam, the Netherlands; [b] Department of Public and Occupational Health, Amsterdam Movement Sciences, Amsterdam Public Health, Amsterdam UMC, University of Amsterdam, Meibergdreef 9, 1105 AZ Amsterdam, the Netherlands; [c] Academic Center for Evidence-based Sports Medicine (ACES), Amsterdam UMC, Meibergdreef 9, 1105 AZ Amsterdam, the Netherlands; [d] Amsterdam Collaboration for Health and Safety in Sports (ACHSS), International Olympic Committee (IOC) Research Center, Amsterdam UMC, Meibergdreef 9, 1105 AZ Amsterdam, the Netherlands
* Corresponding author.
E-mail address: k.m.beekman@amsterdamumc.nl

Radiol Clin N Am 61 (2023) 307–318
https://doi.org/10.1016/j.rcl.2022.10.006
0033-8389/23/© 2022 Elsevier Inc. All rights reserved.

especially in basketball, and plantar fasciitis in running.[6]

In the work-related context, overuse injuries of the ankle and foot receive little attention compared with the more prevalent overuse injuries of the upper extremities and low back.[9,10] Overuse injuries in work are often qualified as work-related injuries or as occupational disease if work is seen as the primary cause.[11] Similar as in sports, reliable incidence figures are hard to find given heterogeneous methods including case definitions and populations. For instance, based on data from the European Union, the percentage of self-reported work-related complaints of the ankle and foot varied between 0 and 18% compared with the other body regions such as upper extremity or low back among economic sectors in Spain.[12] The annual percentage of workers with a physician-diagnosed occupational disease of the ankle and foot varied between 3% and 4% compared with the total number of occupational diseases of the musculoskeletal system in Denmark for the period 2013 to 2017.[12] For the Netherlands, this percentage of workers was 2% during a 10-year period.[13] For the United States of America, the number of overuse injuries of the ankle and foot are based on the 2018 data of the US Bureau of Labor Statistics on cases with an injury or illness involving days away from work for the private industry. Excluding trauma, the percentage of cases with a musculoskeletal system and connective tissue disease of the ankle and foot was 5%.[14] Reported work-related injuries are metatarsal stress fractures in military personnel,[15] Achilles tendinopathy in newspaper carriers,[16] and plantar fasciitis in workers who spent the majority of their workday on their feet.[17]

Overuse injuries can occur due to repetitive trauma of bone and soft tissues (ie, tendons, ligaments, fat pads). The main overuse injury in bone is a stress fracture. Strictly speaking, stress fractures include both insufficiently and fatigue fractures, with the first occurring in an elderly population with osteopenia or osteoporosis, caused by normal loading of abnormal bone. In this overview, we discuss stress fractures in the context of fatigue fractures that occur after abnormal loading of normal bone.[18] Due to repetitive loading on a focal area of the bone, remodeling occurs, and with persistent repetitive loading, osteoblasts are unable to appropriately repair microfractures, and accumulation of these microfractures can cause a macroscopic stress fracture.[19] Fatigue fractures generally occur in a young active population, such as athletes and military recruits. Stress fractures have a female predominance[18] because postmenopausal women are more prone to develop osteoporosis, and in young female athletes, a combination of relative energy deficiency, menstrual cycle disturbance, and the development of osteopenia, also known as the female athlete triad, cause an increased risk of stress fractures.[20] However recently, a similar situation has been described in male athletes, including relative energy deficiency, hormonal disturbances and low bone mineral density, especially in male athletes participating in sports that encourage leanness (esthetic, endurance, and antigravitation sports) or requiring weight-control behaviors (wrestling, judo, rowing, or horse-racing).[21,22] Contributing risk factor for stress fractures can be divided into extrinsic factors such as training schedule, footwear, and type of activity and intrinsic factors such as subject's age, gender, and physical condition.[18]

Overuse tendinopathy is the most frequently reported overuse injury of the soft tissues. It leads to decreased load tolerance and function and is associated with pain and swelling of the affected tendon. Overuse tendinopathy is characterized by a change in the structure of the tendon, caused by scarring and healing response of the tendon, and only minimal inflammation; hence, the term tendinitis is abandoned.[23] On histopathological level, different types of tendon degeneration have been described: hyaline, mucoid, fibrinoid, lipoid and fibrocartilaginous degeneration, calcification, and bony metaplasia. Failed healing response of the tenocytes is hypothesized to be the cause of overuse tendinopathy, which causes degeneration and proliferation of tenocytes, disruption of collagen fibers, and deposition of noncollagenous matrix.[24]

NORMAL MR IMAGING ANATOMY

MR imaging is the most used imaging modality for diagnosis of overuse injuries of the ankle and foot; therefore, we discuss the normal anatomy in this article illustrated by MR images. Recently, interest has increased in radiology for structured reporting, which uses a checklist approach and uniform terminology. Structured reporting is key to minimize errors,[25] accomplish increased homogeneity and consistency in reporting, and improve interdisciplinary communications and quality improvement.[26] Furthermore, structured reporting allows for efficient data mining to facilitate big data research.[26] We would like to advocate the use of structured reporting for MR imaging of the ankle and foot from a clinical perspective. Patients have ankle pain located lateral, medial, anterior, posterior or deep or have complains of the midfoot, lateral, or medial side of the forefoot. If the report is structured according to these departments, for example discussed in a clockwise manner, this could help the clinician extract the most important information more easily from the report.

On the lateral side, the fibula is connected to the tibia by the anterior tibiofibular ligament (ATiFL), this ligament has a distal fascicle (distal fascicle of the anterior tibiofibular ligament: ATiFL-DF), and in neutral position of the ankle, the ATiFL-DF is in contact with the anterolateral part of the talus, this contact is increased in plantarflexion, and disappears in maximum dorsiflexion.[27] The ATiFL-DF is thought to be involved in anterolateral soft tissue impingement; however, this structure is difficult to appreciate on MR imaging. The anterior talofibular ligament (ATFL) and posterior talofibular ligament connect the fibula to the talus. The ATFL consists of 2 fascicles, the superior fascicle is located intra-articular, whereas the inferior fascicle lies extra-articular, and is connected by arciform fibers with the calcaneofibular ligament, which connects the fibula to the calcaneus.[28,29] Furthermore, the peroneal tendons can be found on the lateral side of the ankle, with the peroneus longus tendon running laterally of the peroneus brevis tendon, covered by the superior and inferior peroneal retinaculum. The superior peroneal retinaculum also runs from the fibula to the calcaneus and creates a sleeve for the peroneal tendons.

Posteriorly, the ankle joint is covered by the posterior joint capsule. More superficially the Kager's fat pad can be found with the small plantaris tendon and the large Achilles tendon. The Achilles tendon is the largest tendon in the body and is vulnerable due to limited blood supply, especially 2 to 6 cm from the insertion on the calcaneus.[30]

On the medial side, the medial malleolus is stabilized by the deltoid ligament, which consists of a deep part and a superficial part. The deep component consists of the anterior and posterior tibiotalar ligament. The superficial component consists of the tibio-calcaneal ligament, which runs from the tibia to the sustentaculum tali of the calcaneus, and the tibionavicular ligament. The plantar calcaneonavicular or spring ligament is also located laterally and runs from the calcaneus (sustentaculum tali) to the os naviculare. The flexor tendons run on the medial side of the ankle joint, from medial to lateral, the tibialis posterior, the flexor digitorum longus, and the flexor hallucis longus, covered by the flexor retinaculum.

On the anterior side of the ankle, the joint capsule can be found. Anterior of the joint capsule, the extensor tendons run, from medial to lateral, the extensor tibialis anterior, the extensor hallucis longus and on the lateral side the extensor digitorum longus, covered by the superior and inferior extensor retinaculum.

The anatomy of the foot in complex, containing 26 bones, and 33 joints. Anatomically it is divided in the hindfoot, containing the talus and the calcaneus, the midfoot, containing the bones of the tarsus, that is, os naviculare, os cuboid, and cuneiforms, the forefoot comprises of the metatarsals and the phalanges. Chopart joint divides the hindfoot and the forefoot and consists of the calcaneocuboid joint, and the talocalcaneonavicular joint. The Lisfranc joint separates the midfoot and the forefoot and comprises the tarsometatarsal joints. The cuboids articulate with metatarsal 1, 2, and 3, and the cuboid articulates with metatarsal 4 and 5.

Longitudinally the foot can be divided into the medial column, which consist of ray 1, 2, and 3 of the metatarsal bones and the related phalanges, and the lateral column, consisting of ray 4 and 5.

The extensor muscles and tendons run on the dorsal side of the ankle and foot: from medial to lateral the tibialis anterior, the extensor hallucis longus and brevis, and the extensor digitorum longus. The peroneus longus and brevis run laterally. On the medial and plantar side, the tibialis posterior runs medially, followed by the flexor digitorum longus and the flexor hallucis longus laterally of the tibialis posterior tendon. On the plantar side of the foot, the plantar aponeurosis or plantar fascia, it runs from the tuberosity of the calcaneus to the heads of the metatarsals. Profound of the plantar fascia, from medial to lateral the abductor hallucis, the flexor digitorum brevis and the abductor digiti minimi muscles can be found. This layer is followed by a layer containing the quadratus plantae muscle and the lumbrical muscles, followed by a third layer containing the flexor hallucis brevis medially, the adductor hallucis muscle with a transvers head and an oblique head, and laterally the flexor digiti minimi brevis. The hallux sesamoids are located within the flexor hallucis brevis tendon. The fourth layer consists of the plantar and dorsal interosseous muscles. On the posterior of the ankle, the soleus and the gastrocnemius tendon merge into the calcaneal or Achilles tendon.

IMAGING TECHNIQUE

MR imaging is the main imaging technique in the diagnosis of overuse injuries in our practice because it excellently depicts soft tissues and is able to detect early signs of overuse injuries such as edema. However, in general practice, MR imaging is often limitedly available, and therefore, radiographs are most often the first step in imaging of a patient with a suspected overuse injury. Radiograph allows assessment of the osseous structures, as well as soft tissue swelling and is often used to rule out frank fractures and tumors as a cause of the pain. Early stages of stress fractures and soft tissue injuries can be missed on plain film, therefore, 3-dimensional imaging, preferably with MR imaging, can be warranted. If necessary, osseous structures can be further assessed by computed tomography (CT) and when available, dual energy CT or even weight-bearing cone beam CT. The advantage of CT is the detailed assessment of the osseous structures and the potential to assess bone marrow edema using dual energy CT (DECT).[31,32] Furthermore, CT is widely available and often readily accessible. A disadvantage is the exposure to ionizing radiation; however, with modern CT scanners, the dosage to which the patient is exposed during CT scanning of the extremities is very low. Weight-bearing cone beam CT can be used to assess osseous anatomy in a 3-dimensional way during weight bearing, with even lower radiation exposure. Upcoming photon-counting detector CT will cause a revolution in CT imaging because higher resolutions can be achieved.[33,34] Trabecular structure of the cancellous bone can be visualized; therefore, this new technique might provide diagnostic improvement in the diagnosis of stress fractures. The soft tissue of the ankle and foot can be assessed using ultrasonography, which also allows dynamic assessment of the structures; however, for this review, we will not discuss ultrasonography of the ankle and foot in detail.

PROTOCOLS

MR imaging protocols for the assessment of overuse injuries of the foot at least contain proton density (PD) or T1-weighted images and T2 fat-suppression images, preferably in axial, sagittal, and coronal planes. On T1-weighed images, structural assessment of the ankle and foot can be performed, and especially bones and tendons can be assessed. PD-weighed images can be used both for structural assessment and to assess joint cartilage. On the T2 fat-suppressed images, pathologic condition can be assessed because most pathologic condition is accompanied by increased fluids locally, shown by high signal on the fat-suppressed T2 images. Furthermore, Dixon sequences can be used for the assessment of the ankle and foot. The Dixon technique creates in-phase and out-of-phase images (IP and OP, respectively), using the difference in resonance frequency between water and fat molecules, causing their spins to go in-phase and out-of-phase with each other over time. The signal acquired when the spins are in-phase is the sum of the signal of the water and fat molecules, whereas

the signal acquired when the spins are out-of-phase represents the difference between the signal from the water and the fat molecules. With these IP and OP images, water only and fat only images can be created during postprocessing. The water only images can be used as fat-suppressed images, providing more homogenous fat suppression compared with fat-suppressing techniques, such as short tau inversion recovery, with a higher signal to noise ratio.[35,36] The Dixon technique is versatile and can be applied with T1, T2, or PD weighing and with gradient echo and spin echo sequences. In our practice, we use TSE Dixon to acquire high-resolution images of the ankle and foot. When peroneal tendinopathy is expected, we would like to advocate the use of additional oblique peroneus views, which allow for the assessment of the peroneal tendons in one plane,[37] and making assessment less prone to the magic angle effect, causing increased signal intensity of a tendon orientated at, or close to an angle of 55° compared with the main magnetic field, and could be mistaken for tendinopathy.[38,39] T2 images without fat suppression could be useful in analyzing the calcaneal fat pad.

DECT protocols can be used to visualize bone marrow edema, besides from the detailed osseous structures of the ankle and foot. Images are obtained using 2 different radiograph energy spectra, with a low tube voltage, usually between 70 and 100 kVp and a high tube voltage, usually between 140 and 150 kVp, with an added tin filter to absorb low energy photons of the spectrum and to improve spectral separation. During postprocessing, 3-material decomposition technique uses the difference in attenuation of different tissues, such as calcium within the bone and water and fat in the bone marrow, at the high and low tube voltage, to subtract the osseous components and to generate virtual noncalcium images (VNCa), which allows the assessment of the attenuation of the bone marrow and bone marrow edema.[32]

IMAGING FINDINGS IN OVERUSE INJURIES OF THE ANKLE AND FOOT
Bone

The growing skeleton
In children and adolescents, the growing skeleton is prone to specific overuse injuries, as the growing skeleton contain growth plates, apophysis and epiphysis, which are the weakest links in the chain.[40] *Calcaneal apophysitis*, also known as *Sever disease*, is a traction apophysitis and is one of the most common overuse injuries of the hindfoot in the growing skeleton. The calcaneal

apophysis develops in girls around the age of 6 years and in boys around the age of 8 and exists for approximately 3 to 4 years; therefore, the mean age of presentation ranges from 8 to 13 years of age in girls and from 11 to 15 years of age in boys.[41] Boys are more often affected than girls, and the disease is bilateral in 60% of the cases.[41] Children who perform sports that involve jumping or running, such as basketball, soccer, gymnastics, and track/running are more prone to develop calcaneal apophysitis. Physical therapy or shoe in-lays can help; however, it is a self-limiting disease, and children are able to return to sports within 2 months.[41] Although calcaneal apophysitis is a clinical diagnosis and imaging is normally not necessary, radiographs can be used to diagnose other causes of heel pain like avulsions, stress fractures, or tumors.[42] Radiographs can show fragmentation of the apophysis or increased opacity of the apophysis; however, these findings are nonspecific and can also be present in asymptomatic children[42,43](Fig. 1). On MR imaging, edema of the calcaneus, surrounding tissue, or of the Achilles tendon can be seen.[44]

Apophysitis of the base of the fifth metatarsal, also known as *Iselin disease*, is a less common overuse injury of the growing skeleton, caused by microtrauma to the apophysis of the base of the fifth metatarsal due to traction of the peroneus brevis tendon.[45] On radiographs, widening of the apophysis or fragmentation can be seen; however, as with apophysitis of the calcaneus, this finding is nonspecific. Main differential diagnosis is a fracture of the base of the fifth metatarsal.[45] MR imaging is usually not indicated but can show edema of the base of the fifth metatarsal and the apophysis.[42]

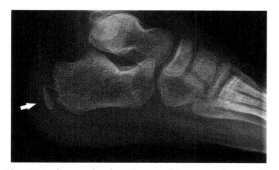

Fig. 1. Radiograph of an 8-year-old soccer player with right heel pain, showing a normal calcaneal apophysitis (*arrow*), that is, not sclerotic and nonfragmented and no alternative explanation for the heel pain. This boy had a previous episode of left heel pain, Sever disease was diagnosed, which improved after cast immobilization.

Pearls and pitfalls—overuse injuries of the growing skeleton:

- Apophysis and epiphysis are the weakest links in the chain of the growing skeleton, and therefore prone to overuse injuries.
- Apophysitis is a clinical diagnosis, imaging findings are nonspecific, radiographs can be used to exclude alternative diagnosis, and MR imaging is usually not indicated.

Stress fractures

Stress fractures can occur with prolonged repetitive loading of a bone, especially when there is an increase in the intensity, duration, or frequency of the activity.[18] Stress fractures have a female predominance,[18] other risk factors are malalignment of the foot (pes planus/cavus, hyperpronation or hypopronation, hindfoot or forefoot varus/valgus), tarsal coalition, limb surgery to the same or opposite limp, muscle weakness or joint instability.[18,46] Stress fractures of the ankle and foot can be divided into low-risk and high-risk fracture sites. Low-risk sites are more common and tend to heal with modification of exposure to activities. These include fractures of the posteromedial tibia, second/third metatarsal and the calcaneus, by far the most common stress fractures of the ankle and foot, and less common sites such as the distal fibula, cuboid, and cuneiforms.[47] Stress fractures at high-risk sites require more aggressive treatment restricted weight-bearing or even surgery. High-risk sites include the anterior tibial cortex, medial malleolus, navicular, talus, base of the fifth metatarsal, base of the second metatarsal, and hallux sesamoids.[47] Stress fractures of the talus are in 60% to 78% associated with a fracture of the calcaneus or the navicular.[48] Stress fractures of the hallux sesamoid bone occur mostly at the medial sesamoid, and can be difficult to distinguish from a bipartite sesamoid, which also occur more often in the medial sesamoid. In this case, prior exams and clinical information can help with diagnosis. Furthermore, bipartite sesamoids, can be seen in 10% to 33% of the general population, 10 times more common in the medial sesamoid, whereas stress fractures of the sesamoids account for less than 4% of the foot and ankle injuries.[47]

Plain radiograph is the imaging method in the evaluation of a suspected stress fracture, although early stress fractures can be missed on plain radiographs because clinical symptoms of pain precede radiographic findings approximately 2 to 3 weeks.[47] An early sign of a stress fracture in cortical bone is the gray cortex sign, showing a focal decreased opacity of the cortex.[49] In cancellous bone, subtle blurring of the trabeculae and faint sclerotic areas, caused by peritrabecular callus formation, can be seen in the earliest stages of a stress fracture.[49] Linear sclerosis, often perpendicular to the major trabeculae, focal periosteal and endosteal reactions can be seen before a, often subtle cortical fracture line, usually first though one cortex.[18] The differential diagnosis of focal cortical thickening includes, normal variant, osteoid osteoma, and chronic osteomyelitis. For periosteal reaction and sclerosis, infection and osteosarcoma can be considered as a differential diagnosis. Linear lucencies can be seen at locations of normal nutrient vessel channels.[18] In the early stage of the stress fracture, sensitivity of the plain radiograph may be as low as 10%, increasing up to 30% to 70% at follow-up. With high clinical suspicion, MR imaging imaging is mandatory. In early cortical stress fractures, endosteal edema and bone marrow edema in early cancellous stress fractures can be seen on T2-weighted fat-suppressed images. In later stages, a hypointense fracture line can be seen on T1-weighted and T2-weighted images, with adjacent bone marrow and soft tissue edema.[18] The differential diagnosis of bone marrow edema on MR imaging, without a visible fracture line, includes transient bone marrow edema syndrome, early avascular necrosis, osteomyelitis, and tumor but also in asymptomatic adults and children, bone marrow edema can be seen on MR imaging.[18] Higher resolution imaging, to detect a fracture line can be considered or dynamic postcontrast MR imaging perfusion imaging can be considered to allow early differentiation from avascular necrosis.[18] CT images can provide more clear imaging of the bone and, when available, DECT can be obtained to assess bone marrow edema. In some cases of stress fractures, imaging of both extremities can show subtle differences in cortical thickness between the symptomatic and asymptomatic side, even in the absence of bone marrow edema. In these cases, markers placed at the location of the pain, comparison to the contralateral extremity, and adjustment of window-level are important (**Fig. 2**).

Pearls and pitfalls of stress fractures of the ankle and foot:

- Signs of stress fractures can be very subtle.
- Do not only look for bone marrow edema but also look for cortical changes and asymmetries.
- Adjust window-level settings when looking at cortical bone.

Soft Tissue

Tendinopathy

Tendinopathy is common overuse injury. Tendinopathy indicates a nonrupture injury of the tendon, exacerbated by mechanical loading.[50] Clinically, it is characterized by pain, swelling, and impaired performance of the injured tendon.[51] Ultrasound may show thickening of the tendon, with hypoechoic areas. On MR imaging, tendinopathic tendons may show intermediate T2 signal intensity, caused by increased blood flow and increased amounts of proteoglycans,[50] whereas normal tendons show a uniform hypointense signal.[38]

The Achilles tendon is the largest tendon in the body, and a common subject to overuse injuries especially during activities that involve running, jumping, and abrupt changes in acceleration and deceleration. *Achilles tendinopathy* is a common overuse injury of the ankle, it is thought to be a degenerative, noninflammatory condition,[52] clinically defined as a combination of pain, swelling, and impaired performance,[51] and divided into midportion Achilles tendinopathy, paratendinopathy, and insertional Achilles tendinopathy.[53] Achilles tendinopathy is a clinical diagnosis; however, imaging can be requested in cases with an atypical clinical presentation, an unexpected course of symptoms or during a preoperative workup.[54] Radiograph can be acquired in cases of insertional tendinopathy, to exclude bony deformities, and can show deviation of soft tissue contours in midportions Achilles tendinopathy. Ultrasound is the preferred imaging modality,[54] and it shows an enlarged diameter of the tendon, heterogeneous aspect of the tendon, and increased color Doppler signal.[53] On MR imaging, fusiform expansion of the tendon can be appreciated (**Fig. 3**), administration of intravenous contrast agents is not necessary but if administrated, central enhancement can be seen, consistent with intratendinous neovascularization.[53] As the Achilles tendon lacks a tendon sheath, overuse can cause inflammation in the paratenon and the surrounding soft tissue called paratendinopathy. Again, although the diagnosis is mainly clinical, on MR imaging, thickening of the paratenon and edema of the Kager's fat pad can be seen.[38] Differential diagnostically retrocalcaneal bursitis and calcaneal apophysitis in young athletes can be considered for hindfoot pain.

Tenosynovitis

Tenosynovitis can be seen as an acute or subacute overuse injury of the tendons of the ankle. Inflammation of the tendons sheath causes fluid accumulation around the tendon. It can be difficult to

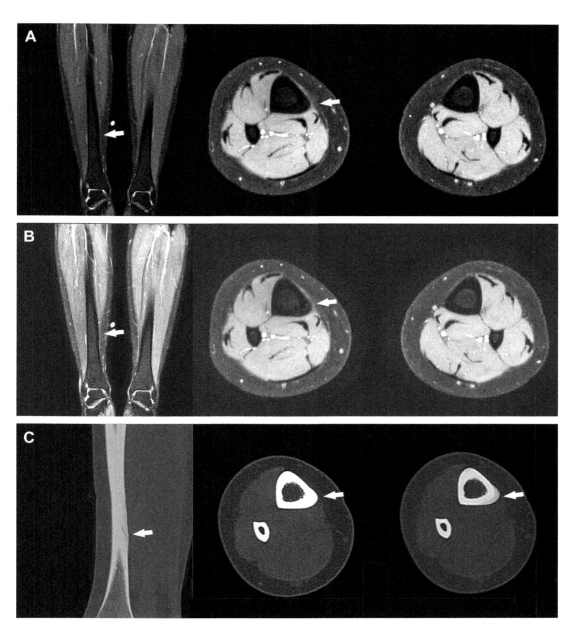

Fig. 2. An 18-year-old professional female marathon runner, fitting the female athlete triad profile, with pain at the posteromedial tibia (A) Coronal MR imaging T2 Dixon water image and axial PD Dixon water image. Marker placed on the skin at the location of the pain. No bone marrow edema present; however, subtle thickening of the cortex on the posteromedial cortex of the distal diaphysis of the right tibia (arrow), compared with the contralateral tibia is present. (B) Same images as (A) with window-level adjustments, which shows slightly increased signal intensity of the thickened part of the cortex at the same location. (C) Additional CT image of the same patient showing a stress fracture of the posteromedial tibia, in the first panel axial CT image without window-level adjustments, only subtle cortical thickening can be appreciated, the second panel shows the same image with window level adjustment, showing periosteal reaction and in the third panel showing a sagittal image showing the fracture line.

distinguish physiological amounts of fluid in the tendon sheaths around the ankle from tenosynovitis. Circumferential amounts of fluid are usually pathological,[38] and fluid around the extensor tendons is mostly pathological, whereas physiological amounts of fluid can be seen around the flexor tendons. On MR imaging, tenosynovitis can be easily detected on fluid-sensitive sequences.

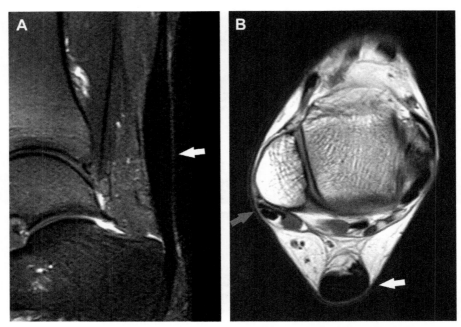

Fig. 3. Case: A 53-year-old woman with pain at the Achilles tendon. (*A*) Sagittal T2 TSE FS and axial PD TSE FS images of the hindfoot, showing fusiform thickening of the Achilles tendon (*white arrow*), consistent with Achilles tendinopathy. (*B*) Axial PD TSE of the same patient, also note the split rupture of the peroneus brevis tendon (*gray arrow*).

Pearls and pitfalls overuse injuries of tendons:

- Tendinopathy indicates a nonrupture injury of the tendon, exacerbated by mechanical loading.
- Achilles tendinopathy is a clinical diagnosis characterized by pain, swelling, and impaired performance.
- Tenosynovitis can be difficult to differentiate from physiological fluid accumulation around tendons.
- Circumferential amounts of fluid and fluid around the extensor tendons are mostly pathological, whereas physiological fluid can be seen around the flexor tendons.

Plantar fasciitis

Plantar fasciitis or *plantar fasciopathy* is a common overuse injury of the plantar fascia (**Fig. 4**) in the community, in occupational settings, in military recruits, and in athletes.[55] Especially in running plantar fasciitis is common, affecting up to 17.4% of the running population. As with tendinopathy, plantar fasciitis, is considered a degenerative disease, and the term plantar fasciopathy is increasingly used in the literature.[56] The main symptom is heel pain, exacerbated by weight-bearing, in a chronic setting, with symptoms lasting more than a year.[56] Increasing body mass index (BMI) is a risk factor of plantar fasciitis in the nonathletic population; however, in the athletic population, BMI is not associated with plantar fasciitis.[56] Furthermore, there seems to be an association between occupational weight-bearing activities such as standing or walking and plantar fasciitis.[17,57] The main imaging feature of plantar fasciitis is plantar plate thickening. It can be measured on plain film, ultrasound or with MR imaging (see **Fig. 4**), with the average plantar plate thickness of 3 mm in control subjects, and an increased thickness of the plantar fascia of 2.3 mm (95% CI 1.86–2.79 mm).[55]

Impingement

Impingement of the ankle is a common overuse injury in athletes. It often occurs in individuals with a history of ankle trauma, and imaging of ankle impingement syndromes has been reviewed by LiMarzi and coworkers.[58] It is caused by soft tissue or osseous abnormities around the tibiotalar joint and extra-articular tissues and causes pain and constrained motion in the ankle joint. Impingement of the ankle can be divided into anterior, anterolateral, anteromedial, posteromedial, and posterior impingement. Ankle impingement is mainly a clinical diagnosis; however, imaging can help confirming the diagnosis or reveal alternative diagnosis. Plain radiograph and CT may reveal osseous abnormalities that predispose ankle impingement, such as bony spurs anterior **Fig. 5** and

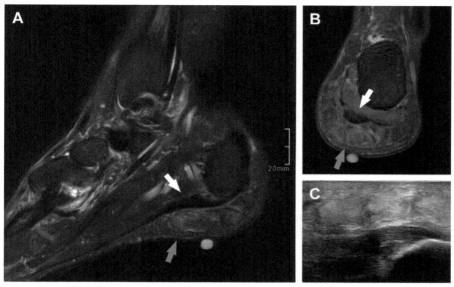

Fig. 4. Case: A 57-year-old woman with heel pain. (*A*) Sagittal T2 Dixon water and (*B*) Coronal PD Dixon water images showering thickening of the plantar fascia, until 8 mm, more pronounced on the medial side (*white arrow*). Furthermore, there is increased T2-signal intensity of the calcaneal fat pad, consistent with a fat pad contusion (*gray arrow*). (*C*) Ultrasound image showing thickening (8 mm) of the planter fascia and increased echogenicity of the calcaneal fat pad.

anteromedial impingement, posttraumatic ossicles in anterolateral impingement and elongated posterior talar process (Stieda process), or os trigonum (although seen in 14–25% of the asymptomatic population[58]) for posterior impingement. Anterolateral impingement is thought to be associated with friction of the ATiFL-DF with the anterolateral talus. However, a recent anatomy study by Dalmau-Pastor and coworkers has shown that ATiFL-DF contact with the talus is physiological in neutral position of the ankle and increases during plantarflexion and disappears in maximum dorsiflexion.[27]

Pearls and pitfalls ankle impingement:

- Ankle impingement is a clinical diagnosis.
- Differentiate bony from soft tissue ankle impingement.

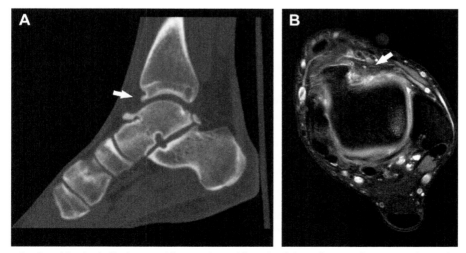

Fig. 5. A professional basketball player, with anterior ankle pain. (*A*) CT showing bony spur (arrow) at the anterior distal tibia, with preservation of the joint space, and (*B*) PD Dixon water image showing increased signal intensity in the soft tissues at the anterior side of the ankle consistent with anterior impingement (*arrow*).

SUMMARY

Overuse injuries of the ankle and foot are common injuries in athletes but also in the working population. MR imaging is the main imaging modality in suspected overuse injuries of the ankle and foot. When available, new techniques such as DECT and weight-bearing CT can give valuable information on osseous structures, bone marrow edema, and osteoarticular communications in weight-bearing position. Imaging findings of overuse injuries of the ankle and foot can be subtle; therefore, the clinical and epidemiological contexts are important to keep in mind. By using structured reporting, increased homogeneity, consistency in reporting and quality can be achieved. Furthermore, structured reporting can facilitate future data mining research. Using structured reporting from a clinical perspective, that is, by location of the pain, could help the clinician extract the most important information more easily from the report, and helps building differential diagnosis. Imaging findings can be subtle and sometimes nonspecific; therefore, high-resolution MR imaging and appropriate window-levels settings are important. Furthermore, clinical and epidemiological context are essential in imaging of overuse injuries of the ankle and foot.

ACKNOWLEDGMENTS

The authors would like to thank Simon Goedegebuure and Gino Kerkhoffs, as respected clinical team partners.

DISCLOSURE

The authors have nothing to disclose.

REFERENCES

1. Beck BR, Bergman AG, Miner M, et al. Tibial stress injury: relationship of radiographic, nuclear medicine bone scanning, MR imaging, and CT Severity grades to clinical severity and time to healing. Radiology 2012;263(3):811–8.
2. Nattiv A, Kennedy G, Barrack MT, et al. Correlation of MRI grading of bone stress injuries with clinical risk factors and return to play: a 5-year prospective study in collegiate track and field athletes. Am J Sports Med 2013;41(8):1930–41.
3. Conti SF, Silverman L. Epidemiology of foot and ankle injuries in the workplace. Foot Ankle Clin 2002;7(2):273–90.
4. Hoch CP, Caughman A, Griffith A, et al. A detailed analysis of workplace foot and ankle injuries. Foot Ankle Orthop 2022;7(1). 2473011421S0024.
5. Herring SA, Nilson KL. Introduction to overuse injuries. Clin Sports Med 1987;6(2):225–39.
6. Sobhani S, Dekker R, Postema K, et al. Epidemiology of ankle and foot overuse injuries in sports: a systematic review. Scand J Med Sci Sports 2013;23(6):669–86.
7. van Tiggelen D, Wickes S, Stevens V, et al. Effective prevention of sports injuries: a model integrating efficacy, efficiency, compliance and risk-taking behaviour. Br J Sports Med 2008;42(8):648–52.
8. Bahr R. No injuries, but plenty of pain? On the methodology for recording overuse symptoms in sports. Br J Sports Med 2009;43(13):966–72.
9. Trepman E, Yodlowski ML. Occupational disorders of the foot and ankle. Orthop Clin North Am 1996;27(4):815–29.
10. Tamminga SJ, Kuijer PPFM, Badarin K, et al. Towards harmonisation of case definitions for eight work-related musculoskeletal disorders - an international multi-disciplinary Delphi study. BMC Musculoskelet Disord 2021;22(1):1018.
11. van der Molen. Frings-Dresen. Occupational Diseases: From Cure to Prevention. J Clin Med 2019;8(10):1681.
12. European Agency for Safety and Health at Work II. Work-related musculoskeletal disorders – facts and figures Synthesis report (of 10 national reports). Publications Office of the European Union. https://data.europa.eu/doi/10.2802/443890. Accessed 9 August 2022.
13. www.beroepsziekten.nl. Accessed 9 August 2022.
14. https://www.bls.gov/iif/oshwc/osh/case/cd_r13_2018.htm#iif_cd_r13p.f.1. Accessed 9 August 2022.
15. MacGregor AJ, Fogleman SA, Dougherty AL, et al. Sex differences in the incidence and risk of ankle–foot complex stress fractures among U.S. military personnel. J Womens Health 2022;31(4):586–92.
16. Torkki M, Malmivaara A, Reivonen N, et al. Individually fitted sports shoes for overuse injuries among newspaper carriers. Scand J Work Environ Health 2002;28(3):176–83.
17. Riddle DL, Pulisic M, Pidcoe P, et al. Risk factors for Plantar fasciitis: a matched case-control study. J Bone Joint Surg Am 2003;85(5):872–7.
18. Matcuk GR, Mahanty SR, Skalski MR, et al. Stress fractures: pathophysiology, clinical presentation, imaging features, and treatment options. Emerg Radiol 2016;23(4):365–75.
19. Welck MJ, Hayes T, Pastides P, et al. Stress fractures of the foot and ankle. Injury 2017;48(8):1722–6.
20. Mountjoy M, Sundgot-Borgen J, Burke L, et al. The IOC consensus statement: beyond the Female Athlete Triad—Relative Energy Deficiency in Sport (RED-S). Br J Sports Med 2014;48(7):491–7.
21. Mountjoy M, Sundgot-Borgen JK, Burke LM, et al. IOC consensus statement on relative energy deficiency in sport (RED-S): 2018 update. Br J Sports Med 2018;52(11):687–97.

22. Tenforde AS, Barrack MT, Nattiv A, et al. Parallels with the female athlete triad in male athletes. Sports Med 2016;46(2):171–82.

23. Opdam KTM, Zwiers R, Wiegerinck JI, et al. Increasing consensus on terminology of Achilles tendon-related disorders. Knee Surg Sports Traumatol Arthrosc 2021;29(8):2528–34.

24. Aicale R, Tarantino D, Maffulli N. Overuse injuries in sport: a comprehensive overview. J Orthop Surg Res 2018;13(1):309.

25. Vosshenrich J, Nesic I, Cyriac J, et al. Revealing the most common reporting errors through data mining of the report proofreading process. Eur Radiol 2021;31(4):2115–25.

26. Kohli A, Castillo S, Thakur U, et al. Structured reporting in musculoskeletal radiology. Semin Musculoskelet Radiol 2021;25(5):641–5.

27. Dalmau-Pastor M, Malagelada F, Kerkhoffs GMMJ, et al. The anterior tibiofibular ligament has a constant distal fascicle that contacts the anterolateral part of the talus. Knee Surg Sports Traumatol Arthrosc 2020;28(1):48–54.

28. Vega J, Malagelada F, Manzanares Céspedes M-C, et al. The lateral fibulotalocalcaneal ligament complex: an ankle stabilizing isometric structure. Knee Surg Sports Traumatol Arthrosc 2020;28(1): 8–17.

29. Dalmau-Pastor M, Malagelada F, Calder J, et al. The lateral ankle ligaments are interconnected: the medial connecting fibres between the anterior talofibular, calcaneofibular and posterior talofibular ligaments. Knee Surg Sports Traumatol Arthrosc 2020; 28(1):34–9.

30. Winnicki K, Ochała-Kłos A, Rutowicz B, et al. Functional anatomy, histology and biomechanics of the human Achilles tendon - A comprehensive review. Ann Anat 2020;229:151461.

31. Suh CH, Yun SJ, Jin W, et al. Diagnostic performance of dual-energy CT for the detection of bone marrow oedema: a systematic review and meta-analysis. Eur Radiol 2018;28(10):4182–94.

32. Gosangi B, Mandell JC, Weaver MJ, et al. Bone marrow edema at dual-energy CT: a game changer in the emergency department. RadioGraphics 2020; 40(3):859–74.

33. Peña JA, Klein L, Maier J, et al. Dose-efficient assessment of trabecular microstructure using ultra-high-resolution photon-counting CT. Z Med Phys 2022. https://doi.org/10.1016/j.zemedi.2022.04.001.

34. Baffour FI, Rajendran K, Glazebrook KN, et al. Ultra-high-resolution imaging of the shoulder and pelvis using photon-counting-detector CT: a feasibility study in patients. Eur Radiol 2022. https://doi.org/10.1007/s00330-022-08925-x.

35. Pezeshk P, Alian A, Chhabra A. Role of chemical shift and Dixon based techniques in musculoskeletal MR imaging. Eur J Radiol 2017;94:93–100.

36. Guerini H, Omoumi P, Guichoux F, et al. Fat suppression with dixon techniques in musculoskeletal magnetic resonance imaging: a pictorial review. Semin Musculoskelet Radiol 2015;19(4):335–47.

37. Park HJ, Lee SY, Kim E, et al. Peroneal tendon pathology evaluation using the oblique sagittal plane in ankle MR imaging. Acta Radiol 2016;57(5): 620–6.

38. Peduto AJ, Read JW. Imaging of ankle tendinopathy and tears. Top Magn Reson Imaging 2010;21(1): 25–36.

39. Erickson SJ, Cox IH, Hyde JS, et al. Effect of tendon orientation on MR imaging signal intensity: a manifestation of the "magic angle" phenomenon. Radiology 1991;181(2):389–92.

40. Kraan RBJ, Kox LS, Oostra RJ, et al. The distal radial physis: Exploring normal anatomy on MRI enables interpretation of stress related changes in young gymnasts. Eur J Sport Sci 2020;20(9):1197–205.

41. Micheli LJ, Ireland ML. Prevention and management of calcaneal apophysitis in children. J Pediatr Orthopaedics 1987;7(1):34–8.

42. Achar S, Yamanaka J. Apophysitis and osteochondrosis: common causes of pain in growing bones. Am Fam Physician 2019;99(10):610–8.

43. Kose O. Do we really need radiographic assessment for the diagnosis of non-specific heel pain (calcaneal apophysitis) in children? Skeletal Radiol 2010; 39(4):359–61.

44. Gao Y, Liu J, Li Y, et al. Radiographic study of Sever's disease. Exp Ther Med 2020;20(2):933–7.

45. Forrester RA, Eyre-Brook AI, Mannan K. Iselin's disease: a systematic review. J Foot Ankle Surg 2017; 56(5):1065–9.

46. Muthukumar T, Butt SH, Cassar-Pullicino VN. Stress fractures and related disorders in foot and ankle: plain films, scintigraphy, CT, and MR imaging. Semin Musculoskelet Radiol 2005;09(03):210–26.

47. Mandell JC, Khurana B, Smith SE. Stress fractures of the foot and ankle, part 2: site-specific etiology, imaging, and treatment, and differential diagnosis. Skeletal Radiol 2017;46(9):1165–86.

48. Sormaala MJ, Niva MH, Kiuru MJ, et al. Bone stress injuries of the talus in military recruits. Bone 2006; 39(1):199–204.

49. Kiuru MJ, Pihlajamäki HK, Ahovuo JA. Bone stress injuries. Acta Radiol 2004;45(3). https://doi.org/10.1080/02841850410004724.

50. Scott A, Backman LJ, Speed C. Tendinopathy: update on pathophysiology. J Orthop Sports Phys Ther 2015;45(11):833–41.

51. Maffulli N. Overuse tendon conditions: time to change a confusing terminology. Arthroscopy 1998;14(8):840–3.

52. Magnan B, Bondi M, Pierantoni S, et al. The pathogenesis of Achilles tendinopathy: a systematic review. Foot Ankle Surg 2014;20(3):154–9.

53. van Dijk CN, van Sterkenburg MN, Wiegerinck JI, et al. Terminology for Achilles tendon related disorders. Knee Surg Sports Traumatol Arthrosc 2011; 19(5):835–41.

54. de Vos R-J, van der Vlist AC, Zwerver J, et al. Dutch multidisciplinary guideline on Achilles tendinopathy. Br J Sports Med 2021;55(20):1125–34.

55. van Leeuwen KDB, Rogers J, Winzenberg T, et al. Higher body mass index is associated with plantar fasciopathy/'plantar fasciitis': systematic review and meta-analysis of various clinical and imaging risk factors. Br J Sports Med 2016;50(16):972–81.

56. Rhim HC, Kwon J, Park J, et al. A systematic review of systematic reviews on the epidemiology, evaluation, and treatment of plantar fasciitis. Life (Basel) 2021;11(12). https://doi.org/10.3390/life11121287.

57. Waclawski ER, Beach J, Milne A, et al. Systematic review: plantar fasciitis and prolonged weight bearing. Occup Med (Chic III 2015; 65(2):97–106.

58. LiMarzi GM, Khan O, Shah Y, et al. Imaging manifestations of ankle impingement syndromes. Radiol Clin North Am 2018;56(6):893–916.

Imaging of Acute Ankle and Foot Sprains

Luis S. Beltran, MD[a],*, Nicolas Zuluaga, MD[b], Anna Verbitskiy, MD[c], Jenny T. Bencardino, MD[b]

KEYWORDS

• Ankle • Sprain • Traumatic • Anatomy • Ligament

KEY POINTS

- Ankle sprains can be a source of significant financial burden, time lost to injury, and long-term disability.
- The normal ankle anatomy, ligamentous injuries of the ankle, and associated conditions of ankle sprains are well depicted on MR imaging.
- The following are MR findings often found in the setting of acute ligamentous injury: discontinuity, detachment, irregular contour, thinning, increased intraligamentous signal on T2-weighted images indicative of edema, or hemorrhage.

INTRODUCTION

Epidemiology

Ankle sprains are characterized by the stretching or tearing of the ankle ligaments and are one of the most common musculoskeletal injuries. In the United States, approximately 2 million acute ankle sprains occur each year.[1] Data from emergency department visits indicate an incidence rate of two-to-seven acute ankle sprains per 1000 person-years[1,2]; however, it is believed that this is likely a significant underestimation because many people do not report to the emergency department or seek medical care at all.[3] Populations at increased risk of ankle sprain include athletes, military personnel, and other populations that are predisposed to this injury from running, jumping, and cutting motions,[4] such as is seen in basketball, football, soccer, and volleyball.

A sprain of the lateral ankle ligament complex is the most common type of ankle sprain,[3] accounting for more than three-quarters of all acute ankle sprains, and approximately 73% of these involve an injury to the anterior talofibular ligament (ATFL)[5,6] The remaining ~25% of ankle sprains involve the deltoid ligament or syndesmotic ligaments.[7]

The high incidence rate of acute ankle sprains is in part thought to be due to frequent reinjury after an initial sprain.[6,8] One study demonstrated that recurrent injuries accounted for 46% of acute ankle sprains that occurred in volleyball, 43% in American football, 28% in basketball, and 19% in soccer.[8]

Chronic ankle instability (CAI), which is characterized by laxity and mechanical instability that interfere with activity, is associated with high reinjury rate after an acute lateral ankle sprain.[3] Up to 70% of individuals who sustain an acute lateral ankle sprain may develop CAI over a short time period after the initial injury.[2]

The most significant long-term outcome of ankle sprain injuries can be the development of osteoarthritis. In one study by Gribble and colleagues, lateral ankle sprains contributed to 13% to 22% of all osteoarthritis cases involving the ankle and 80% of post-traumatic osteoarthritis cases.[2] Post-traumatic osteoarthritis can also result from

[a] Department of Radiology, Harvard Medical School, Brigham and Women's Hospital, 75 Francis Street, Boston, MA 02115, USA; [b] Department of Radiology, University of Pennsylvania Health System, 3737 Market Street, Philadelphia, PA 19104, USA; [c] Department of Radiology, NYU Grossman School of Medicine, New York, NY 10016, USA
* Corresponding author.
E-mail address: lbeltran@bwh.harvard.edu

Radiol Clin N Am 61 (2023) 319–344
https://doi.org/10.1016/j.rcl.2022.10.015
0033-8389/23/© 2022 Elsevier Inc. All rights reserved.

other injuries such as fractures and osteochondral lesions, which are often also associated with ankle sprains.[9] Post-traumatic osteoarthritis of the ankle may develop at a younger age than is seen in idiopathic osteoarthritis, with the mean age of onset in the fifth decade of life and an age range that includes patients in their 20s.[2]

Clinical Considerations

Clinical examination can only accurately diagnose the ligaments involved in 50% of acute lateral ankle sprains.[10] Once the pain and swelling have diminished at around a week post-injury, the sensitivity and specificity of the physical examination increases to 96% and 84%, respectively.[11] Ankle sprains can cause a significant financial burden, time lost to injury and long-term disability.[5,12] Van Rijn and colleagues reported residual symptoms in 33% of patients 1 year following an ankle sprain, and recurrent ankle sprains ranged from 3% to 34% within 2 weeks to 96 months after the initial injury.[13] Post-traumatic ankle arthrosis is a known sequela of recurrent sprains.[14]

Diagnostic Imaging

MR imaging, MR arthrography, conventional arthrography, ultrasound, computed tomography (CT) scan, and radiography have all been described in the imaging of ankle sprain.[15] MR imaging and CT are generally not routinely performed in the setting of an acute ankle sprain. MR imaging is usually reserved for highly competitive athletes and ballet dancers in whom primary ligamentous repair is contemplated and people with CAI.[16–19]

MR imaging can depict complex ankle anatomy, ligamentous injuries of the ankle, and associated injuries occurring in conjunction with ankle sprains.[20] On MR images, normal ankle ligaments are seen as low-signal intensity structures connecting nearby bones, usually delimited by surrounding fat signal.[21] Signal heterogeneity, striations, and apparent areas of discontinuity may be noted in normal ligaments such as the posterior talofibular ligament (PTFL), posterior tibiotalar component of the deltoid ligament, and anterior inferior tibiofibular ligament.[19,22] This appearance typically results from fat interposed between the ligament fascicles.[23]

On MR imaging, discontinuity, detachment, contour irregularity, thinning, and increased intraligamentous signal on T2-weighted images (WI) indicative of edema or hemorrhage can be demonstrated in the setting of acute ligamentous injuries.[24,25] Secondary findings on T2-WI include extravasation of joint fluid or hemorrhage into the adjacent soft tissues, joint effusion, tenosynovial effusion, bone avulsion at the ligamentous insertion, and bone contusion.[26–28] In the setting of subacute or chronic injury, the edema and hemorrhage have typically reabsorbed, and only direct morphologic changes can be seen. Common findings include signal heterogeneity, waviness, thickening, thinning, elongation, and poor or nonvisualization of the ligament.[20,25] Decreased signal of the surrounding fat on both T1 and T2-WI is often seen due to scarring or synovial proliferation.[19]

Numerous MR protocols have been advocated for optimal visualization of the ligaments including three-dimensional (3D) imaging[27] as well as imaging the ankle with the foot in varying degrees of dorsiflexion, plantar flexion, and/or the neutral position.[18,24,29] A routine ankle MR imaging is performed in the axial, coronal, and sagittal planes. Generally, axial and coronal imaging with the foot in dorsiflexion and plantar flexion allow visualization of the ligaments in their entirety.[22] The sagittal images are rarely useful for visualizing the ligaments. The ligaments are almost consistently seen on routine orthogonal ankle imaging as long as the foot is mildly plantar flexed and thin slices of 3 mm thickness are obtained. The foot is imaged in the oblique axial plane (ie, parallel to the long axis of the metatarsal bones), the oblique coronal plane (ie, perpendicular to the long axis of the metatarsals), and the oblique sagittal plane.[19]

BIOMECHANICS
Functional Anatomy

The ankle joint has three articulations (tibiotalar, subtalar, and distal tibiofibular syndesmosis) supported by three ligamentous groups (lateral collateral, medial collateral, and syndesmosis).[30] The joints are stabilized by the congruity of the articular surfaces (loaded joint), static ligamentous restraints, and dynamic muscle–tendon units.[31] The coupled motion of the ankle and subtalar joints allows for simultaneous motions in all three planes resulting in inversion, eversion, protonation, and supination.[32,33] During non-weight-bearing protonation can be described as dorsiflexion, eversion, and abduction/external rotation, whereas supination is plantar flexion, inversion, and adduction/internal rotation. During weight-bearing protonation can be defined as plantar flexion, eversion, and adduction/internal rotation, whereas supination is dorsiflexion, inversion, and abduction/external rotation.[32] Inversion at the subtalar joint occurs when the medial border of the foot elevates and the lateral border of the foot depresses, ranging from 20° to 30°, whereas eversion is the elevation of the lateral border and depression of the medial border of the foot, ranging from 5° to 15°.[33]

CLINICAL SYNDROMES
High Ankle Sprain

Epidemiology
High ankle or tibiofibular syndesmotic sprains compose approximately 7% of ankle sprains.[7] In athletes, the incidence has been reported as high as 40%.[34] American football, skiing, running/jumping, ice hockey, and soccer players are among those more commonly affected.[33–35]

Functional anatomy
The interosseous membrane limits lateral displacement of the fibula during weight-bearing and load sharing with the fibula.[33,36] The distal interosseous (tibiofibular) ligament acts as a spring during dorsiflexion of the ankle joint, allowing for minimal separation of the medial and lateral malleoli.[37]

Clinical considerations and mechanism of injury
The two most common causes of syndesmotic injury are excessive external rotation and hyperdorsiflexion. External rotation forces the talus laterally, which pushes the fibula laterally from the mortise.[33] Isolated external rotation usually leads first to rupture of the anterior aspect of the deltoid ligament or fracture of the medial malleolus. This is followed by the involvement of the anterior inferior tibiofibular ligament (AITFL), the superficial posterior inferior tibiofibular ligament (PITFL), the inferior transverse ligament (ITL), the interosseous membrane, and lastly a spiral fracture to the fibula, or Maisonneuve fracture.[38] In football players, the main mechanism is a direct blow to the lateral leg of a downed player or a blow to the lateral knee, whereas the foot is planted in external rotation and the body is rotating in the opposite direction. In skiing injuries, the foot is fixed in place when the external rotational and forces are applied.[33]

The PITFL is usually injured concomitantly with the AITFL.[38]

Diagnostic imaging
On radiography, the talotibial angle is normally 83 ± 4°, the medial clear space is less than 3 mm, and the talar tilt difference is 2 mm.[39] The height of the tibiofibular recess in normal patients is 0.54 ± 0.68 cm (**Fig. 1**). In acute injury, the tibiofibular recess measures 1.2 ± 0.92 cm, as compared with 1.4 ± 0.57 cm in chronic injury.[40] Isolated AITFL injuries may have no associated swelling making clinical diagnosis difficult.

Vogl and colleagues reported that the sensitivity and specificity of contrast-enhanced T1-weighted MR imaging sequences in detecting disruption of the AITFL was 100% and 83%, respectively.[41] Oae and colleagues compared MR imaging with arthroscopy, using arthroscopy as the gold standard, based on two criteria[1]: ligament discontinuity and[2] wavy/curved contour or nonvisualization of the ligament.[42] The accuracy of MR imaging has been reported to be 100% in diagnosing syndesmotic disruption compared with 64% by mortise radiography and 48% by anteroposterior (AP) radiography.[39]

Blurring, lateral fibular subluxation, fibular shortening, tibiofibular diastasis, and fluid-like signal are MR findings associated with trauma to the syndesmotic ligaments. Interosseous membrane injuries are seen as linear hyperintensity at the level of the distal tibia and fibula on heavily T2-weighted, fat saturated proton density (FS PD) fast spin echo (FSE), or short tau inversion recovery (STIR) images. Low-signal-intensity foci can represent hemosiderin, fibrosis, or calcifications.[30] Brown and colleagues reported that distal tibiofibular syndesmosis sprains are highly associated with ATFL injury (74%), tibiofibular joint incongruity in chronic injury (33%), bone bruise in acute injury (24%), and osteochondral lesion of the talar dome in both acute and chronic injury (28%).[40]

AITFL/PITFL The AITFL and PITFL are usually seen on two or more sequential axial and coronal MR images at the level of the tibial plafond and talar dome. On axial images they often appear striated and discontinuous. The morphology of the talus and the distal fibula can be used to distinguish the anterior and posterior inferior tibiofibular ligaments from the ATFL and PTFL on axial MR images (T1- and T2-weighted). The talar dome at the level of the tibiofibular ligaments is somewhat squared in shape. In addition, the tibiofibular ligaments insert into the fibula above the malleolar fossa where the cross-section of the fibula is round.[20]

The AITFL is trapezoidal in shape and composed of multiple bands.[20,24,28] It originates from the longitudinal tubercle of the lateral malleolus, courses superomedially, and attaches on the anterolateral tubercle of the tibia (**Fig. 2**).[33] In the horizontal plane, the AITFL makes a 35° angle with the coronal axis of the tibial plafond and a 65° angle with its sagittal axis.[43] The AITFL is 20% intra-articular and makes contact with the lateral ridge of the trochlear surface of the talus in plantar flexion.[30]

The anatomic variations of the AITFL can be classified into five categories based on the number

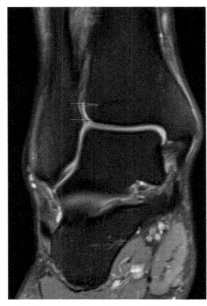

Fig. 1. Tibiofibular recess. Coronal PD with fat saturation MR image showing the height of the tibiofibular recess to be 7.0 mm, which is within normal limits.

of fascicles, presence or absence of separations between the fascicles, attachment of inferior fascicle to the main portion of the ligament, and presence of a separate accessory inferior

fascicle.[44] The accessory AITFL ligament, also referred to as the distal fascicle or Bassett's ligament, is present in 21% to 92% of human ankles in cadaveric and MR imaging studies. This accessory ligament is a triangular-shaped horizontal band, which is separated from the other AITFL bands by a triangular fat-filled space. It usually runs inferior and parallel to the AITFL.[37] The PITFL is triangular-shaped and has a broad tibial insertion (see **Fig. 2**). It originates from the posterior tubercle of the tibia and courses inferolaterally to the posterior lateral malleolus.

Attenuation, laxity, or discontinuity of the ligament are MR features of sprain injuries of the AITFL. Other findings include periarticular edema or hemorrhage in the subcutaneous tissues anterior to the torn ligament, which may extend between the torn ends of the ligament in continuity with the tibiofibular recess of the ankle joint. Injuries of the PITFL can also have this appearance (**Figs. 3** and **4**).[41] The AITFL can be thick or thin in the absence of pathology, a known pitfall. Both the AITFL and PITFL can mimic intraarticular loose bodies on the sagittal plane due to their transverse course. Therefore, it is important to find associated morphologic and signal changes of the ligaments supportive of sprain.[45]

Inferior transverse ligament/intermalleolar ligament/interosseous ligament The ITL is a strong,

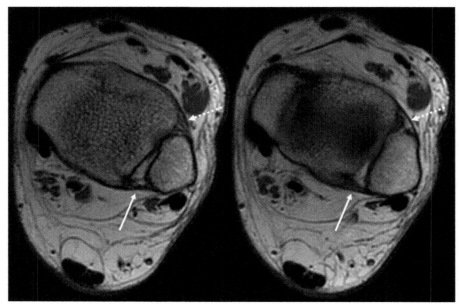

Fig. 2. Normal tibiofibular ligaments. Consecutive axial intermediate-weighted MR images at the level of the tibiotalar joint. The syndesmotic ligaments are demonstrated as hypointense bands and include the anterior inferior tibiofibular ligament or AITFL (*dashed arrows*) and the posterior inferior tibiofibular ligament or PITFL (*solid arrows*).

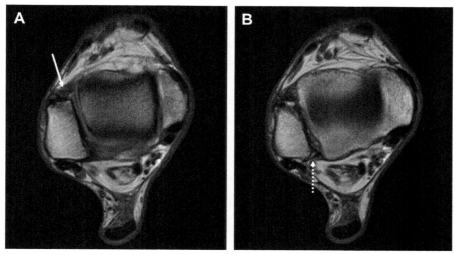

Fig. 3. Remote high ankle sprain. (*A* and *B*) Consecutive axial PD MR images through the tibial plafond demonstrate an irregular wavy contour and signal heterogeneity of both the AITFL (*solid arrow* in *A*) and the PITFL (*dashed arrow* in *B*). The findings are compatible with a remote partial tear of the AITFL and PITFL.

thick deep component of the PITFL. Whether the ITL and distal PITFL form one anatomic unit or are two distinct structures is controversial.[33] The ITL can be considered a labrum-like extension of the tibial articular surface with more horizontal orientation compared with the remainder of the PITFL fibers.[23] It attaches to the osteochondral junction on the posteromedial aspect of the distal fibula.[33] During plantar flexion, the ITL is tightly positioned between the posterior tibial margins and the PTFL.[46] It functions to limit the talus from posterior translation and increases stability of the joint.[33] This ligament is best visualized on coronal

and axial oblique planes parallel to the PITFL.[23,30,47] However, the labrum-like characteristics are best seen on the sagittal plane (**Fig. 5**). On coronal plantarflexion images, the ITL and PTFL ligaments approximate and may overlap.[24]

The intermalleolar ligament (IML), or the posterior IML, is a normal variant of the posterior ankle joint. The reported frequency of the IML is 19% on MR imaging and 56% to 82% on dissected anatomic specimens. The IML may appear as a thick hypointense band or as two-to-three parallel strips traversing between the ITL and PTF. The IML originates within the malleolar fossa, superior to

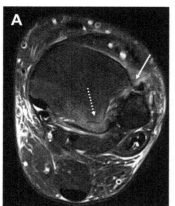
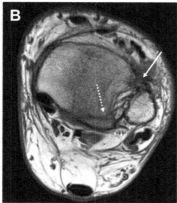
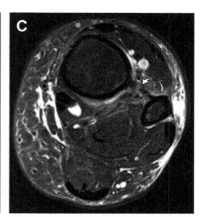

Fig. 4. Recent high ankle sprain and tibial fracture. (*A*) Axial fat-saturated T2 and (*B*) Axial T1 MR images at the level of the tibiotalar joint demonstrate a lax wavy contour of the AITFL which is torn and avulsed from the tibial attachment with surrounding edema (*solid arrows*). Fracture of the posterior tibial malleolus outlined by marrow edema (*dashed arrows*) is also seen. (*C*) Axial fat-saturated T2 image shows a tear of the oblique/syndesmotic ligament which is disrupted (*curve arrow*).

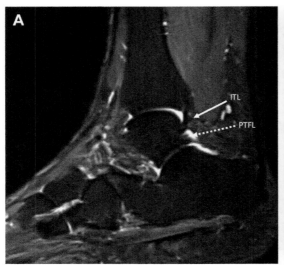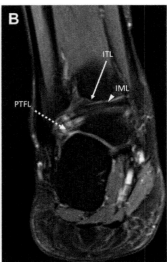

Fig. 5. Inferior transverse ligament. (*A*) Fat-saturated T2 sagittal and (*B*) coronal images of the ankle. White arrow is pointing to the inferior transverse ligament (ITL). This ligament is best visualized parallel to the intermalleolar ligament (IML) in this case. However, the labrum-like characteristics are best seen on the sagittal plane (*solid arrow*). The dashed arrow represents the posterior talofibular ligament (PTFL).

the origin of the PTFL, and courses obliquely to insert into the posteromedial tibial cortex, medial to the site of insertion of the ITL.[47,48] The interosseous ligament (IOL) is the lowest end of the interosseous membrane as it thickens.[33] The IOL is a multi-fascicular broad ligament that originates in the fibular notch of the tibia and courses obliquely to attach on the anteroinferior triangular segment of the distal medial fibular shaft above the tibiotalar joint.[23] This ligament may be completely absent.[20]

Lateral Ankle Sprains: Inversion Injuries

Epidemiology
Lateral ankle injuries account for up to 20% of all sports injuries and up to 45% of injuries in basketball.[49] Out of these, the ATFL is injured in 83%, the calcaneofibular ligament (CFL) in 67%, and the PTFL in 34%.[50] Avulsion fractures of the lateral ankle ligaments are not infrequent and can be seen in up to 26% of severe inversion injuries.[51] The CFL has 2 to 3.5 times greater maximum load compared with the ATFL, which likely explains the high prevalence and incidence of ATFL injuries.[52]

Functional anatomy
The lateral ligament complex acts as a static stabilizer of the ankle, limiting excessive inversion-type motion.[53] A recent study by de Asla and colleagues showed that the ATFL elongates during plantar flexion and supination, whereas the CFL increases in length with dorsiflexion and protonation [56]. The two ligaments appear to have opposing

movements—one shortens while the other one elongates. They concluded that under excessive loading conditions, the ATFL may be more susceptible to injury in plantar flexion and supination, whereas the CFL may be more susceptible to injury in dorsiflexion and protonation.[54]

Clinical considerations and mechanism of injury
Patients usually localize tenderness over the ATFL at 4 to 7 days following injury.[55] The integrity of the lateral ligaments, specifically the ATFL and the CFL, can be tested with provocative maneuvers including the anterior drawer and talar tilt tests.[56] Residual symptoms after lateral ankle sprain affect 37% of patients at 6 months.[35] Approximately 20% of acute ankle sprains develop functional or mechanical instability, resulting in a diagnosis of CAI.[55] CAI is defined as mechanical and/or functional instability.[31] CAI is associated with a history of ≥ two ankle sprains, difficulty walking with uneasiness/apprehension on uneven surfaces, and/or a history of the ankle "giving way."[35,55]

Injury to the lateral complex typically occurs during forced plantar flexion and inversion.[55] When the center of gravity is shifted to the lateral border of the leg, the ankle rolls inward at a high velocity.[57] The mechanism is usually of the twisting type with both dorsiflexion and internal rotation resulting in a mid-substance rupture of the ATFL, CFL, and the intervening capsule.[30] The predictable pattern of injury involves first the ATFL, followed by the CFL, and then the PTFL.[58]

Table 1
Imaging modalities that can be used in the assessment of lateral ankle sprains

Imaging of the Lateral Ankle Ligaments	
Ultrasound	Ultrasound accuracy is reported as high as 95% and 90% for acute sprains of the ATFL and CFL, respectively. Findings include discontinuity, hypoechogenicity, or lack of visualization.[117,118]
Radiography	Talar tilt test is evaluated on stress AP radiographs and is considered positive if there is a 5° difference compared with the uninjured ankle or a 10° absolute value.[55]
CT scan	3D CT is useful in the evaluation of ATFL lesions, particularly chronic injury. Accuracy in diagnosing ATFL sprain is reported as high as 94%.[119]
Arthrography	Arthrography within 48 h of acute injury has a sensitivity and specificity of 96% and 71%, respectively.[120]
MR arthrography	MR arthrography may be superior to MR imaging for the assessment of lateral collateral ligament injuries. In a series of 17 patients with chronic ankle instability, Magnetic Resonance Arthrography was found to be 100% and 82% accurate, whereas conventional MR imaging was only 59% and 63% accurate in detecting ATFL and CFL tears, respectively.[121]
MR imaging	MR imaging has a reported sensitivity and specificity of 83% and 77% when compared with arthrography, for the detection of CFL tears.[63] 3D FISP imaging has a reported accuracy of 94% for detecting ATFL and CFL tears. Compared with operative findings, the sensitivity and specificity for diagnosing rupture of the ATFL and the CFL was 100/50%, and 92/100%, respectively.[27]

Diagnostic imaging

Various imaging modalities have been studied in imaging the lateral ankle ligaments (**Table 1**). On MR imaging, defects within the substance of the ATFL can be seen within 2 weeks after trauma.[25] During the remodeling phase (15–28 days), the ligament forms collagen fibers that align longitudinally and cross-link.[57] By this time, the edema and hemorrhage have usually resolved and the ligament's altered morphology is better visualized. Observed changes include attenuation, thickening, thinning, elongation, or waviness. Periarticular edema is commonly present until up to the seventh week after injury; however, edema associated with ATFL and CFL injuries usually resolve by the fourth week.[25,59] After 7 weeks, the visualized defect closes, leaving either a thin hypoplastic or thick hyperplastic ligament.[25]

Anterior talofibular ligament The ATFL is best imaged on axial T1 or high-resolution PD MR images, appearing as a flat, thin, homogeneous band of low-signal intensity arising from the anterior margin of the lateral malleolus and coursing anteromedially downward to attach onto the neck of the talus, just anterior to the fibular articular cartilage (**Fig. 6**).[21,24,60] At the level of the talofibular ligaments, the talus is oblong in shape and the sinus tarsi (ST) is partially visualized, serving as landmarks in localization. The lower portion of the fibular malleolus has a crescentic configuration, which forms the malleolar fossa.[19] When the foot is positioned in neutral or plantar flexion, the orientation of the ATFL is 45° to the coronal plane of the tibia.[30] Studies have shown that the ATFL is 13 to 25 mm in length, 7 to 11 mm in width, and 2 to 3 mm thick.[60,61]

ATFL tears are usually associated with a capsular rupture and extravasation of joint fluid into the anterolateral soft tissues, and on fluid-sensitive sequences, native joint fluid outlines the ATFL.[19,24,30] On axial T1 or PD MR images, the ligament may be indistinct or thickened, with associated signal heterogeneity. On FS T2 FSE, fluid-like

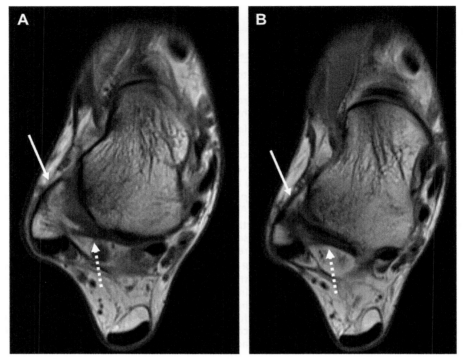

Fig. 6. Normal talofibular ligaments. (*A* and *B*) Consecutive axial PD MR image depicts a taut ATFL measuring 2 mm in thickness (*solid arrow*). The PTFL has a striated appearance due to interspersed fat (*dashed arrow*).

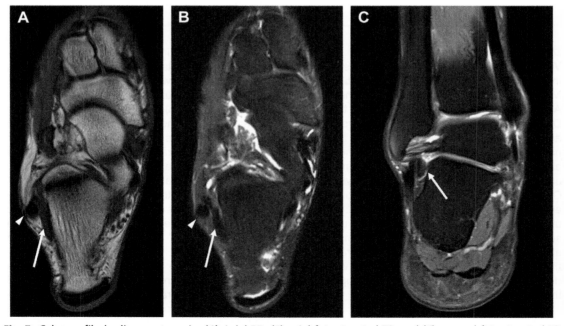

Fig. 7. Calcaneofibular ligament sprain. (*A*) Axial PD, (*B*) axial fat-saturated T2, and (*C*) coronal fat-saturated T2 demonstrate acute on chronic sprain of the CFL (*solid arrow*) with thickened and edematous fibers paralleling the lateral calcaneal wall, deep to the peroneal tendons (*arrowheads*), a reliable anatomic landmark.

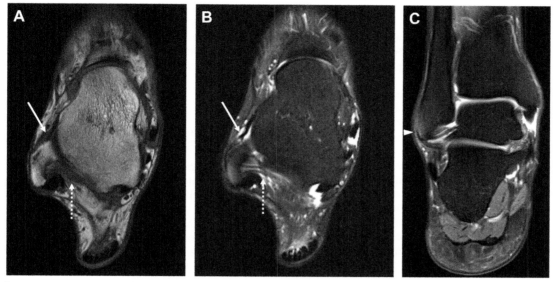

Fig. 8. Acute anterior talofibular ligament avulsion. (*A*) Axial PD1, (*B*) axial fat-saturated T2, and (*C*) coronal fat-saturated intermediate MR images demonstrate near complete disruption of the ATFL (*solid white arrows*) at its fibular insertion site. The PTFL (*dashed arrow*) shows hyperintense signal and an irregular wavy contour consistent with a partial tear. Marrow edema is noted at the site of avulsion of the CFL from the fibula (*arrowhead*).

signal intensity is often seen within the torn ATFL fibers (**Fig. 7**).[30] A complete tear of the ATFL can be seen as a fluid-filled defect across the ruptured ligament with retraction of wavy/lax fibers. Intrasubstance tears can be seen as abnormal

increased STIR or T2 signal within the ligament, indicative of edema or hemorrhage.[62] Chronic tears may manifest either as severe attenuation or as thickening secondary to scarring. In chronic injuries, granulation/scar tissue beneath the ATFL

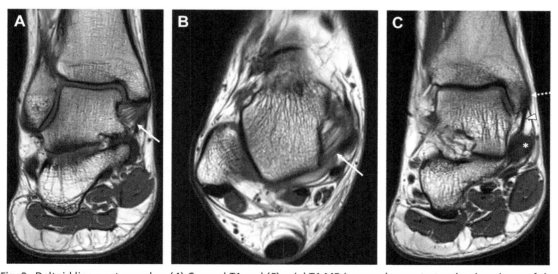

Fig. 9. Deltoid ligament complex. (*A*) Coronal T1 and (*B*) axial T1 MR images demonstrates the deep layer of the deltoid ligament complex (*arrows*), which consists of the anterior tibiotalar ligament (aTTL) and the posterior tibiotalar ligament (pTTL). (*C*) Coronal T1 MR image shows the takeoff of the superficial layer of the deltoid ligament from the anterior colliculus (*dashed arrow*) of the medial malleolus. This layer consists of the tibionavicular ligament (TNL), tibiospring ligament (TSL), and tibiocalcaneal ligament (TCL). The TSL (*arrowhead*), which is best visualized in this image, converges with the superomedial calcaneonavicular ligament (smCNL) component of the spring ligament complex deep to the posterior tibial tendon (*asterisk*).

in the anterolateral gutter can form a triangular shape, which is often referred to as a "meniscoid" lesion due to its similar morphology to a meniscus in the knee, and this tissue can be a cause of impingement in the ankle (**Figs. 8** and **9**).[19]

CFL The CFL is large, strong, and cordlike. It arises from the deep aspect of the inferior tip of lateral malleolus and courses posteroinferiorly to attach to the lateral aspect of the calcaneus, just about the retrotrochlear eminence. The CFL crosses both the tibiotalar and subtalar joints and is located deep to the peroneal tendons.[24,30,60] It is best seen on axial and coronal images (see **Fig. 8**).[19] On axial images, the peroneal retinaculum can sometimes be mistaken for the CFL, although the peroneal retinaculum is located superficial to the peroneal tendons.[24] On sequential T1-weighted coronal images, the CFL is depicted in cross-section as a thin, homogenous low-signal intensity structure deep to the peroneal tendons.[19,21] The ligament is best depicted on axial images in plantar flexion.[20] The CFL should be clearly identified to avoid confusing it with a loose body or an avulsion fracture of the calcaneus, particularly in the coronal plane.[63] The CFL has an average length of 36 mm, a width of 5 mm, and a thickness of 2 mm.[60]

CFL tears are characterized by indistinctness of the ligament fibers and signal heterogeneity. The ligament is frequently thickened with obliteration of the surrounding fat planes (see **Fig. 8**).[19,30] Thickening of the superior peroneal retinaculum and peroneal tenosynovial effusions is also commonly seen with CFL tears due to a communication between the tibiotalar joint and the peroneal tendon sheath.[25]

Posterior talofibular ligament The PTFL is inhomogeneous, thick, multi-fascicular and considered the strongest and deepest ligament of the lateral collateral complex.[21,30] The PTFL is intracapsular but extrasynovial.[30] On axial and coronal images, the PTFL has a fan-shaped configuration, extending inferomedially from the deep aspect of the lateral malleolus to attach on the mid to posterior aspect of the talus.[20,24,21]

The PTFL often shows marked signal heterogeneity and thickening due to the presence of fat striations, which should not be misinterpreted as a tear.[20] Sprains involving the PTFL manifest as high T2 signal within the ligament, which has an irregular wavy contour. The PTFL and the posterior IML course transversely behind the tibiotalar joint and frequently are seen as punctuate low signal intensity structures posteriorly in the

sagittal plane, potentially mimicking intraarticular bodies in the posterior ankle (see **Fig. 5**). It is important to carefully track each of these ligaments from their origin to their insertions on orthogonal imaging planes to avoid this pitfall.[45]

Medial Ankle Sprains: Eversion Injury

Epidemiology

Injuries of the deltoid ligament complex accounted for approximately 5% of ankle sprains in a study by Waterman and colleagues.[7] Medial ankle sprains were more commonly seen in men's rugby, gymnastics, and soccer. Male athletes are three times more likely to experience medial ankle sprains than female athletes. Up to 10% of deltoid ligament complex sprains are associated with syndesmotic injuries (**Fig. 4**).[30]

The ligamentous complex is triangular/deltoid-shaped and can be subdivided into two, obliquely oriented, parallel groups. The more superficial ligaments include the tibionavicular ligament (TNL), tibiospring ligament (TSL), and tibiocalcaneal ligament (TCL), whereas the deeper ligaments include the anterior tibiotalar ligament (aTTL) and posterior tibiotalar ligament (pTTL) (see **Fig. 11**).[24] The deep portion of the deltoid ligament is intra-articular and surrounded by synovium.[64] The pTTL is considered the strongest component, followed by the TSL, TNL, and TCL.[65] The deltoid ligament complex stabilizes the ankle against valgus, protonation, and external rotational forces on the talus.[64,66–68]

Clinical considerations and mechanism of injury

Medial ankle sprains are usually more painful than their lateral counterpart, and mechanical instability is characteristic.[30] The eversion stress test is considered a reliable clinical examination.[67] Acute injuries are usually clinically apparent with hematoma and tenderness over the medial ankle.[64] Chronic sprains are characterized by chronic insufficiency, pain, medial gutter tenderness, and hindfoot valgus during weight bearing and protonation. Complete tears can sometimes be seen in conjunction with lateral malleolar and bimalleolar fractures.[67]

Acute injury usually occurs with eversion forces resulting in valgus stress and/or internal rotation forces causing protonation stress.[67] Deep ligament tears are more common than superficial tears, and partial tears are more common than full-thickness tears.[30,64] Sprains of the deep components of the deltoid ligament are frequently noted in patients after inversion injuries.[19,20]

Diagnostic imaging

On routine MR imaging, positioning the foot in dorsiflexion optimizes visualization of the more posterior components of the deltoid ligament in the coronal plane, such as the TSL and deep tibiotalar ligament (TTL).[20] Most of the ligaments are best seen in the coronal plane (see **Fig. 9**A,C). Axial images are reserved for evaluating the tendons and surrounding neurovascular structures, which may be injured in association with deltoid ligament injury.[24] The 3D Fourier transform gradient-recalled echo MR images are useful for visualizing the various components along their orthogonal plane.[20] With this MR sequence, the foot position is not critical. Reformatting images in coronal oblique planes along the expected course of each ligament, obtained from a paramedia sagittal plane, are considered useful to better delineate the ligaments.[65] Ultrasonography has been shown to be a highly accurate diagnostic modality in assessing deltoid ligament injury in the setting of supination external rotation fractures of the ankle.[69]

Superficial The superficial group of ligaments arises from the anterior colliculus of the medial malleolus and fans out anteriorly and posteriorly (see **Fig. 9**C).[30,65] The TNL is a homogeneous, thin, low signal band that attaches at the talus and crosses both the ankle and talonavicular joints inferiorly to insert on the medial navicular tuberosity.[21,24] This ligament shares a distal attachment with the posterior tibial tendon (PTT) and superior part of the spring (plantar calcaneonavicular) ligament. The TNL and aTTL form part of the tibiotalar and talonavicular joints.[24] The TNL is sometimes difficult to discern on routine coronal images due to its oblique forward course and may require oblique coronal planes to be visualized on a single image.[20] The TNL has a mean thickness of 1 to 2 mm.[70]

The full length of the TCL is frequently seen on a single routine coronal image, appearing as a homogeneous band of low signal intensity attached to the posterior sustentaculum tali.[21,24,70] It may be difficult to distinguish TCL from TSL due to its close proximity.[70] The TSL courses downward, across the ankle and anterior subtalar joints, to attach to the lateral aspect of the superomedial (SM) oblique band of the spring ligament (SL).[64,67,70] Mengiardi and colleagues reported the TSL to be the second largest component of the deltoid ligament with an average thickness of 2 mm (1–4 mm). Both the TSL and the TNL were found to be significantly thicker in men compared with women.[70] The PTT and its sheath course posteromedial to the deltoid ligament and come in direct contact with the TSL and pTTL.[24] The

PTT serves to maintain the medial arch of the foot and is often associated with SL and TSL pathology related to medial ankle instability.[64]

Deep The deep components of the deltoid complex are shorter and arise from the intercollicular/malleolar groove.[30,65] The aTTL is thin, multifascicular, and has a broad insertion more anteriorly on the talar body and neck. This ligament is best seen on coronal images in 50% to 84% of normal asymptomatic ankles.[65,70] The pTTL is a low signal, thick band with a rectangular shape (see **Fig. 9**B). It courses posteroinferiorly and broadly attaches to the medial surface of the talus as far posteriorly as the posteromedial talar tubercle.[21,30,65] This ligament is generally regarded as the thickest ligament ranging in thickness from 6 to 11 mm.[70] It is normal for this ligament to have a heterogeneous appearance and striations due to interposed fat.[20,65,70]

In medial ankle sprains, high T2 signal can be seen on fat-saturated PD or T2-weighted MR images with associated fluid-filled gaps or complete discontinuity of the ligament (**Figs. 10** and **11**).[64] Findings include intermediate signal intensity on T1 or PD-WI, amorphous hyperintensity on FS PD FSE, indistinct margins and loss of fiber striation in the TTL, or mass-like morphology with associated hemorrhage and edema (**Fig. 12**).[30] A potential pitfall is that asymptomatic patients over 45 years of age have variable increased T2-weighted signal in the anterior TTL, TNL, and TSL.[70]

Other associated injuries include medial malleolar fractures, distal avulsion fractures, osteochondral lesions of the talus, lateral collateral, and syndesmotic ligament injuries, SL, and PTT injuries.[64] Over 60% of posterior TTL injuries are due to avulsion.[65]

Post-Traumatic Sinus Tarsi Syndrome

Epidemiology

ST syndrome (STS) is caused by trauma in 70% of cases.[71,72] Klein and Spreitzer reported that lateral collateral ligament tears were found to be present in about 79% of cases of STS, and lateral collateral ligament injuries had abnormal signal within the region of the ST in 39% of cases.[73]

Functional anatomy

The ST ligaments, nerves, and vessels play an important role in stabilization and proprioception of the subtalar joint.[62] The ST can be divided into the superficial, intermediate, and deep layers. The superficial layer includes the lateral root of the inferior extensor retinaculum (IER), lateral talocalcaneal (TL) ligament, CFL, posterior TL

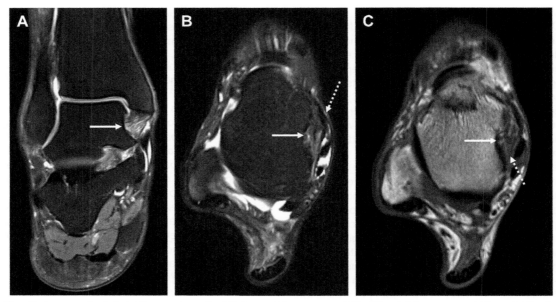

Fig. 10. Low-grade deltoid ligament sprain. (*A*) Coronal fat-saturated PD, (*B*) axial fat-saturated T2, and (*C*) axial T1 MR images show fluid-like hyperintense signal of the deep (*solid arrows*) with low-grade partial tear. Mild sprain of the superficial deltoid ligament fibers (*dashed arrows*) is noted. There is also loss of the normal striated appearance of the posterior tibiotalar component of the deep deltoid ligament complex (*solid arrow* in *C*).

ligament, and the medial TL ligament. The intermediate layer includes the cervical ligament and intermediate root of the IER. The deep layer contains the interosseous TL ligament and medial root of the IER.[30] The interosseous TL and cervical ligaments are important in the overall function of the lateral ankle and hindfoot complex. The cervical ligament also acts to limit inversion.[71]

Clinical considerations and mechanism of injury
Patients with STS present with pain exacerbated with weight bearing along the lateral aspect of the foot.[29] Patients usually have subjective sensation of instability of the hindfoot, especially when walking on uneven ground[71,73] However, there is usually little objective evidence of instability.[73] STS is usually a chronic condition primarily because acute ST injury is confounded by swelling of the entire ankle from other ankle sprains.[72]

ST injury commonly develops after an inversion injury.[29,58,73] The IOL is subject to traction and torsional stresses and is taut in supination and relaxed in protonation of the foot. Progressive inversion of the heel without dorsiflexion or

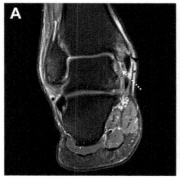
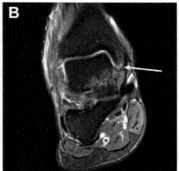
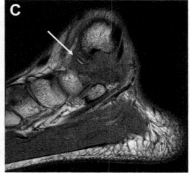

Fig. 11. High-grade deltoid ligament sprain. (*A* and *B*) Coronal fat-saturated PD and (*C*) sagittal T1 MR images demonstrate near complete discontinuity of the deep deltoid fibers outlined by fluid (*dashed arrow*). Remote well-corticated avulsion fracture fragment off the tip of the medial malleolus (*solid arrows*). Also noted is acute avulsion (*arrowhead*) of the superficial deltoid fibers from the medial malleolus with associated marrow edema. The findings are compatible with acute on chronic injury.

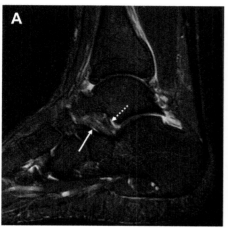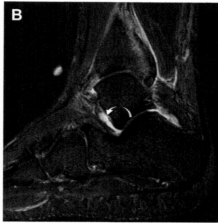

Fig. 12. Post-traumatic sinus tarsi syndrome. (*A* and *B*) Sagittal fat-saturated T2 image shows edema of the cervical (*white arrow*) and the talocalcaneal (*dashed arrow*) ligaments in the sinus tarsi. Associated posterior subtalar joint effusion with distension of the anterior joint recess (*curved arrow*). Incidentally noted is fracture of the posterior tibial malleolus (*arrowhead*).

extension induces rupture of the ATFL and CFL ligaments, followed by the interosseous TL ligament.[71]

Diagnostic imaging

Before the advent of MR imaging, the only techniques for diagnosing STS were arthrography, which showed the lack of filling of the anterior recesses of the subtalar joint or clinically with relief of pain following local anesthetic or steroid injection.[71,73] MR imaging has dramatically improved our ability to demonstrate normal anatomy and pathology of the ST.[29,62] The ST is a wedge-shaped space in the lateral aspect of the ankle, between the inferior aspect of the talus and the superior aspect of the calcaneus.[29,71] The osseous walls of the ST are irregular and covered by multiple vascular foramina.[29,71]

The TL, or interosseous, ligament is broad and strong and is composed of a single band medially. The posterior and medial fibers extend from the inferior aspect of the ST laterally to the superior aspect of the deepest portion of the tarsal canal. Laterally, two bands are seen separated by fat, vessels, and nerves. The most anterior division of the TL ligament is the cervical ligament, which extends from a small tubercle on the inferior lateral aspect of the neck of the talus onto the dorsal surface of the calcaneus. This can be seen as a low signal intensity band, which is better appreciated on sagittal MR images rather than coronal. On T1-weighted MR imaging, the TL ligament is seen deep within the tarsal canal as a fan-like structure.[71] The cervical ligament can be seen as a medial structure within the ST extending from the inferior aspect of the talus to the superior aspect of the calcaneus and is best seen on sagittal and coronal planes.[29]

STS can be diagnosed on T1 and PD-weighted MR imaging by effacement of the ST fat with or without injury to the ligaments (see **Fig. 12**).[30] Osteoarthritis of the subtalar joint with subchondral cysts, bone marrow edema of the talus or calcaneus at the level of the ligament, PTT tear, and contrast enhancement of hypertrophied synovium are among associated findings.[20,58,71,73,74]

Post-Traumatic Flat Foot Deformity: Spring Ligament Complex

Epidemiology

SL injury is usually associated with PTT dysfunction in middle-aged women.[75]

Functional anatomy

The SL complex, or plantar calcaneonavicular ligament (CNL), is a hammock-like structure that extends from the sustentaculum tali of the calcaneus to the posteromedial process of the navicular.[76,77] Despite its name, the SL is not elastic.[78] The complex consists of three ligaments: SM, inferior plantar longitudinal (IPL), and medioplantar oblique (MPO) (see **Fig. 14**).[76,77,79] The SM component is the most often torn and plays the most impact on the stability of the SL.[77] The SL along with the anterior and middle facets of the calcaneus and the proximal articular surface of the navicular comprise the acetabulum pedis.[78] This complex supports the talar head and is thus critical for static stabilization of the medial longitudinal arch of the foot and for supporting the head of the talus.[77]

Clinical considerations and mechanism of injury
SL dysfunction causes talar plantar flexion and hindfoot valgus, resulting in acquired flatfoot deformity (pes planovalgus) due to the loss of support of the longitudinal arch of the foot.[76,77] It has been observed that hindfoot deformity is most severe when both the SL and the PTT are injured.[80]

Tears of the plantar components of the SL complex as a result of macrotrauma can be seen in the young athletic population in association with talar head impaction injuries.[81]

Diagnostic imaging
The sensitivity and specificity of detecting SL rupture or laxity with MR imaging has been reported to be 54% to 77% and 100%, respectively.[82] Rule and colleagues described the SL as a low signal intensity band on T2-WI, which overall is best seen in the oblique sagittal and axial planes.[83] However, other studies have noted that the SM band is particularly best viewed in the coronal and axial planes.[77] In between the PTT and the SM band of the SL, there is a gliding zone composed of fibrocartilage, which measures 1 to 3 mm.[64,70] Sometimes, it is difficult to differentiate the PTT, the gliding zone, and the SM band of the SL. The SM originates from the superomedial aspect of the sustentaculum tali and travels obliquely, wrapping around the tuberosity of the navicular, to attach in a fan-like fashion to the superomedial navicular bone. The SM band runs immediately deep to the distal PTT, and the SM fibers merge with the superficial tibiospring fibers of the deltoid ligament complex, close to their insertion on the sustentaculum tali.[76,79] The average thickness of the SM is 3 mm (2–5 mm).[79]

The MPO and IPL bands of the SL complex are located more inferior than the SM band and are considered weaker than the SM band.[28,83] The MPO band originates from a notch located between the anterior and middle articular facets of the calcaneus, referred to as the coronoid fossa. It fans out to attach to the medial plantar aspect of the navicular bone. This band is generally long and best seen on axial and coronal images.[78,79,84] The IPL ligament is short, thick, and originates from the coronoid fossa of the calcaneus, anterior to the MPO band. It courses obliquely to attach on the inferior beak of the navicular bone and is best seen on sagittal, coronal, or coronal oblique planes. The average thickness of the IPL is 4 mm (2–6 mm).[79]

On MR imaging, findings of sprains of the SL can include heterogeneous or increased signal on fluid-sensitive sequences, thickening, ligament laxity, waviness or a full-thickness gap (**Fig. 13**).[62,76,77] PTT tendinopathy, surrounding edema, and impaction injuries of the talar head can also be seen.[77] Desai and colleagues described the SL recess, a fluid-filled space that communicates with the talocalcaneonavicular joint between the MPO and IPL components of the SL (**Fig. 14**).[78] The average size of the recess is 0.4 cm (0.2–0.9 cm) × 0.8 cm (0.4–1.5 cm) in transverse and craniocaudal dimensions, respectively. The SL recess is best visualized on axial images when the tibiotalar joint is distended with fluid and has a teardrop shape on coronal and sagittal images. The SL recess should not be misinterpreted as a tear of the SL, synovial cyst, or ganglion cyst.[78]

Midtarsal (Chopart) Joint Sprain

Epidemiology
A less recognized injury that is often associated with an ankle sprain is a midtarsal sprain, which is a sprain of the talonavicular and calcaneocuboid joints, and is also known as a Chopart joint sprain.[85] It was generally considered a relatively rare injury accounting for only 5.5% of ankle and foot sprains in some reports, especially when occurring in isolation.[86,87] However, other reports suggest that it is a much more common injury accounting for up to 33% of inversion ankle injuries and in isolation in up to 24% of inversion injuries.[87,88] The disparity in the reported frequencies of this injury is likely secondary to the clinical underdiagnosis because the symptoms and signs of Chopart joint injury can be easily mistaken for or overshadowed by the more common injury of the lateral collateral ligament complex of the ankle.[89,90]

Functional anatomy
The midtarsal joint, or Chopart joint, is the articulation between the hindfoot (calcaneus and talus) and the midfoot (navicular and cuboid) which provides both midfoot flexibility and stability and is critical to normal gait and weight bearing.[91] The Chopart joint is composed of two articulations, the calcaneocuboid joint and the talonavicular joint, and is stabilized by several ligaments (see **Fig. 16**). The dorsal calcaneocuboid ligament and the short and long plantar ligaments stabilize the calcaneocuboid joint; the dorsal talonavicular and SLs stabilize the talonavicular joint.[92] Both joints are also stabilized by the bifurcate ligament, which has a calcaneocuboid component (also called medial calcaneocuboid component) and calcaneonavicular component (also called lateral calcaneonavicular component).

The dorsal calcaneocuboid ligament has its origin at the dorsolateral calcaneus and inserts approximately 0.5 to 1.0 cm distal to the

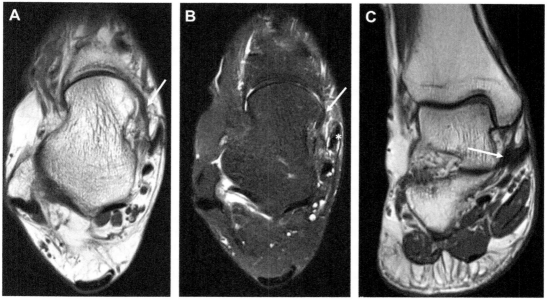

Fig. 13. Sprain of the spring ligament. (*A*) Axial T1, (*B*) axial T2 FS, and (*C*) coronal T1 images show thickening and hyperintense signal in the superomedial band of the spring ligament (*arrow*) with surrounding edema. Grade 1 posterior tibial tendon dysfunction with tendinosis and mild tenosynovitis (*asterisk*).

calcaneocuboid joint.[93] It can have substantial anatomic variation with either a single band, multiple bands, upward-, or downward-pointing bundles, a prominent lateral band, fusion with the

calcaneocuboid component of the bifurcate ligament, and a meniscoid variant.[93,94]

The long plantar ligament originates from the plantar aspect of the calcaneus and has deep

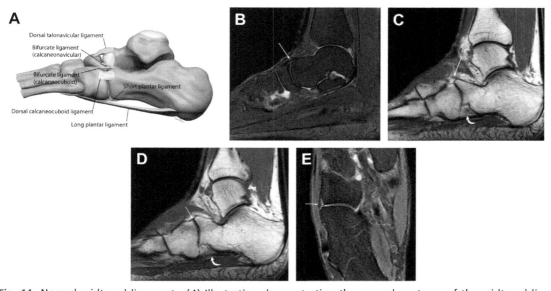

Fig. 14. Normal midtarsal ligaments. (*A*) Illustration demonstrating the normal anatomy of the midtarsal ligaments. (*B*) Sagittal T2 FS MR image shows a normal dorsal talonavicular ligament (*arrow*). (*C*) Sagittal T1 MR image shows a normal calcaneonavicular component of the bifurcate ligament (*arrow*) which is highlighted by the surround fat and the short plantar ligament (*curved arrow*) which has a normal striated appearance. (*D*) Sagittal T1 MR image located slightly more lateral shows a normal calcaneocuboid component of the bifurcate ligament (*arrow*) and the long plantar ligament (*curved arrow*). (*E*) Axial PD FS MR image shows a normal dorsal calcaneocuboid ligament (*arrow*).

fibers that inset on the cuboid ridge and superficial fibers that insert more distally along the plantar aspect of the second through fourth metatarsal bases.[92] It can also have variable attachments to the adjacent peroneus longus tendon sheath.[95,96] The short plantar ligament originates from the anterior calcaneal tubercle and inserts at the plantar aspect of the cuboid.[92,95,96]

The two bifurcate ligament components originate from the dorsolateral anterior process of the calcaneus and form a V-shaped configuration, with the more lateral calcaneocuboid component inserting on the dorsomedial cuboid and the more medial calcaneonavicular component inserting on the dorsal navicular.[95]

The SL complex anatomy was already described in the previous section. It is also an important stabilizer of the Chopart joint.[92]

The dorsal talonavicular ligament is also considered a thickening of the dorsal talonavicular joint capsule. It originates at the dorsal aspect of the talar neck and inserts along the dorsal navicular bone.[92]

Clinical considerations and mechanism of injury

Midtarsal sprain is an injury of the Chopart joint and its supporting ligaments, which can sometimes include an avulsion fracture or less commonly an impaction fracture.[92] On physical examination, it is suspected when there is pain and tenderness located along the Chopart joint associated with joint laxity or instability, which is often confirmed with stress radiographs to evaluate for Chopart and subtalar joint instability.[97] As the clinical presentation of midtarsal sprain and ankle sprain can be similar and often both injuries can occur simultaneously, it is thought that midtarsal sprains can be overlooked or misdiagnosed as lateral ankle sprains which are much more common.[98]

The most common mechanism of injury in midtarsal sprain is an inversion of the ankle with or without plantar flexion.[87,89] The resulting varus force applied to the lateral and dorsolateral aspect of the calcaneocuboid joint can cause tensile distraction forces with ligamentous avulsion along the dorsolateral aspect of the joint.[88] The injuries that occur with this mechanism include avulsion of the dorsal calcaneocuboid ligament and calcaneocuboid component of the bifurcate ligament as well as extensor digitorum brevis origin avulsion.[85,99] Impaction injuries occur medially along the talonavicular joint producing contusions or fractures of the talar head and navicular body.[85,99] Furthermore, distraction forces across the Chopart joint complex may cause avulsions of the plantar components of the SL.[85,99] When

an ankle inversion is accompanied by plantar flexion, this can also cause distraction forces at the talonavicular joint with dorsal talonavicular ligament avulsion injury, plantar talonavicular impaction due to rotation of the talar head, and plantar calcaneocuboid impaction.[99] Distraction forces at the medial calcaneocuboid joint may also produce joint capsule and short plantar ligament avulsion injuries.[85,99]

A less common mechanism of injury in midtarsal sprain is an ankle eversion, which is associated with compressive impaction forces along the lateral aspect of the calcaneocuboid joint, producing impaction fractures of the anterior process of the calcaneus and posterolateral cuboid, which are referred to as a "nutcracker injuries,"[100] and are often comminuted and depressed. Distraction forces along the medial aspect of the talonavicular joint can cause navicular tuberosity avulsion fractures due to traction by the PTT.[99]

It is important to note that a midtarsal sprain is distinct from a Chopart fracture–dislocation injury which also occurs in the Chopart joint but is a more severe and obvious injury, usually as a result of high-energy impact trauma, such as a fall from height or road traffic collision, associated with fractures of the calcaneus, cuboid, and navicular and superior medial dislocation at the Chopart joint when the foot is inverted, or lateral dislocation when the foot is everted.[101]

Diagnostic imaging

The normal anatomy of the midtarsal ligaments is best evaluated on MR imaging (see **Fig. 14**). The dorsal calcaneocuboid ligament is best seen on axial MR images, where the commonly present lateral band can be readily seen originating from the anterior process of the calcaneus and inserting 0.5 to 1.0 cm distal to the calcaneocuboid joint.[92] Visualization of the dorsal calcaneocuboid ligament on sagittal MR images can vary in difficulty because of its thin dorsal component and volume averaging with the extensor digitorum brevis muscle.[92] When visible in the sagittal plane, the ligament can be detected on the first or second slice where the anterior calcaneal process is also visible while scrolling through the MR images from lateral to medial.[92] The calcaneonavicular component of the bifurcate ligament is well visualized on sagittal MR images due to the fat surrounding the ligament, which increases its conspicuity.[92] The dorsal talonavicular ligament is best visualized on sagittal MR images at the level of the mid-talar head, where the ligament blends with the dorsal joint capsule of the talonavicular joint. It is important to note that isolated thickening of the dorsal talonavicular ligament, without abnormality of the other ligaments at the Chopart joint, was seen in 44% of normal control subjects in one study by Walter and colleagues[92] and thus should not be misinterpreted as a sprain when it occurs in isolation. The long plantar ligament is best visualized on sagittal images at the mid-plantar aspect of the calcaneocuboid joint, and similar the short plantar ligament is best visualized on sagittal images at the medial plantar aspect of the calcaneocuboid joint.[92]

The initial imaging evaluation for acute ankle trauma is radiography, which is sometimes followed by CT if the injury is complicated or surgery is contemplated. Midtarsal sprain can sometimes be occult at radiography as it may only involve a soft tissue ligamentous injury, however, if an avulsion fracture is associated with the injury which is most commonly the case, small avulsion fracture fragments at typical locations can help to make the diagnosis.[88]

MR imaging may be indicated in the subacute to chronic setting after trauma, particularly when patients have persistent pain that has failed conservative management and the clinical suspicion is that there is more extensive injury than initially suspected at the time of acute trauma. Tiny displaced avulsion fractures which frequently occur with midtarsal sprains may be better detected on radiography or CT; however, MR imaging is the optimal modality for the detection of midtarsal ligament sprains and tears and associated foci of marrow edema related to avulsion, impaction, or contusion.[88] The high sensitivity of MR imaging in the detection of bone marrow edema can aid in detecting non-displaced avulsion fracture lines and minimally impacted fractures that can be easily missed on radiography. This highlights the importance of interpreting MR imaging studies in conjunction with radiography and CT studies, which are often performed before MR imaging.

As with MR imaging of ligament injuries elsewhere in the body, midtarsal ligament injuries are best seen on fluid-sensitive fat-suppressed proton density or T2-WI, which can demonstrate areas of discontinuity or edema in the ligaments. A sprain of the midtarsal ligament will appear as thickening with intermediate signal from intrasubstance edema and surrounding edema in the periligamentous soft tissues.[88] A partial ligament tear will demonstrate attenuated appearance and hyperintense intrasubstance signal of the ligament due to partial disruption of the ligament fibers with surrounding edema.[88] A complete rupture of a ligament will appear as complete discontinuity of the ligament with a fluid-filled gap separating the torn and distracted ligament fibers.[19,102]

Inversion and plantar flexion midtarsal injuries In the setting of inversion mechanism of injury in midtarsal sprain, midtarsal fractures and the associated ligamentous injuries can be subdivided into three major categories, which often occur simultaneously: (1) avulsion fractures of the lateral column of the foot, (2) impaction fractures along the medial column, and (3) plantar flexion-related avulsion fractures.[88]

Lateral column avulsion fractures from inversion injury most commonly occur at the anterior process of the calcaneus and along the dorsolateral cuboid, which involve the origins and insertions of the dorsal calcaneocuboid ligament and the calcaneocuboid component of the bifurcate ligament[88] (**Fig. 15**). Avulsion fractures of the anterior process of the calcaneus are best seen on oblique and lateral radiographs of the foot and ankle and sagittal images on CT and MR imaging. Avulsion fracture of the extensor digitorum brevis muscle origin at the anterior calcaneal process may also occur and may be difficult to distinguish from an avulsion fracture of the dorsal calcaneocuboid or bifurcate ligaments, although extensor digitorum brevis (EDB) avulsion typically produces a large fracture fragment.[88] Fractures of the anterior process of the calcaneus may occasionally also be seen on the AP radiograph of the ankle, where there will be associated soft-tissue swelling distal to the fibular tip, raising suspicion for this fracture and the possibility of midtarsal sprain.[88] Small avulsion fractures along the plantar surfaces of the lateral calcaneus and cuboid may also occur in the lateral column, which are attributed to calcaneocuboid joint capsule avulsion or long plantar ligament avulsion. These injuries are best seen on AP radiographs of the foot and axial CT and MR images of the foot or ankle. In addition, tiny plantar navicular avulsion fractures may occur at the plantar SL insertion, which are best seen on lateral radiographs of the foot or ankle and on sagittal CT and MR images.

Impaction injuries of the medial column from inversion injury usually occur at the medial aspect of the talonavicular joint producing contusions or osteochondral impaction fractures of the talar head and navicular body. These injuries may be subtle and are best seen on AP and oblique radiographs of the foot and on axial CT and MR images.[88]

Plantar-related avulsion fractures which often occur concurrently with that inversion injuries described previously occur at the dorsal aspect of the talonavicular joint, with the avulsed osseous fragment arising from the dorsal talar head or the dorsal navicular at the origin and insertion of the dorsal talonavicular ligament. These fractures are

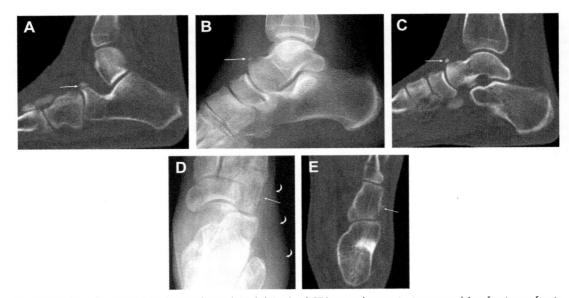

Fig. 15. Midtarsal sprain on Radiography and CT. (*A*) Sagittal CT image demonstrates an avulsion fracture of anterior process of calcaneus (*arrow*) which was not visible on radiographs. (*B*) Lateral radiograph and (*C*) sagittal CT images show an avulsion fracture of the dorsal talar head (*arrows*). (*D*) AP radiograph and (*E*) axial CT images show an avulsion fracture of the dorsolateral cuboid (*straight arrows*). Note the prominent soft tissue swelling in the lateral hindfoot and midfoot on the radiograph which is a clue to the subtle diagnosis (*curved arrows* in *D*).

best seen on lateral radiographs of the foot and ankle and on sagittal CT and MR images (see **Fig. 15**).

Midtarsal sprain injuries are often associated with small avulsion fractures as discussed previously, which can be very subtle on radiography and sometimes CT as well. Therefore, MR imaging may be used in these circumstances to diagnose the associated ligamentous injuries that occur and to detect areas of bone marrow edema with or without associated fractures (**Fig. 16**).

Eversion midtarsal injuries With the less common eversion mechanism of injury in midtarsal sprain, the fractures that occur can also be subdivided into two categories: (1) avulsion fractures of the medial column of the foot and (2) impaction fractures of the lateral column.[88] Medial column avulsion fractures involve the navicular tuberosity and are due to tensile force applied by the PTT and superomedial SL and are best seen on AP radiographs of the foot and axial CT and MR images.[88] Lateral column nutcracker-type impaction fractures occur at the lateral aspect of the calcaneocuboid joint, producing impaction fractures of the anterior process of the calcaneus and posterolateral cuboid, and are best seen on lateral and oblique radiographs of the foot and lateral radiographs of the ankle and on sagittal or axial CT and MR images.[88]

Lisfranc Ligament

Epidemiology
Midfoot sprains are more common in athletes and have been reported to occur in up to 4% of American football.[103] Low impact injures of the midfoot may result in a Lisfranc ligament sprain. High-impact injures result in Lisfranc fracture subluxation/dislocation, accounting for 0.2% of all fractures and less than 1% of dislocations.[30] The importance of recognizing this injury lies in its poor long-term prognosis when treatment is inadequate, inappropriate, or delayed.[104] Chronic pain, functional loss, and arthrosis are the potential sequelae of delayed or inappropriate treatment.[104,105] The rate of missed diagnosis of Lisfranc injuries is as high as 35%.[106]

Functional anatomy
The Lisfranc joint, also known as the tarsometatarsal (TMT) joint, is a complex system composed of osseous (TMT, intertarsal, and intermetatarsal), articular surfaces, and soft tissue components (articular capsules, TMT ligaments, and tendons).[107] The intermetatarsal and TMT ligaments are part of the thick joint capsule, whereas the Lisfranc ligament is a discrete structure, which has been somewhat variably described in the literature as consisting of plantar and dorsal bundles.[108] One classification system described by De Palma and colleagues and used by Castro and colleagues includes dividing the complex into three

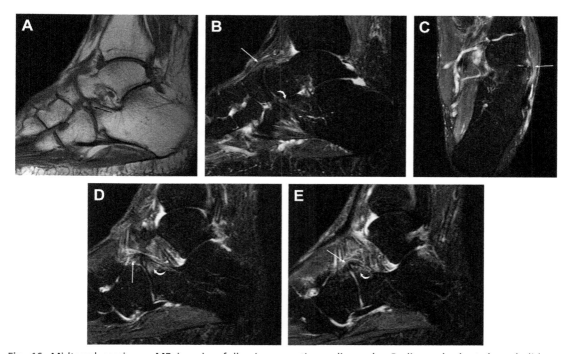

Fig. 16. Midtarsal sprain on MR imaging following negative radiographs. Radiographs (not shown) did not demonstrate any evidence of fracture. (*A*) Sagittal T1 MR image demonstrates a non-displaced avulsion fracture of anterior process of calcaneus (*arrow*). (*B*) Sagittal STIR MR image demonstrates a sprain of the dorsal talona-vicular ligament (*straight arrow*) and bone marrow edema in the anterior calcaneal process (*curved arrow*). (*C*) Axial T2 FS MR image shows a sprain of the dorsal calcaneocuboid ligament (*arrow*). (*D*) Sagittal STIR MR image demonstrates a sprain of the calcaneonavicular component of the bifurcate ligament (*straight arrow*) with bone marrow edema in anterior process of calcaneus (*curved arrow*). (*E*) Sagittal STIR MR image located slightly more lateral demonstrates a sprain of the calcaneocuboid component of the bifurcate ligament (*straight arrow*) with bone marrow edema in anterior process of calcaneus (*curved arrow*).

groups: dorsal, interosseous, and plantar compo-nents.[107] In general, the dorsal components are weaker than the plantar components.[104,105,109]

Five metatarsal bases and the distal row of tarsal bones, connected by TMT ligaments, make up the Lisfranc joint. The TMT ligaments are composed of dorsal, interosseous, plantar, inter-metatarsal, and intertarsal ligaments. There are seven dorsal TMT ligaments, which appear as short, flat, homogeneous, low signal strips, best seen on sagittal or coronal MR images.[107] The Lis-franc ligament, the first of three interosseous TMT ligaments, originates from the lateral cortex of the first/medial cuneiform and connects to the medial cortex of the second metatarsal base plantarly.[105,107,109,110]

The second plantar TMT ligament (also termed the plantar Lisfranc ligament) originates from the inferolateral surface of the medial cuneiform below the Lisfranc ligament, splitting into two bands. The superficial short thin band attaches to the base of second metatarsal and a thicker longer band courses to attach to third metatarsal.

This ligament is best visualized on the long axis axial and transverse oblique imaging planes, but can also be seen in the short axis coronal plane. Both the Lisfranc ligament and the plantar Lis-franc ligament have an oblique anterolateral orientation.[107]

Clinical considerations and mechanism of injury
Patients with Lisfranc injuries present with pain at the TMT joint of the midfoot and cannot bear weight on the affected foot. Popping or snapping, midfoot edema, shortening of the foot, limited forefoot abduction or adduction, and/or plantar ecchymosis can be seen.[30,109] The functional sta-tus can be evaluated by assessing gait, the medial arch, weight bearing on toes, or the pronation-abduction test.[109]

The mechanisms of injury can be divided into direct and indirect trauma. Direct trauma from a blow or a crush injury such as dropping a weight on the foot is less common than indirect trauma.[30,62,111] Indirect forces include forced plantar flexion and forefoot abduction.[105] Plantar

Table 2 Classification of Lisfranc injuries	
Classification of Lisfranc Injury[112]	
Type A	Total incongruity of the tarsometatarsal joint with homolateral or dorsoplantar displacement of the first to fifth metatarsals
Type B	Partial incongruity with medial dislocation of the first metatarsals and lateral dislocation of the second to the fifth metatarsals
Type C	Divergent, with partial or total displacement of the first metatarsal medially and the lesser metatarsals laterally

flexion injuries are more common in the setting of Lisfranc fracture dislocations.[111] In this position, the forefoot acts as an extension of the entire lower extremity. When the full body weight force is applied on the Lisfranc joint and the TMT can no longer support the tension across the dorsum of the midfoot, the joint gives way.[105,111] Specifically, the weaker dorsal components are the first to give way.[111] This is similar to the mechanisms of a misstep from a curb with the forefoot "rolled over" by the entire body.[105] The dorsal band maintains plantar flexion and often develops partial tears.[62] Forefoot abduction injuries occur in players with cleats when the foot is planted and rotates to change direction.[105] A similar mechanism is a fall from a horse when the foot is caught in the stirrup.[109]

Diagnostic imaging

Lisfranc injuries are associated with fractures in up to 90% of cases, most commonly involving the medial aspect of the second metatarsal base or the distal lateral aspect of the middle cuneiform.[106,112] Myerson described small cortical avulsions as the "fleck sign" on radiography.[112] CT is considered a good diagnostic tool in detecting fractures not seen on radiography and/or MR imaging, and subtle misalignment not seen on radiographs.[104] MR is more sensitive than CT in identifying the extent of post-traumatic bone marrow edema and the number of bones of the tarsus affected but is similar to CT in detecting malalignment.[30,62]

MR imaging is superior in demonstrating the ligaments of the midfoot.[104] Lisfranc ligament disruption is demonstrated on MR imaging even in the setting of normal weight-bearing radiographs.[113] On radiography, diastasis between the base of the first and second metatarsal greater than 2 mm on weight-bearing is suggestive of Lisfranc injury.[62] Complete tears are seen as displacement of the second metatarsal and medial cuneiform.[62] It has been suggested that non-weight-bearing radiographs miss up to 10% of TMT injuries.[114] Other positive radiographic findings include malalignment of the lateral margins of the first metatarsal and medial cuneiform and the medial margins of the fourth metatarsal and cuboid.[104]

There are two types of Lisfranc injuries: homolateral and divergent.[30] Myerson and colleagues described a classification system based on segmental pattern of injury (**Table 2**) On MR imaging, the Lisfranc ligament is usually well seen on oblique axial long axis MR images of the foot.[104] The short axis oblique coronal and oblique sagittal

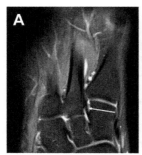
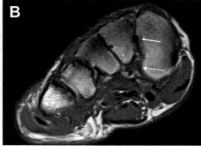
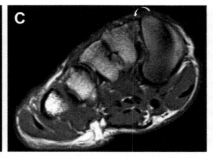

Fig. 17. Normal Lisfranc ligament. (*A*) Fat-saturated T2 MR image in the long axis plane and (*B* and *C*) short axis coronal PD MR images showing the Lisfranc ligament complex. The dorsal band (*curved arrow*) originates along the dorsolateral aspect of the medial cuneiform and inserts along the dorsomedial aspect of the base of the second metatarsal. The interosseous band (*solid arrow*) originates along the central lateral aspect of the medial cuneiform and inserts along the central medial aspect of the base of the second metatarsal. The plantar band (*dashed arrow*) originates at the plantar lateral aspect of the medial cuneiform and inserts into the plantar medial aspect of the base of the second and third metatarsals.

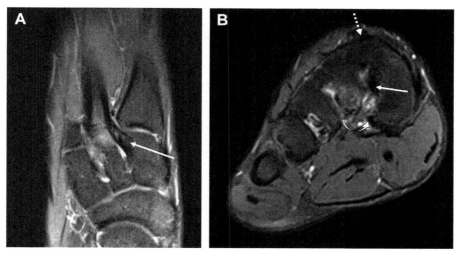

Fig. 18. Partial tear of the Lisfranc ligament. (A) Long axis fat-saturated PD and (B) short axis coronal fat-saturated T2 images showing partial intrasubstance tear of the interosseous component (*white arrow*) of the Lisfranc ligament complex. Low-grade sprain of the plantar component of the Lisfranc ligament (*curved arrow*). The dorsal component (*dashed arrow*) is also intact. Note marrow contusion in the second metatarsal base.

images are less effective in visualizing the ligament. The ligament is depicted as a homogenous band of low signal intensity, which courses obliquely from the medial cuneiform to the base of the second metatarsal (**Fig. 17**).[20] The length, width, and thickness range for the interosseous Lisfranc ligament was 7 to 11 mm, 4 to 8 mm, and 5 to 9 mm, respectively.[107]

MR imaging affords detection of Lisfranc ligament tears, which were depicted as either partial or complete absence or fragmentation of the ligament (**Figs. 18 and 19**).[115] Commonly associated fractures occur at the base of second or third metatarsals, the medial aspect of the medial and middle cuneiforms, or the navicular bone. Other findings include fraying or tearing of the Lisfranc ligament with or without synovitis, subchondral bone marrow edema at the TMT joints suggestive of a chip fracture or trabecular fracture, capsular edema and tears, lateral column shortening,

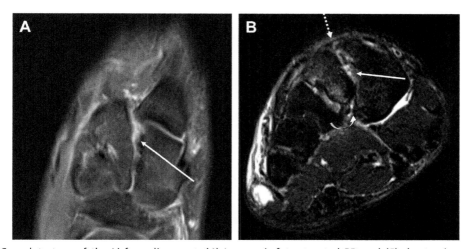

Fig. 19. Complete tear of the Lisfranc ligament. (A) Long axis fat-saturated PD and (B) short axis coronal fat-saturated T2 images showing complete discontinuity and avulsion of the interosseous component (*white arrow*) of the Lisfranc ligament complex with surrounding edema. The plantar component of the Lisfranc ligament (*arrowhead*) is also discontinuous and replaced by fluid-like signal consistent with a high-grade tear (*arrowhead*). The dorsal component (*dashed arrow*) is also torn. Note marrow edema in the second metatarsal base related to fracture in this location (not shown).

disruption of the dorsal arch, arterial injury, and marrow edema in the displaced metatarsals, or medial and middle cuneiforms.[26]

TREATMENT IMPLICATIONS

Immediate management of ligament sprains involves RICE (Rest, Ice, Compression, Elevation).[15,116] Ice-cooling, or cryotherapy, and the use of nonsteroidal anti-inflammatory drugs may enhance the healing process and speed up the recovery. Low-grade sprains (Grades I–II) are treated conservatively, with preference for functional rehabilitation over immobilization. Strengthening exercises and motion restoration are used as functional rehabilitation tools[116]: air cast, elastic brace, elastic support bandage, training on wobble board, ankle disk training, imagery, and resistive walking boot. The treatment of severe sprain (Grade III) is controversial in the literature; a suggested approach is to treat with conservative functional measures and if this fails, surgical repair may be performed.[15]

In summary, current MR imaging technology provides exquisite delineation of the ankle ligaments. In particular, clear depiction of the normal anatomy and the typical morphologic changes involving the ligamentous structures of the ankle following sprain injury is widespread in today's MR clinical practice.

CLINICS CARE POINTS

- Populations at increased risk of ankle sprain include athletes, military personnel, and other populations that are predisposed to this injury from running, jumping, and cutting motions.

- Clinical examination is often limited in ability to accurately diagnose the ligaments involved in acute ankle sprains therefore MR imaging can play a singificant role in making the correct diganosis when patients do not respond to conservative management.

- Treatment of ankle sprains depends on the severity of injury. Low-grade ankle sprains are treated conservatively, with preference for functional rehabilitation over immobilization. The treatment of severe sprain varies but a suggested approach is to treat with conservative functional measures and if this fails, surgical repair may be performed.

DISCLOSURE

The authors have nothing to disclosure.

REFERENCES

1. Waterman BR, Owens BD, Davey S, et al. The epidemiology of ankle sprains in the United States. J Bone Joint Surg Am 2010;92(13):2279–84.
2. Gribble PA, Bleakley CM, Caulfield BM, et al. Evidence review for the 2016 International Ankle Consortium consensus statement on the prevalence, impact and long-term consequences of lateral ankle sprains. Br J Sports Med 2016;50(24):1496–505.
3. Herzog MM, Kerr ZY, Marshall SW, et al. Epidemiology of ankle sprains and chronic ankle instability. J Athl Train 2019;54(6):603–10.
4. McCriskin BJ, Cameron KL, Orr JD, et al. Management and prevention of acute and chronic lateral ankle instability in athletic patient populations. World J Orthop 2015;6(2):161–71.
5. Fong DT, Hong Y, Chan LK, et al. A systematic review on ankle injury and ankle sprain in sports. Sports Med 2007;37(1):73–94.
6. Roos KG, Kerr ZY, Mauntel TC, et al. The epidemiology of lateral ligament complex ankle sprains in national collegiate athletic association sports. Am J Sports Med 2017;45(1):201–9.
7. Waterman BR, Belmont PJ Jr, Cameron KL, et al. Risk factors for syndesmotic and medial ankle sprain: role of sex, sport, and level of competition. Am J Sports Med 2011;39(5):992–8.
8. Attenborough AS, Hiller CE, Smith RM, et al. Chronic ankle instability in sporting populations. Sports Med 2014;44(11):1545–56.
9. Valderrabano V, Hintermann B, Horisberger M, et al. Ligamentous posttraumatic ankle osteoarthritis. Am J Sports Med 2006;34(4):612–20.
10. Raatikainen T, Putkonen M, Puranen J. Arthrography, clinical examination, and stress radiograph in the diagnosis of acute injury to the lateral ligaments of the ankle. Am J Sports Med 1992;20(1):2–6.
11. van Dijk CN, Lim LSL, Bossuyt PMM, et al. Physical examination is sufficient for the diagnosis of sprained ankles. J Bone Joint Surg Br 1996;78-B(6):958–62.
12. Yeung MS, Chan KM, So CH, et al. An epidemiological survey on ankle sprain. Br J Sports Med 1994;28(2):112–6.
13. van Rijn RM, van Os AG, Bernsen RMD, et al. What Is the Clinical Course of Acute Ankle Sprains? A Systematic Literature Review. Am J Med 2008;121(4):324–31. e7.
14. Harrington KD. Degenerative arthritis of the ankle secondary to long-standing lateral ligament instability. J Bone Joint Surg 1979;61(3):354–61.

15. Fong DT, Chan Y-Y, Mok K-M, et al. Understanding acute ankle ligamentous sprain injury in sports. BMC Sports Sci Med Rehabil 2009;1(1):14.

16. Hamilton WG. Foot and ankle injuries in dancers. Clin Sports Med 1988;7(1):143–73.

17. Kannus P, Renström P. Treatment for acute tears of the lateral ligaments of the ankle. Operation, cast, or early controlled mobilization. J Bone Joint Surg 1991;73(2):305–12.

18. Griffith JF, Brockwell J. Diagnosis and Imaging of Ankle Instability. Foot Ankle Clin 2006;11(3): 475–96.

19. Rosenberg ZS, Beltran J, Bencardino JT. MR Imaging of the Ankle and Foot. RadioGraphics 2000; 20(suppl_1):S153–79.

20. Rosenberg Z, Beltran J. Magnetic resonance imag- ing and computed tomography of the ankle and foot. In: Myerson MS, editor. Foot and ankle disorders1. Philadelphia: Saunders1; 1998. p. 123–56.

21. Muhle C, Frank LR, Rand T, et al. Collateral liga- ments of the ankle: high-resolution MR imaging with a local gradient coil and anatomic correlation in cadavers. RadioGraphics 1999;19(3):673–83.

22. Mesgarzadeh M, Schneck CD, Tehranzadeh J, et al. Magnetic resonance imaging of ankle liga- ments. Magn Reson Imaging Clin N Am 1994; 2(1):39–58.

23. Boonthathip M, Chen L, Trudell DJ, et al. Tibiofibu- lar syndesmotic ligaments: mr arthrography in ca- davers with anatomic correlation. Radiology 2010; 254(3):827–36.

24. Schneck CD, Mesgarzadeh M, Bonakdarpour A, et al. MR imaging of the most commonly injured ankle ligaments. Part I. Normal anatomy. Radiology 1992;184(2):499–506.

25. Labovitz J, Schweitzer M, Larka U, et al. Magnetic resonance imaging of ankle ligament injuries corre- lated with time. J Am Podiatr Med Assoc 1998; 88(8):387–93.

26. Labovitz JM, Schweitzer ME. Occult osseous in- juries after ankle sprains: incidence, location, pattern, and age. Foot Ankle Int 1998;19(10): 661–7.

27. Verhaven EFC, Shahabpour M, Handelberg FWJ, et al. The accuracy of three-dimensional magnetic resonance imaging in the diagnosis of ruptures of the lateral ligaments of the ankle. Am J Sports Med 1991;19(6):583–7.

28. Schneck CD, Mesgarzadeh M, Bonakdarpour A. MR imaging of the most commonly injured ankle ligaments. Part II. Ligament injuries. Radiology 1992;184(2):507–12.

29. Beltran J, Munchow AM, Khabiri H, et al. Ligaments of the lateral aspect of the ankle and sinus tarsi: an MR imaging study. Radiology 1990;177(2):455–8.

30. Stoller D, Ferkel R. Magnetic Resonance Imaging in Orthopaedics and Sports Medicine2007. 733- 1050 p.

31. Hertel J. Functional anatomy, pathomechanics, and pathophysiology of lateral ankle instability. J Athl Train 2002;37(4):364–75.

32. Rockar PA. The subtalar joint: anatomy and joint motion. J Orthop Sports Phys Ther 1995;21(6): 361–72.

33. Norkus SA, Floyd RT. The anatomy and mecha- nisms of syndesmotic ankle sprains. J Athl Train 2001;36(1):68–73.

34. Boytim MJ, Fischer DA, Neumann L. Syndesmotic ankle sprains. Am J Sports Med 1991;19(3):294–8.

35. Gerber JP, Williams GN, Scoville CR, et al. Persis- tent disability associated with ankle sprains: a pro- spective examination of an athletic population. Foot Ankle Int 1998;19(10):653–60.

36. Skraba JS, Greenwald AS. The role of the inteross- eous membrane on tibiofibular weightbearing. Foot & Ankle 1984;4(6):301–4.

37. Hermans JJ, Beumer A, De Jong TAW, et al. Anat- omy of the distal tibiofibular syndesmosis in adults: a pictorial essay with a multimodality approach: Anatomy of the distal tibiofibular syndesmosis. J Anat 2010;217(6):633–45.

38. Dattani R, Patnaik S, Kantak A, et al. Injuries to the tibiofibular syndesmosis. J Bone Joint Surg Br 2008;90-B(4):405–10.

39. Takao M, Ochi M, Naito K, et al. Arthroscopic diag- nosis of tibiofibular syndesmosis disruption. J Arthroscopic Relat Surg 2001;17(8):836–43.

40. Brown KW, Morrison WB, Schweitzer ME, et al. MRI findings associated with distal tibiofibular syndes- mosis injury. Am J Roentgenol 2004;182(1):131–6.

41. Vogl TJ, Hochmuth K, Diebold T, et al. Magnetic resonance imaging in the diagnosis of acute injured distal tibiofibular syndesmosis. Invest Ra- diol 1997;32(7):401–9.

42. Oae K, Takao M, Naito K, et al. Injury of the tibiofib- ular syndesmosis: value of MR imaging for diag- nosis. Radiology 2003;227(1):155–61.

43. Ebraheim NA, Taser F, Shafiq Q, et al. Anatomical evaluation and clinical importance of the tibiofibu- lar syndesmosis ligaments. Surg Radiol Anat 2006;28(2):142–9.

44. Ray RG, Kriz BM. Anterior inferior tibiofibular liga- ment. Variations and relationship to the talus. J Am Podiatr Med Assoc 1991;81(9):479–85.

45. Gyftopoulos S, Bencardino JT. Normal variants and pitfalls in MR imaging of the ankle and foot. Magn Reson Imaging Clin N Am 2010;18(4):691–705.

46. Muhle C, Frank LR, Rand T, et al. Tibiofibular syn- desmosis: high-resolution MRI using a local gradient coil. J Comput Assist Tomogr 1998; 22(6):938–44.

47. Rosenberg ZS, Cheung YY, Beltran J, et al. Posterior intermalleolar ligament of the ankle: normal anatomy and MR imaging features. Am J Roentgenol 1995;165(2):387–90.

48. Oh CS, Won HS, Hur MS, et al. Anatomic variations and MRI of the intermalleolar ligament. AJR Am J Roentgenol 2006;186(4):943–7.

49. Sandelin J, Santavirta S, Lättilä R, et al. Sports injuries in a large urban population: occurrence and epidemiological aspects. Int J Sports Med 1988;9(1):61–6.

50. Fallat L, Grimm DJ, Saracco JA. Sprained ankle syndrome: prevalence and analysis of 639 acute injuries. J Foot Ankle Surg 1998;37(4):280–5.

51. Haraguchi N, Toga H, Shiba N, et al. Avulsion fracture of the lateral ankle ligament complex in severe inversion injury: incidence and clinical outcome. Am J Sports Med 2007;35(7):1144–52.

52. Attarian DE, McCrackin HJ, DeVito DP, et al. Biomechanical Characteristics of Human Ankle Ligaments. Foot & Ankle. 1985;6(2):54–8.

53. Safran MR, Benedetti RS, Bartolozzi AR, et al. Lateral ankle sprains: a comprehensive review Part 1: etiology, pathoanatomy, histopathogenesis, and diagnosis. Med Sci Sports Exerc 1999; 31(Supplement):S429–37.

54. de Asla RJ, Kozánek M, Wan L, et al. Function of anterior talofibular and calcaneofibular ligaments during in-vivo motion of the ankle joint complex. J Orthopaedic Surg Res 2009;4(1):7.

55. Chan KW, Ding BC, Mroczek KJ. Acute and chronic lateral ankle instability in the athlete. Bull NYU Hosp Jt Dis 2011;69(1):17–26.

56. Bahr R, Pena F, Shine J, et al. Mechanics of the anterior drawer and talar tilt tests: A cadaveric study of lateral ligament injuries of the ankle. Acta Orthop Scand 1997;68(5):435–41.

57. Dubin JC, Comeau D, McClelland RI, et al. Lateral and syndesmotic ankle sprain injuries: a narrative literature review. J Chiropractic Med 2011;10(3):204–19.

58. Bencardino J, Rosenberg ZS, Delfaut E. MR imaging in sports injuries of the foot and ankle. Magn Reson Imaging Clin N Am 1999;7(1):131–49.

59. Rijke AM, Goitz HT, McCue FC, et al. Magnetic resonance imaging of injury to the lateral ankle ligaments. Am J Sports Med 1993;21(4):528–34.

60. Dimmick S, Kennedy D, Daunt N. Evaluation of thickness and appearance of anterior talofibular and calcaneofibular ligaments in normal versus abnormal ankles with MRI. J Med Imaging Radiat Oncol 2008;52(6):559–63.

61. Milner CE, Soames RW. Anatomy of the collateral ligaments of the human ankle joint. Foot Ankle Int 1998;19(11):757–60.

62. Cheung Y, Rosenberg ZS. MR imaging of ligamentous abnormalities of the ankle and foot. Magn Reson Imaging Clin N Am 2001;9(3):507–31.

63. Bencardino JT, Rosenberg ZS. Normal variants and pitfalls in mr imaging of the ankle and foot. Magn Reson Imaging Clin N Am 2001;9(3):447–63.

64. Chhabra A, Subhawong TK, Carrino JA. MR imaging of deltoid ligament pathologic findings and associated impingement syndromes. RadioGraphics 2010;30(3):751–61.

65. Klein MA. MR imaging of the ankle: normal and abnormal findings in the medial collateral ligament. Am J Roentgenol 1994;162(2):377–83.

66. Rasmussen O. Stability of the Ankle Joint: Analysis of the Function and Traumatology of the Ankle Ligaments. Acta Orthop Scand 1985;56(sup211):1–75.

67. Hintermann B, Knupp M, Pagenstert GI. Deltoid ligament injuries: diagnosis and management. Foot Ankle Clin 2006;11(3):625–37.

68. Rasmussen O, Kromann-Andersen C, Boe S. Deltoid ligament: functional analysis of the medial collateral ligamentous apparatus of the ankle joint. Acta Orthop Scand 1983;54(1):36–44.

69. Henari S, Banks LN, Radovanovic I, et al. Ultrasonography as a diagnostic tool in assessing deltoid ligament injury in supination external rotation fractures of the ankle. Orthopedics 2011;34(10):e639–43.

70. Mengiardi B, Pfirrmann CW, Vienne P, et al. Medial collateral ligament complex of the ankle: MR appearance in asymptomatic subjects. Radiology 2007;242(3):817–24.

71. Beltran J. Sinus tarsi syndrome. Magn Reson Imaging Clin N Am 1994;2(1):59–65.

72. Breitenseher MJ, Haller J, Kukla C, et al. MRI of the sinus tarsi in acute ankle sprain injuries. J Comput Assist Tomogr 1997;21(2):274–9.

73. Klein MA, Spreitzer AM. MR imaging of the tarsal sinus and canal: normal anatomy, pathologic findings, and features of the sinus tarsi syndrome. Radiology 1993;186(1):233–40.

74. Lowy A, Schilero J, Kanat IO. Sinus tarsi syndrome: a postoperative analysis. J Foot Surg 1985;24(2):108–12.

75. Balen PF, Helms CA. Association of Posterior Tibial Tendon Injury with Spring Ligament Injury, Sinus Tarsi Abnormality, and Plantar Fasciitis on MR Imaging. Am J Roentgenol 2001;176(5):1137–43.

76. Toye LR, Helms CA, Hoffman BD, et al. MRI of Spring Ligament Tears. Am J Roentgenol 2005;184(5): 1475–80.

77. Ting AYI, Morrison WB, Kavanagh EC. MR Imaging of Midfoot Injury. Magn Reson Imaging Clin N Am 2008;16(1):105–15.

78. Desai KR, Beltran LS, Bencardino JT, et al. The spring ligament recess of the talocalcaneonavicular joint: depiction on MR images with cadaveric and histologic correlation. Am J Roentgenol 2011;196(5):1145–50.

79. Mengiardi B, Zanetti M, Schöttle PB, et al. Spring ligament complex: MR imaging–anatomic correlation and findings in asymptomatic subjects. Radiology 2005;237(1):242–9.

80. Gazdag AR, Cracchiolo A. Rupture of the posterior tibial tendon. evaluation of injury of the spring ligament and clinical assessment of tendon transfer and ligament repair. J Bone Joint Surg (American Volume) 1997;79(5):675–81.

81. Kavanagh EC, Koulouris G, Gopez A, et al. MRI of rupture of the spring ligament complex with talocuboid impaction. Skeletal Radiol 2007;36(6):555–8.

82. Yao L, Gentili A, Cracchiolo A. MR imaging findings in spring ligament insufficiency. Skeletal Radiol 1999;28(5):245–50.

83. Rule J, Yao L, Seeger LL. Spring ligament of the ankle: normal MR anatomy. Am J Roentgenol 1993;161(6):1241–4.

84. Taniguchi A, Tanaka Y, Takakura Y, et al. Anatomy of the spring ligament. J Bone Joint Surgery-American Volume 2003;85(11):2174–8.

85. Andermahr J, Helling H-J, Maintz D, et al. The Injury of the Calcaneocuboid Ligaments. Foot Ankle Int 2000;21(5):379–84.

86. Lohrer H, Nauck T. Augmented periosteal flap repair of the chronically unstable calcaneocuboid joint: a series of six cases. JBJS 2006;88(7): 1596–601.

87. Søndergaard L, Konradsen L, Hølmer P, et al. Acute Midtarsal Sprains: Frequency and Course of Recovery. Foot Ankle Int 1996;17(4):195–9.

88. Walter WR, Hirschmann A, Alaia EF, et al. JOURNAL CLUB: MRI Evaluation of Midtarsal (Chopart) Sprain in the Setting of Acute Ankle Injury. AJR Am J Roentgenol 2018;210(2):386–95.

89. Thiounn A, Szymanski C, Lalanne C, et al. Prospective observational study of midtarsal joint sprain: Epidemiological and ultrasonographic analysis. Orthop Traumatol Surg Res 2016;102(5):657–61.

90. van Dorp KB, de Vries MR, van der Elst M, et al. Chopart joint injury: a study of outcome and morbidity. J Foot Ankle Surg 2010;49(6):541–5.

91. Blackwood CB, Yuen TJ, Sangeorzan BJ, et al. The midtarsal joint locking mechanism. Foot Ankle Int 2005;26(12):1074–80.

92. Walter WR, Hirschmann A, Alaia EF, et al. Normal anatomy and traumatic injury of the midtarsal (chopart) joint complex: an imaging primer. RadioGraphics 2018;39(1):136–52.

93. Patil V, Ebraheim N, Wagner R, et al. Morphometric dimensions of the dorsal calcaneocuboid ligament. Foot Ankle Int 2008;29(5):508–12.

94. Lohrer H, Nauck T, Arentz S, et al. Dorsal calcaneocuboid ligament versus lateral ankle ligament repair: a case-control study. Br J Sports Med 2006;40(10): 839–43.

95. Melao L, Canella C, Weber M, et al. Ligaments of the transverse tarsal joint complex: MRI-anatomic correlation in cadavers. AJR Am J Roentgenol 2009;193(3):662–71.

96. Ward KA, Soames RW. Morphology of the plantar calcaneocuboid ligaments. Foot Ankle Int 1997; 18(10):649–53.

97. Zwipp H, Rammelt S, Grass R. Ligamentous injuries about the ankle and subtalar joints. Clin Podiatr Med Surg 2002;19(2):195–229.

98. Lee SW, Kim DD, Buskanets A, et al. Midtarsal Sprain Misdiagnosed as Ankle Sprain: Role of Ultrasonography in Diagnosis. Am J Phys Med Rehabil 2016; 95(3):e44–5.

99. Main BJ, Jowett RL. Injuries of the midtarsal joint. J Bone Joint Surg Br 1975;57-B(1):89–97.

100. Hermel MB, Gershon-Cohen J. The nutcracker fracture of the cuboid by indirect violence. Radiology 1953;60(6):850–4.

101. Rammelt S, Schepers T. Chopart injuries: when to fix and when to fuse? Foot Ankle Clin 2017;22(1): 163–80.

102. Hirschmann A, Walter WR, Alaia EF, et al. Acute fracture of the anterior process of calcaneus: does it herald a more advanced injury to chopart joint? Am J Roentgenol 2018;210(5):1123–30.

103. Meyer SA, Callaghan JJ, Albright JP, et al. Midfoot sprains in collegiate football players. Am J Sports Med 1994;22(3):392–401.

104. Gupta RT, Wadhwa RP, Learch TJ, et al. Lisfranc injury: imaging findings for this important but often-missed diagnosis. Curr Probl Diagn Radiol 2008;37(3):115–26.

105. Hatem SF. Imaging of lisfranc injury and midfoot sprain. Radiol Clin North Am 2008;46(6):1045–60.

106. Vuori J-P, Aro HT. Lisfranc joint injuries. trauma mechanisms and associated injuries. J Trauma Inj Infect Crit Care 1993;35(1):40–5.

107. Castro M, Melão L, Canella C, et al. Lisfranc joint ligamentous complex: MRI with anatomic correlation in cadavers. Am J Roentgenol 2010;195(6):W447–55.

108. MacMahon PJ, Dheer S, Raikin SM, et al. MRI of injuries to the first interosseous cuneometatarsal (Lisfranc) ligament. Skeletal Radiol 2009;38(3):255–60.

109. Mullen JE, O'Malley MJ. Sprains—residual instability of subtalar, Lisfranc joints, and turf toe. Clin Sports Med 2004;23(1):97–121.

110. Kura H, Luo Z-P, Kitaoka HB, et al. Mechanical Behavior of the Lisfranc and Dorsal Cuneometatarsal Ligaments: In Vitro Biomechanical Study. J Orthop Trauma 2001;15(2):107–10.

111. Curtis MJ, Myerson M, Szura B. Tarsometatarsal joint injuries in the athlete. Am J Sports Med 1993;21(4):497–502.

112. Myerson MS, Fisher RT, Burgess AR, et al. Fracture Dislocations of the Tarsometatarsal Joints: End Results Correlated with Pathology and Treatment. Foot & Ankle 1986;6(5):225–42.

113. Hatem SF, Davis A, Sundaram M. The case: Your diagnosis? Orthopedics 2005;28(1):2–77.

114. Arntz CT, Veith RG, Hansen ST. Fractures and fracture-dislocations of the tarsometatarsal joint. J Bone Joint Surg 1988;70(2):173–81.

115. Resnick D, Niwayama G. Diagnosis of bone and joint disorders. 1995.

116. Ivins D. Acute ankle sprain: an update. Am Fam Physician 2006;74(10):1714–20.

117. Peetrons P, Creteur V, Bacq C. Sonography of ankle ligaments. J Clin Ultrasound 2004;32(9): 491–9.

118. Campbell DG, Menz A, Isaacs J. Dynamic Ankle Ultrasonography: A New Imaging Technique for Acute Ankle Ligament Injuries. Am J Sports Med 1994;22(6):855–8.

119. Nakasa T, Fukuhara K, Adachi N, et al. Evaluation of Anterior Talofibular Ligament Lesion Using 3-Dimensional Computed Tomography. J Comput Assist Tomogr 2006;30(3):543–7.

120. van Dijk CN, Molenaar AHM, Cohen RH, et al. Value of arthrography after supination trauma of the ankle. Skeletal Radiol 1998;27(5):256–61.

121. Chandnani VP, Harper MT, Ficke JR, et al. Chronic ankle instability: evaluation with MR arthrography, MR imaging, and stress radiography. Radiology 1994;192(1):189–94.

Imaging of Rheumatic Diseases Affecting the Lower Limb

Aurea Valeria Rosa Mohana-Borges, MD[a], Christine B. Chung, MD[a,b],*

KEYWORDS

- Imaging • MR imaging • Ultrasound • CT • Conventional radiography • Osteoarthritis
- Rheumatoid arthritis • Gout

KEY POINTS

- MR imaging and ultrasonography can identify early findings of joint inflammation and structural damage associated with arthritis and are of paramount importance in the management of inflammatory rheumatic diseases.
- MR imaging is the best imaging modality for assessment of whole organ abnormalities associated with osteoarthritis.
- Ultrasonography and dual-energy computed tomography are biomarkers for evaluation of gouty arthritis.

INTRODUCTION
Discussion of Problem/Clinical Presentation

The successful use of disease-modifying antirheumatic drugs, which interrupt the inflammatory cascade, provided strong motivation for identification of biomarkers of inflammation, subclinical disease, and earliest objective findings of active disease. In this context, imaging methods capable of detecting inflammation, such as MR imaging and ultrasound (US), are of paramount importance in rheumatic disease management, not only for diagnostic purposes but also for monitoring disease activity and treatment response. The purpose of this review is to provide an overview of imaging of some of the most prevalent inflammatory rheumatic diseases affecting the lower limb (osteoarthritis [OA], rheumatoid arthritis [RA], and gout) and up-to-date recommendations regarding imaging diagnostic workup.

OSTEOARTHRITIS
Background

OA is the most prevalent form of arthritis, with a chronic and progressive course. In the 2019 Global Health Data Exchange, OA had an estimated global prevalence of more than 527.8 million cases surpassing common conditions of the modern world, such as depression, anxiety, and interpersonal violence. A large proportion of the OA burden is caused by involvement of joints of the lower limbs, such as knee and hip, which account for approximately 60.6% and 5.5%, respectively, of years lived with disability attributed to the disease.[1] OA can lead to undesirable long-term opioid addiction as a "side effect" of chronic pain therapy and to joint replacement at end stage of the disease.[2] As we might expect, joint replacement surgeries have become one of the most common orthopedic procedures worldwide, especially total knee arthroplasty.[3]

[a] Department of Radiology, University of California San Diego, 9427 Health Sciences Drive, La Jolla, CA 92093, USA; [b] Department of Radiology, VA San Diego, 3350 La Jolla Village Drive, La Jolla, CA 92161, USA
* Corresponding author. Department of Radiology, University of California San Diego, 9427 Health Sciences Drive, La Jolla, CA 92093
E-mail address: cbchung@health.ucsd.edu

Radiol Clin N Am 61 (2023) 345–360
https://doi.org/10.1016/j.rcl.2022.10.007
0033-8389/23/Published by Elsevier Inc.

OA was traditionally considered a degenerative articular disease, caused by "wear and tear." However, new molecular biology techniques in association with findings of advanced imaging methods progressively changed the way the scientific community has come to view the disease. It is now considered a much more complex condition affecting the whole joint, with both biomechanical and inflammatory drivers.[4] Several risk factors are implicated to trigger a low-grade inflammation in the joint inducing structural damage. They include, but are not limited to, age, female gender, prior joint injury, obesity, genetic predisposition, and mechanical factors, such as malalignment and abnormal joint shape.[5]

Imaging Findings

Findings of inflammation and structural damage can be identified by several imaging methods (**Fig. 1**). Joints often compromised in the lower limb are knee, hip, and first metatarsophalangeal joint. Osteoarthritic changes elsewhere in the foot, such as the subtalar joint, are usually caused by altered mechanics from congenital or acquired abnormalities (eg, pes planus, coalition, trauma) or are secondary to another underlying arthropathy (eg, psoriasis, reactive arthritis).[6]

Radiography

Radiography in OA can directly identify structural damage by the presence of osteophytes (bone

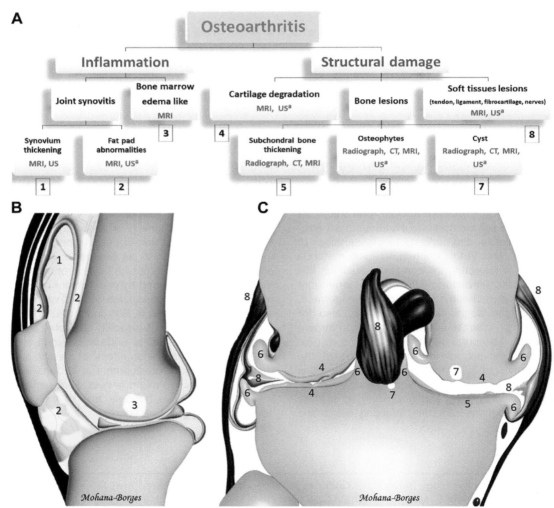

Fig. 1. (*A*) Flowchart of alterations observed in OA with best imaging methods for diagnosis. Accompanying diagrams in (*B*) lateral and (*C*) anterior views. Note. There are limitations in the use of US in the evaluation of deep-seated structures. However, US can be reliably used to evaluate superficial joint pathologies such as marginal erosions and marginal synovial cysts.

outgrowths), subchondral bone sclerosis, and bone cysts. Joint space narrowing is another important radiographic finding but should be considered the indirect and nonspecific sequelae of cartilage loss, meniscal volume reduction, and/or meniscus extrusion. In OA, joint space narrowing is usually asymmetric as opposed to the symmetric joint reduction observed in RA. In the knee, asymmetric distribution more often predominates in the medial compartment. In the hip, superior joint space narrowing predominates (Fig. 2). On weight-bearing knee radiographs, a finding of joint space greater than 5 mm is considered normal and less than 3 mm, an absolute indication of joint space narrowing.

Subchondral sclerosis occurs as cartilage loss increases and appears as an area of increased density on the radiograph. In the advanced stage of the disease, subchondral remodeling with collapse of the joint may occur; however, ankylosis is usually not present in patients with primary OA.[6] Subchondral cysts usually have a sclerotic border and may or may not communicate with the joint space and can occur before cartilage loss.[6] However, the last two findings are best visualized by MR imaging.

In 1952, Kellgren and Lawrence (KL) introduced a 5-grade radiographic classification system for OA[7] (Figs. 3 and 4). In KL classification, the most important radiographic finding for diagnosis is the definite presence of osteophyte, and to

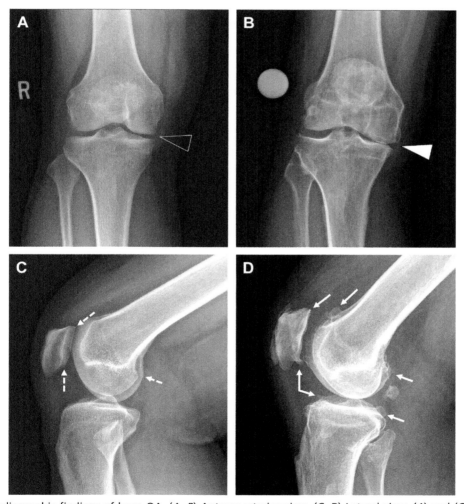

Fig. 2. Radiographic findings of knee OA. (A, B) Anteroposterior view. (C, D) Lateral view. (A) and (C) demonstrate a mild OA, with possible reduction of the medial joint space (open arrowhead) and tiny osteophytes (dotted arrows). (B) and (D) demonstrate a moderate to severe OA with reduction of the medial joint space (arrowhead) and moderate to large-sized osteophytes (arrows in D). Marginal subchondral bone sclerosis is observed in the medial tibial plateau with slight bone deformity associated. Also note irregularity in contour of the femoral trochlea in lateral view (D). This case demonstrates findings of bicompartmental OA, involving the medial femorotibial and patellofemoral compartments.

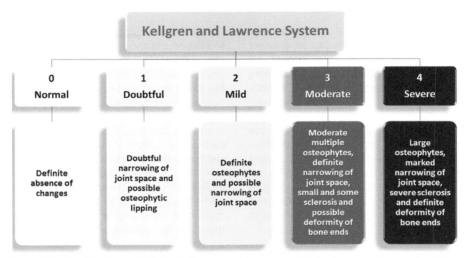

Fig. 3. Radiographic classification of OA by Kellgren and Lawrence. OA is diagnosed in grades ≥2.

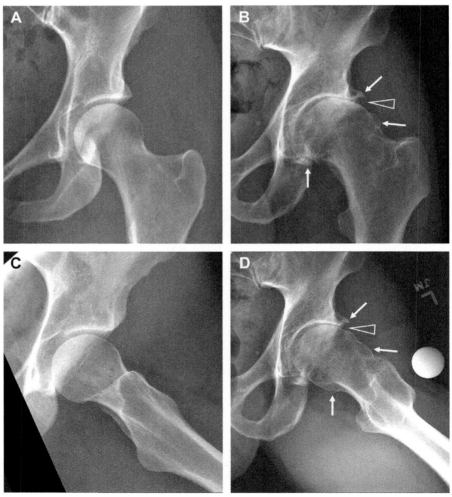

Fig. 4. Radiographic findings of hip OA. (*A, B*) Anteroposterior (AP) view. (*C, D*) Lateral view. (*A*) and (*C*) demonstrate normal hip joint (KG 0) with preservation of joint space and absence of osteophytes. (*B*) and (*D*) show marked osteoarthritic (KG 4) changes with large marginal osteophytes (*arrows*), marked narrowing of the superior joint space (*open arrowhead*), severe sclerosis in the lateral aspect of the femoral head and acetabulum, and femoral head deformity.

Advantages of radiography are low-cost, wide availability, and short imaging time. Disadvantages are the use of ionizing radiation and detection of more advanced disease as it is unable to directly visualize synovium and cartilage as well as insensitive to detect soft tissues abnormalities.[11] Radiographs are also subjected to a lack of reproducibility of joint space measurements in longitudinal assessment.[11]

MR Imaging

MR imaging can directly identify joint inflammation and structural damage, being suitable for diagnosis of both early and advanced OA. Detection of early OA by MR imaging is a window of opportunity to prevent further articular damage and avoid pain sensitization. In addition to the conventional morphologic joint evaluation,[12] MR imaging can also be applied in semi-quantitative (SQ) scoring systems of the whole joint,[13–15] quantitative analysis of the biochemical composition of the joint tissues (compositional MR imaging),[16] and quantitative volumetric analyses of cartilage and other tissues (quantitative MR imaging)[17,18] (**Box 1, Table 1**). Disadvantages of MR imaging are the higher cost and longer time for imaging in comparison with radiographs, US, and computed tomography (CT).

Morphologic MR Imaging

Synovitis is characterized by synovial thickening and enhancement in post-contrast imaging and may be accompanied by variable amounts of joint fluid (effusion).[19,20] On conventional MR imaging, synovitis and synovial fluid can be difficult to distinguish as the synovium typically appears hyperintense on T2-weighted sequences and hypo- to isointense to skeletal muscle and cartilage on T1-weighted sequences.[20] More recently, promising novel non-contrast enhanced assessment of synovitis was proposed with sequences such as fluid attenuated inversion recovery (FLAIR) with fat-saturated, quantitative double-echo in steady state (qDESS), and dual inversion recovery (DIR).[20]

In the knee, synovitis may be associated with areas of edema and contour irregularities in fat pads, such as prefemoral, suprapatellar, and Hoffa's fat pad. However, edema in fat pads seems to be a nonspecific measure of synovitis when contrast enhancement is used as the reference.[19]

Bone marrow lesions (BMLs), also called bone marrow edema (BME), are ill-defined areas of altered signal intensity best seen as hyperintensities on fluid-sensitive sequences.[21] Some authors avoid the term BME because the altered

estimate the severity of the disease, the narrowing of the joint space. KL grading system continues to be used today for diagnosis and disease progression. Additional OA classification systems and atlas were proposed by Ahlbäck,[8] Osteoarthritis Research Society International,[9] and Altman and colleagues.[10]

Table 1
MR imaging sequences for evaluation of (A) synovitis and (B) bone

Synovitis	Bone Lesion

Morphologic
  Fluid-sensitive sequences (fat-saturated PD-
    weighted and T2-weighted and STIR):
    Detects articular fluid produced by synovium
  T1-contrasted enhanced:
    Detects enhancement in areas of synovitis
Compositional
  Diffusion tensor imaging:
    Restricted motion of water in joints as a
      result of inflammatory cell aggregation
Functional
  Dynamic contrast-enhanced MR imaging:
    Characterize the uptake and washout of
      gadolinium-based contrast agents in
      synovium, providing biomarkers of tissue
      perfusion, capillary permeability, and
      blood and interstitial volume
	Morphologic
	  T1-weighted:
	    Detects bone erosion, attrition, and fracture
	  Fluid-sensitive sequences (PD-weighted and
	    T2-weighted and STIR):
	    Detects bone marrow edema-like cysts
	  T1-contrasted enhanced:
	    Detects enhancement in areas of osteitis/
	      bone marrow edema like
	Compositional
	  UTE (quantitative ultrashort echo time) T2*,
	    ZTE, MT:
	    Detects alterations in composition of
	      osteochondral junction and bone

Abbreviations: GAG, glycosaminoglycan; MT, magnetization transfer; PD, proton density; ZTE, zero echo time.

signal in OA is due to a combination of several non-characteristic histologic abnormalities that include bone marrow necrosis, bone marrow fibrosis, and trabeculae abnormalities.[22] In OA, BMLs are frequently detected in conjunction with areas of cartilage damage (**Fig. 5**). The identification of BMLs is relevant because they are associated with pain and greater OA severity. Furthermore, their presence may predict OA progression.[23]

Regarding structural damage, the T1-weighted sequence is the best sequence for evaluation of osteophytes (bone outgrowths) and subchondral bone remodeling. However, cartilage is best evaluated on fluid-sensitive sequences, especially intermediate-weighted fast spin-echo sequences.[24,25] Cartilage lesions usually have higher signal intensity in comparison to normal cartilage signal, which is caused by damage to collagenous ultrastructure and increased free water. This

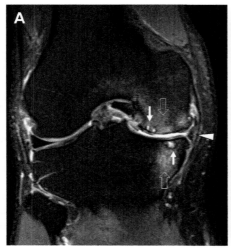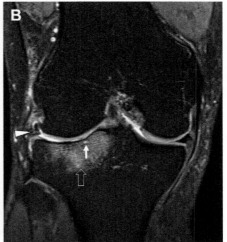

Fig. 5. MR imaging findings of OA in the knee. (*A*) Medial compartment OA and (*B*) lateral compartment OA. Note bone marrow lesions (*open arrows*) with associated subchondral bone cysts (*arrows*). In (*A*) cartilage lesions are more pronounced in the femoral condyle and in (*B*) in the tibial plateau. Note associated meniscal lesions (*arrowhead*) in both cases.

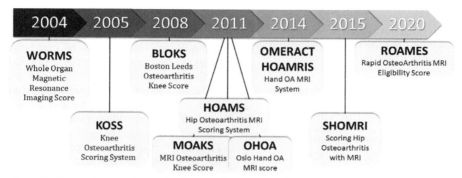

Fig. 6. Timeline of MR imaging semiquantitative grading systems for OA.

mechanism is elegantly exploited in compositional MR imaging.

Semiquantitative MR Imaging

Several SQ MR imaging grading systems have been developed for evaluation of OA in the knee (Whole Organ Magnetic Resonance Score [WORMS], KOSS, BLOKS, MOAKS, ROAMES), hip (HOAMS, SHOMRI), and hand (OHOA, HOAM-RIS)[26,27] (**Fig. 6**). The first comprehensive MR imaging-based SQ scoring system was published in 2004 and received the name WORMS.[13] WORMS is a complex and detailed system with features evaluated in 15 different regions subdivided by anatomic landmarks.[26] WORMS protocol is time-consuming and developed in a research environment. The last published MR imaging grading system, ROAMES, on the other hand, was proposed to be a simplified version of previous systems, with less features to be evaluated and less subdivisions of anatomic regions for analysis. In ROAMES, investigators introduced five different imaging phenotypes (inflammatory, subchondral bone, meniscus/cartilage, atrophic, and hypertrophic), aimed to explore potential targets for clinical trials of disease-modifying OA drug.[28]

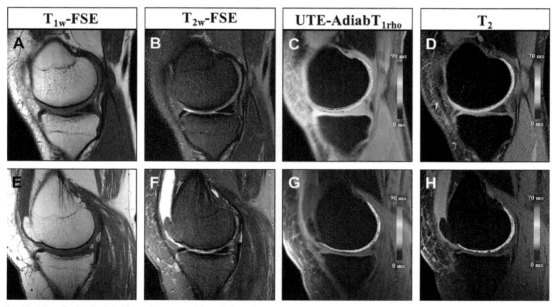

Fig. 7. Morphologic (*A, B*) and compositional (*C, D*) MR imaging in OA. Sagittal images in the medial femorotibial compartment demonstrate cartilage findings in (*A–D*) a 23-year-old male and (*E–H*) 74-year-old female with diagnosis of OA. In both cases, compositional MR imaging can identify changes in the cartilage (*C, D, G, H*) characterized by areas of increased T1-rho and T2 values (*yellow and red*), more pronounced in established OA (*G, H*). Morphologic sequences in (*A*) and (*B*) were insensitive to cartilage abnormalities. (*Courtesy* of Y Ma, PhD, San Diego, California.)

Table 2
Outcome measures in rheumatology clinical ultrasound semiquantitative scoring system for cartilage abnormalities in osteoarthritis

Grade	Classification	Finding
Grade 0	Normal joint	Normal cartilage (anechoic structure, normal margins of cartilage)
Grade 1	Small cartilage loss	Loss of anechoic structure and/or focal thinning of cartilage layer OR irregularities and/or loss of sharpness of at least one cartilage margin
Grade 2	Moderate cartilage loss	Loss anechoic structure and/or focal thinning of cartilage layer AND irregularities and/or loss of sharpness of at least one cartilage margin
Grade 3	Severe cartilage loss	Focal absence or complete loss of the cartilage layer

Compositional MR Imaging

Compositional MR imaging aims to identify early damage and breakdown of cartilage exploring changes that occur in cartilage macromolecules. In OA, proteoglycan and collagen content are reduced. This disrupts the collagen network and results in matrix degradation and increased water content.[29] Compositional MR imaging sequences can be divided into collagen-sensitive, for example, T2 and T2* mapping, and proteoglycan-sensitive, for example, T1-rho and dGEMRIC (delayed gadolinium-enhanced MR imaging of cartilage)[30] (Fig. 7). In T2–T2* mapping and T1-rho, increased values are associated with decreased collagen and proteoglycan content in hyaline cartilage and meniscus.[31]

Ultrasonography

Like MR imaging, US can identify synovitis and much of the structural damage associated with OA. It is cheaper and faster than MR imaging and without nonionizing radiation. However, there are limitations associated with the acoustic window and wave penetration, with only partial visualization of deeper joint tissues. In knee OA, US adds diagnostic information over radiographs primarily by its ability to directly visualize cartilage and meniscus as well as to sensitively depict effusion and synovitis.[27] The Outcome Measures in

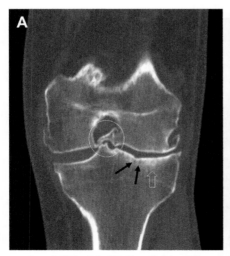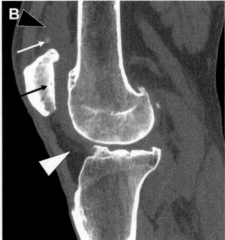

Fig. 8. Conventional CT in OA. CT directly identifies structural damage related to bone and indirectly damage to cartilage and meniscus by means of evaluation of joint space narrowing. Note (A) bridging hypertrophic osteophytes in the region of the intercondylar (*circle*) notch resulting in mass effect on and impingement of the cruciate ligaments. Joint space narrowing in the lateral femorotibial compartment is associated with subchondral sclerosis (*open large arrow*) and cysts (*black arrows*). Subchondral cysts are manifested as well-marginated lucent foci, in this case of small size (*black arrows* in A and B). (B) Joint effusion (black *arrowhead*) and soft tissue abnormalities, such as infiltration of Hoffa's fat pad (*white arrowhead*) are usually better identified by CT than radiography but not as well visualized as by MR imaging. However, small intra-articular bodies (*white arrow*) are better visualized by CT than MR imaging.

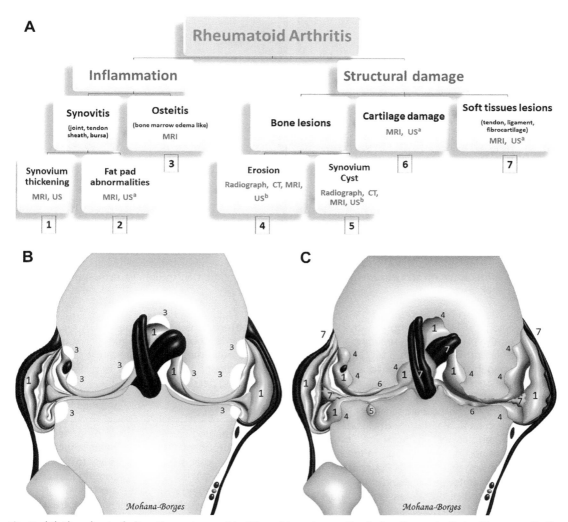

Fig. 9. (*A*) Flowchart of alterations observed in RA and imaging methods for diagnosis. Note. There are limitations in the use of US in the evaluation of deep-seated structures. However, US can be reliably used to evaluate superficial joint pathologies such as marginal erosions and marginal synovial cysts. Accompanying diagrams with findings of (*B*) inflammation and (*C*) inflammation and structural damage. Fat pad abnormalities (2) not shown.

Rheumatology Clinical Trials (OMERACT) of US created a grading system for cartilage loss (**Table 2**) and osteophytes (varying from 0 normal to 3 severe) to assess OA in finger, which can also be applied to other joints.

Computed Tomography

Like radiographs, conventional CT can identify structural damage (**Fig. 8**). Identification of soft tissue abnormalities with CT is better than with radiograph, but less sensitive than with MR imaging. However, techniques such as CT arthrography and PET/CT add value in the investigation of the soft tissues and synovitis. A recent novel use of CT arthrography is the ability to measure sulfated

glycosaminoglycans (GAGs) in a similar way of compositional MR imaging, such as dGEMRIC. Contrast agent uptake and GAG content correlate negatively for anionic agents, that is, the higher the uptake the lower the GAG content, and positively for cationic agents, that is, the higher uptake, the higher the GAG content.[32]

RHEUMATOID ARTHRITIS
Background

RA is the typical synovium-based inflammatory arthritis. RA is a systemic chronic autoimmune disease with production of autoantibodies, such as rheumatoid factor and anti-citrullinated protein antibody. The current understanding of the

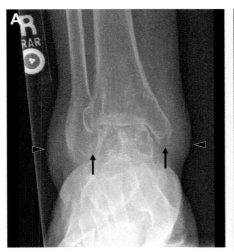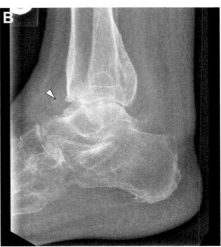

Fig. 10. Radiographic findings in RA. Ankle (*A*) AP and (*B*) lateral views. Note soft tissue swelling (*black arrowheads*), joint effusion (*white arrowhead*) and diffuse osteopenia, in addition to bone structural damage, such as erosions (*black arrows*).

pathophysiology of RA has progressed and proposes a genetic predisposition resulting in autoreactive T cells and B cells, and a triggering event providing antigen-presenting cells to activate the autoreactive lymphocytes.[33]

Unlike OA, which typically affects one specific joint or fewer joints at presentation, RA is classically described as a symmetric small joint polyarthritis with additional involvement of large joints.[34] Joints commonly involved in the feet are metatarsal phalangeal joints (MTPs) and proximal interphalangeal joints. Jacoby and colleagues reported involvement of the knees, ankle, and MTP in 56%, 53%, and 48% of cases, respectively.[35] Positive RF is one of the best predictors of small joint erosions.

Imaging Findings

Imaging methods for RA diagnosis and follow-up that identify early synovial inflammation, such as US and MR imaging, are superior to the ones that only diagnosis later structural damage, such as conventional radiography and CT (**Fig. 9**).

Radiography

Radiographic analysis should start with the location and distribution of radiologic findings, considering that in the feet, RA affects more proximal joints compared with OA and psoriatic arthritis, which predominate in the distal joints. Early radiographic findings identified in RA are soft tissue swelling and osteoporosis. Findings of established disease and advanced damage are erosions, cysts, joint space narrowing, and deformity (**Fig. 10**). Detection

of bone erosions at the time of RA diagnosis is related to a poor long-term functional and radiographic outcome, and the presence of erosions in early undifferentiated arthritis is a risk factor for developing persistent arthritis.[36]

MR Imaging

RA MR imaging scoring system proposed by the working group of OMERACT was initially developed and validated from 1998 to 2002 and updated in 2016.[37] Their recommendations for basic MR imaging sequences are T1-weighted images before and after IV gadolinium-contrast injection for detection of erosions and synovitis, with visualization in two planes. The fluid-sensitive sequence T2-weighted fat-sat and STIR images, on the other hand, are recommended for assessment of BME/osteitis, whereas tenosynovitis can be assessed either by the fluid-sensitive sequences or by precontrast and postcontrast T1-weighted images[37] (**Fig. 11**). Osteitis identified by MR imaging has been shown to be highly predictive of subsequent bone erosion.

Ultrasonography

In 2017, the European League Against Rheumatisms (EULAR) in collaboration with OMERACT US task force published a consensus-based definition for synovitis in RA.[38] The consensus stated that synovial hypertrophy is necessary for synovitis even in the absence of Doppler signal. Greater than 90% of participants agreed not to consider effusion alone (ie, without concomitant synovial hypertrophy) as a sign of synovitis and not to define

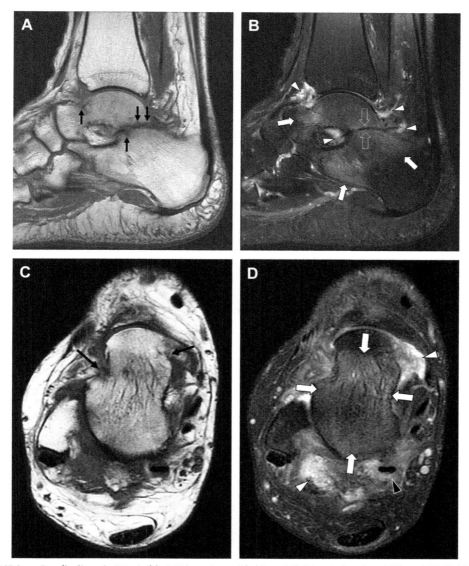

Fig. 11. MR imaging findings in RA. Ankle MR imaging with (*A* and *C*) T1-weighted and (*B*) and (*D*) fluid-sensitive sequences. The inclusion of T1-weighted sequence in the basic protocol for RA aim to improve the detection of erosions (*black arrows*) while the inclusion of fluid sensitive images, the detection of effusion (*white arrowhead*), bone marrow edema (*large white arrow*), and tenosynovitis (*black arrowhead*). Note in (*B*) the well depiction of joint space narrowing (*open large arrows*).

and score joint effusion and synovial hypertrophy together as components of a common process.[38]

Doppler US is used to evaluate soft tissue hyperemia and distinguish active from inactive inflammatory tissue. Ongoing angiogenesis in areas of synovial hypertrophy is responsible for the intra-articular Doppler signal. The continued presence of intensely perfused areas of synovial hypertrophy inside the joint is a reliable indicator of insufficient response to therapy and is predictive of the development of erosions.[39]

Computed Tomography

CT can detect bone erosions more accurately than other techniques, such as MR imaging, US, and radiography but is limited in the detection of synovitis and soft tissue abnormalities.[40] Another disadvantage of CT in routine clinical practice is the radiation exposure. One alternative to conventional CT in the evaluation of peripheral joints is the novel and sensitive technique high-resolution peripheral quantitative CT that is reported to have a

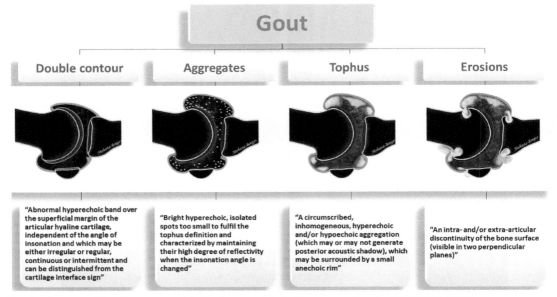

Fig. 12. Gout-specific ultrasonographic findings and definitions according to OMERACT USWG.

very low radiation dose with maintenance of the high accuracy of conventional CT for erosion detection.[40]

GOUT
Background

Gout is the second most prevalent form of arthritis, only behind OA, and is characterized by chronic deposition of monosodium urate (MSU) crystals, which form in the presence of increased urate concentrations. The clinical features of gout occur as a result of the inflammatory response to monosodium urate crystals.[41]

Gout is more common in men than in women with male to female sex ratio varying from 2:1 to 8:1 depending on the population-based studies.[41] The incidence and prevalence of gout also

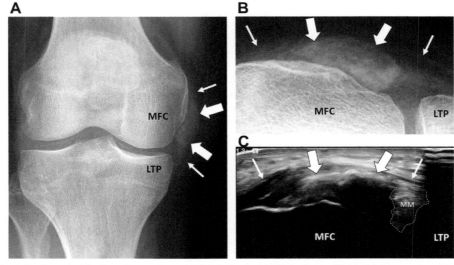

Fig. 13. Gout findings in (*A*, *B*) radiograph and (*C*) US. Radiograph in B was flipped to correspond to US image. Note the tophus (*large arrows*) compressing the joint capsule (*small arrows*). The tophus has a slightly higher density than surrounding soft tissues in radiograph (*A* and *B*). (*C*) The tophi in US have a globular inhomogeneous hyperechoic appearance associated with acoustic shadowing. LTP, lateral tibial plateau; MCF, medial femoral condyle; MM, medial meniscus. (*Courtesy of* Karen Chen, MD, San Diego, California.)

increase with age. Several risk factors are associated with gout, such as genetic, drugs, dietary, and metabolic syndrome.[41]

Acute gouty arthritis is typically of sudden onset, involving one or few joints (less frequently polyarticular), with a preference for inferior limbs (in 85% of cases), particularly for the first metatarsophalangeal space.[42] The predilection for the first MTP joint, a condition known as podagra, is related to local anatomic characteristic of lower temperature and repetitive physical trauma.

Imaging

Imaging in gout is traditionally focused on the detection of tophus, a chronic, foreign-body granulomatous inflammatory response to MSU crystals deposits,[41] and USG and dual-energy CT (DECT) have a high sensitivity and specificity for tophus detection and are the preferred method for diagnosis. Both US and DECT have been incorporated in the American College of Rheumatology (ACR)/EULAR 2015 gout classification criteria.[43]

Radiography

In acute gouty arthritis, radiographs are most of the time normal or display a nonspecific joint effusion and/or periarticular soft tissue edema. Some radiographic features seen in chronic gouty arthritis are intermediate to high-density tophi in subcutaneous or intraosseous location, well-defined, "punched-out" periarticular bone erosions with overhanging edges adjacent to tophus,

with relative preservation of joint space and osseous mineralization.

MR Imaging

MR imaging cannot specifically identify MSU crystals, as in the case of US and DECT, but it provides important information about the presence of synovitis, erosions, and BME.[44] Another advantage of MR imaging is its ability to visualize deeper structures as well as intraosseous deposits, not accessible to US.[44] Some disadvantages of the method are the high cost and time of imaging.

MR imaging features of gout are variable. Tophi may have intermediate or low signal intensity on T1-weighted and heterogeneous signal intensity on fluid-sensitive sequences, depending on the degree of hydration and its calcium concentration.[45] Tophi show intense gadolinium enhancement due to hypervascular soft tissue and granulation tissue that surround tophi. A clue to the diagnosis of gout in the setting of generic inflammatory changes is that BME is uncommon and if present is often mild, the presence of extensive BME on MR imaging should raise the question of infection.[45]

Ultrasonography

Characteristic ultrasonographic findings in gout can be divided into general findings and gout-specific findings. The general ultrasonographic findings include synovitis and tenosynovitis along with subcutaneous edema which are common in

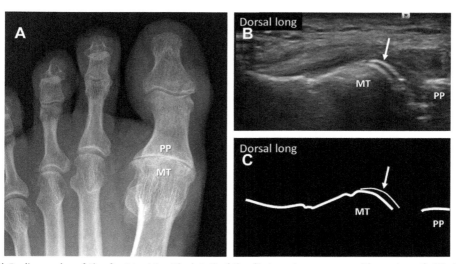

Fig. 14. (A) Radiography of the foot in AP with detail of the first ray in a person with gouty arthritis. Note joint space narrowing in the metatarsophalangeal joint and soft tissue swelling in the distal interphalangeal joint. (B) US of the metatarsophalangeal joint of the hallux demonstrates the double contour (arrow) at the level of the metatarsal head. (C) Corresponding diagram. (Courtesy of Karen Chen, MD, San Diego, California.)

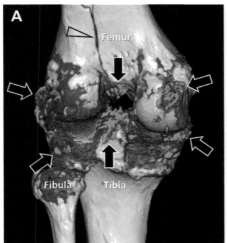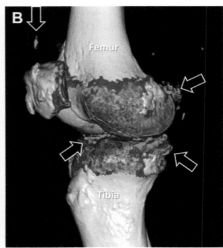

Fig. 15. DECT findings in gout. (*A*) Posterior view. (*B*) Lateral view. Monosodium urate crystal deposits are demonstrated in green (*arrows*). Note incidental fracture in the femur (*arrowhead*). (*Courtesy of* Karen Chen, MD, San Diego, California.)

patients with ongoing joint attacks. The gout-specific findings include visualization of the crystal deposits in both joints and tendons and definitions were provided by OMERACT US working group.[46] They include double contour, aggregated, tophus, and erosion (**Figs. 12–14**).

Computed Tomography and Dual-Energy Computed Tomography

In the early stages of gout, standard CT has little utility because it is not suitable for imaging the soft tissue inflammation that characterizes early gout. Later in the progression of the disease, bone erosions and tophi can be visualized and quantified.[47] Tophi have a characteristic density of around 160 Hounsfield units and volume and density measurements can be performed using CT.

DECT has revolutionized gout imaging. The technology can separate urate and calcium in a highly sensitive way because the tissues have different absorption spectra on 80-keV and 140/150-keV voltage.[48] Thus, DECT has become the recommended modality to diagnose urate distribution around the joint in 3D and even automatically calculate the volume of urate along with any change of urate load after treatment (**Fig. 15**). In addition, with a bone algorithm, conventional CT images can be used to detect potential erosive changes with better sensitivity and in more detail than either radiograph or MR imaging.[48,49] DECT has reduced the need for aspiration of joint fluid and phase-contrast microscopic analysis to make the diagnosis and for these reasons has

become part of the classification system for gout evaluation recommended by both ACR and EULAR.[48]

SUMMARY

The imaging diagnostic workup in arthritis is based on the identification of inflammation and structural damage. In practice, radiographs still a frequent method of investigation not because the ability for detection of abnormalities but availability and cost. MR imaging and US can detect synovium hypertrophy, increased vascularity, bone and cartilage damage, and intra-articular and extra-articular soft tissue abnormalities. However, US have some limitations in visualization of deeper joint tissues caused by bone interference in the acoustic window and the tradeoff of penetration and resolution. US and DECT are recommended as the first line of investigation of tophus because of high sensitivity and specificity in comparison with other imaging methods.

CLINICS CARE POINTS

- Clinicians should be aware of the limitations of radiographs in assessing inflammation in rheumatological diseases and the implications in patient treatment.

- BMLs and synovitis mediate pain in OA, and the best imaging method for the simultaneous evaluation of these findings is MR imaging.

- US and MR imaging can detect early findings of inflammation in RA, which is relevant for the clinical management of patients.
- US and DECT are recommended as the first line of investigation of the gouty tophus.

DISCLOSURE

The authors having nothing to disclosure.

REFERENCES

1. Long H, Liu Q, Yin H, et al. Prevalence trends of site-specific osteoarthritis from 1990 to 2019: findings from the Global Burden of Disease Study 2019. Arthritis Rheumatol 2022. https://doi.org/10.1002/art.42089.
2. Safiri S, Kolahi AA, Smith E, et al. Global, regional and national burden of osteoarthritis 1990-2017: A systematic analysis of the global burden of disease study 2017. Ann Rheum Dis 2020. https://doi.org/10.1136/annrheumdis-2019-216515.
3. Cisternas AF, Ramachandran R, Yaksh TL, et al. Unintended consequences of COVID-19 safety measures on patients with chronic knee pain forced to defer joint replacement surgery. Pain Rep 2020;5(6). https://doi.org/10.1097/PR9.0000000000000855.
4. Mobasheri A, Batt M. An update on the pathophysiology of osteoarthritis. Ann Phys Rehabil Med 2016;59(5–6):333–9.
5. Loeser RF, Goldring SR, Scanzello CR, et al. Osteoarthritis: A disease of the joint as an organ. Arthritis Rheum 2012;64(6):1697–707.
6. Swagerty DL, Hellinger D. Radiographic assessment of osteoarthritis. Am Fam Physician 2001;64(2):279–86. http://www.ncbi.nlm.nih.gov/pubmed/11476273.
7. KELLGREN JH, LAWRENCE JS. Rheumatism in miners. II. X-ray study. Br J Ind Med 1952;9(3):197–207.
8. Ahlbäck S. Osteoarthrosis of the knee. a radiographic investigation. Acta Radiol Diagn (Stockh) 1968;277:7–72. Available at: http://www.ncbi.nlm.nih.gov/pubmed/5706059.
9. Altman RD, Hochberg M, Murphy WA, et al. Atlas of individual radiographic features in osteoarthritis. Osteoarthritis Cartilage 1995;3:3–70.
10. Altman R, Asch E, Bloch D, et al. Development of criteria for the classification and reporting of osteoarthritis: Classification of osteoarthritis of the knee. Arthritis Rheum 1986;29(8):1039–49.
11. Guermazi A, Roemer FW, Burstein D, et al. Why radiography should no longer be considered a surrogate outcome measure for longitudinal assessment of cartilage in knee osteoarthritis. Arthritis Res Ther 2011;13(6). https://doi.org/10.1186/ar3488.
12. Bae W, Du J, Bydder G, et al. Conventional and ultrashort MRI of articular cartilage, meniscus and intervertebral disc. Top Magn Reson Imaging 2010;21(5):275–89. Conventional.
13. Peterfy CG, Guermazi A, Zaim S, et al. Whole-organ magnetic resonance imaging score (WORMS) of the knee in osteoarthritis. Osteoarthr Cartil 2004;12(3):177–90.
14. Kornaat PR, Ceulemans RYT, Kroon HM, et al. MRI assessment of knee osteoarthritis: knee osteoarthritis scoring system (KOSS) - inter-observer and intra-observer reproducibility of a compartment-based scoring system. Skeletal Radiol 2005;34(2):95–102.
15. Hunter DJ, Lo GH, Gale D, et al. The reliability of a new scoring system for knee osteoarthritis MRI and the validity of bone marrow lesion assessment: BLOKS (Boston-Leeds Osteoarthritis Knee Score). Ann Rheum Dis 2008;67(2):206–11.
16. Ariyachaipanich A, Bae WC, Statum S, et al. Update on MRI pulse sequences for the knee: imaging of cartilage, meniscus, tendon, and hardware. Semin Musculoskelet Radiol 2017;21(2):45–62.
17. Wang Y-XJ. Non-invasive MRI assessment of the articular cartilage in clinical studies and experimental settings. World J Radiol 2010;2(1):44.
18. Eckstein F, Wirth W. Quantitative cartilage imaging in knee osteoarthritis. Arthritis 2011;2011:1–19.
19. Guermazi A, Roemer FW, Hayashi D, et al. Assessment of synovitis with contrast-enhanced MRI using a whole-joint semiquantitative scoring system in people with, or at high risk of, knee osteoarthritis: the MOST study. Ann Rheum Dis 2011;70(5):805–11.
20. Thoenen J, MacKay JW, Sandford HJC, et al. Imaging of synovial inflammation in osteoarthritis, from the AJR special series on inflammation. Am J Roentgenol 2022;218(3):405–17.
21. Roemer FW, Frobell R, Hunter DJ, et al. MRI-detected subchondral bone marrow signal alterations of the knee joint: terminology, imaging appearance, relevance and radiological differential diagnosis. Osteoarthr Cartil 2009;17(9):1115–31.
22. Zanetti M, Bruder E, Romero J, et al. Bone marrow edema pattern in osteoarthritic knees: Correlation between MR imaging and histologic findings. Radiology 2000;215(3):835–40.
23. Link T, Li X. Bone marrow changes in osteoarthritis. Semin Musculoskelet Radiol 2011;15(03):238–46.
24. Disler DG, Recht MP, McCauley TR. MR imaging of articular cartilage. Skeletal Radiol 2000;29(7):367–77.
25. Link TM, Stahl R, Woertler K. Cartilage imaging: motivation, techniques, current and future significance. Eur Radiol 2007;17(5):1135–46.
26. Jarraya M, Hayashi D, Roemer FW, et al. MR imaging-based semi-quantitative methods for knee osteoarthritis. Magn Reson Med Sci 2016;15(2):153–64.

27. Roemer FW, Demehri S, Omoumi P, et al. State of the art imaging of osteoarthritis. Radiology 2020;47(3): 2009.

28. Roemer FW, Collins J, Kwoh CK, et al. MRI-based screening for structural definition of eligibility in clinical DMOAD trials: Rapid OsteoArthritis MRI Eligibility Score (ROAMES). Osteoarthr Cartil 2020; 28(1):71–81.

29. Braun HJ, Gold GE. Advanced MRI of articular cartilage. Imaging Med 2011;3(5):541–55.

30. Chang EY, Ma Y, Du J. MR parametric mapping as a biomarker of early joint degeneration. Sports Health 2016;8(5):405–11.

31. Takao S, Nguyen TB, Yu HJ, et al. T1rho and T2 relaxation times of the normal adult knee meniscus at 3T: analysis of zonal differences. BMC Musculoskelet Disord 2017;18(1):1–9.

32. Freedman JD, Ellis DJ, Lusic H, et al. dGEMRIC and CECT comparison of cationic and anionic contrast agents in cadaveric human metacarpal cartilage. J Orthop Res 2020;38(4):719–25.

33. Lin Y-J, Anzaghe M, Schülke S. Update on the pathomechanism, diagnosis, and treatment options for rheumatoid arthritis. Cells 2020;9(4):880.

34. Llopis E, Kroon HM, Acosta J, et al. Conventional radiology in rheumatoid arthritis. Radiol Clin North Am 2017;55(5):917–41.

35. Jacoby RK, Jayson MIV, Cosh JA. Onset, early stages, and prognosis of rheumatoid arthritis: a clinical study of 100 patients with ii-year follow-up. Br Med J 1973;2(5858):96–100.

36. Døhn UM, Ejbjerg BJ, Court-Payen M, et al. Are bone erosions detected by magnetic resonance imaging and ultrasonography true erosions? A comparison with computed tomography in rheumatoid arthritis metacarpophalangeal joints. Arthritis Res Ther 2006;8(4):1–9.

37. Østergaard M, Peterfy CG, Bird P, et al. The OMERACT rheumatoid arthritis magnetic resonance imaging (MRI) scoring system: Updated recommendations by the OMERACT MRI in arthritis working group. J Rheumatol 2017;44(11):1706–12.

38. D'Agostino MA, Terslev L, Aegerter P, et al. Scoring ultrasound synovitis in rheumatoid arthritis: a EULAR-OMERACT ultrasound taskforce - Part 1: Definition and development of a standardised, consensus-based scoring system. RMD Open 2017;3(1):1–9.

39. Šenolt L, Grassi W, Szodoray P. Laboratory biomarkers or imaging in the diagnostics of rheumatoid arthritis? BMC Med 2014;12(1):1–6.

40. Barile A, Arrigoni F, Bruno F, et al. Computed Tomography and MR Imaging in Rheumatoid Arthritis. Radiol Clin North Am 2017;55(5):997–1007.

41. Dalbeth N, Gosling AL, Gaffo A, et al. Gout Lancet 2021;397(10287):1843–55.

42. Jacques T, Michelin P, Badr S, et al. Conventional radiology in crystal arthritis: gout, calcium pyrophosphate deposition, and basic calcium phosphate crystals. Radiol Clin North Am 2017;55(5):967–84.

43. Neogi T, Jansen TLTA, Dalbeth N, et al. 2015 Gout classification criteria: an American college of rheumatology/European league against Rheumatism collaborative initiative. Ann Rheum Dis 2015; 74(10):1789–98.

44. Araujo EG, Manger B, Perez-Ruiz F, et al. Imaging of gout: new tools and biomarkers? Best Pract Res Clin Rheumatol 2016;30(4):638–52.

45. Chowalloor PV, Siew TK, Keen HI. Imaging in gout: A review of the recent developments. Ther Adv Musculoskelet Dis 2014;6(4):131–43.

46. Gutierrez M, Schmidt WA, Thiele RG, et al. International consensus for ultrasound lesions in gout: Results of delphi process and web-reliability exercise. Rheumatol (United Kingdom) 2015;54(10): 1797–805.

47. Buckens CF, Terra MP, Maas M. Computed Tomography and MR Imaging in Crystalline-Induced Arthropathies. Radiol Clin North Am 2017;55(5): 1023–34.

48. Boesen M, Roemer FW, Østergaard M, et al. Imaging of common rheumatic joint diseases affecting the upper limbs. Radiol Clin North Am 2019;57(5): 1001–34.

49. McQueen FM, Doyle A, Dalbeth N. Imaging in gout - what can we learn from MRI, CT, DECT and US? Arthritis Res Ther 2011;13(6):246.

Imaging of Lower Limb Tumors and Tumor-Like Conditions

Sinan Al-Qassab, MBChB, MRCS, FRCR[a], Radhesh Lalam, MBBS, MRCS, FRCR[a,*],
Jaspreet Singh, MRCP, FRCR[a], Prudencia N.M. Tyrrell, MBBCh, BAO, MRCPI, FRCR[a]

KEYWORDS

• Bone tumors • Soft-tissue tumors • Lower limb • Tumor mimics

KEY POINTS

• Generally, bone and soft-tissue tumors are more common in the lower limbs.
• Many lesions are nonneoplastic but may mimic tumors.
• Age, anatomical location, relationship to adjacent structures and clinical history are pivotal in providing a reasonable diagnosis.
• Radiography is the primary imaging modality for bone lesions and ultrasound is the first imaging modality for soft-tissue lesions.

INTRODUCTION

The aim of this article was to deliver practical points to guide in the diagnosis and management of common lower limb tumors and tumor-like conditions. Bone tumors in general have a higher predilection to the lower limb. Knowledge of the patient's age is crucial in reaching the diagnosis as well as limiting the differential diagnosis of soft-tissue tumors according to their anatomic location.

BONE TUMORS

Primary bone tumors tend to show more male predominance. Four crucial parameters are used to give a reasonable differential diagnosis when a bone lesion is encountered. The patient's age (younger or older than 40 years), the anatomic location of the lesion within the bone (epiphyseal, metaphyseal or diaphyseal, cortical or medullary and central or eccentric), radiographic appearances (aggressive or not) and multiplicity. Radiographic features suggestive of a low biological activity (nonaggressive lesion) include a narrow zone of transition, sclerotic margins, absence of or a solid periosteal reaction, intact cortex, and lack of a soft-tissue component. Lesions of low biological activity displaying nonaggressive features are not necessarily benign and vice versa. For example, infections and langerhans cell histiocytosis (LCH) can demonstrate aggressive features on imaging and are clearly nonneoplastic, whereas low-grade osteosarcoma can have nonaggressive features on imaging and are clearly malignant neoplastic lesions.

Radiographically Nonaggressive Tumors

Patients younger than 40 years

Chondroblastomas is a frequently encountered *epiphyseal* lesion seen in children and young adults before 40 years of age with 50% of cases seen before skeletal maturity.[1] They most commonly affect the proximal tibia, followed by the proximal femur and the distal femur.[2] On radiography, they are lobulated eccentric lesions. They usually appear nonaggressive but may

The authors have nothing to disclose.
[a] Radiology Department, Robert Jones and Agnes Hunt Orthopaedic Hospital, Oswestry, SY10 7AG, UK
* Corresponding author.
E-mail address: radhesh.lalam@nhs.net

radiologic.theclinics.com

occasionally demonstrate aggressive features. They may have an aneurysmal bone cyst (ABC) component in 15% of cases.[3] Chondroblastomas can demonstrate internal mineralization in up to 50% of cases. Lesions demonstrating internal mineralization may appear similar to osteoblastomas although the latter are less frequently seen in the epiphysis. A characteristic feature on MR imaging is surrounding marrow and soft-tissue edema and synovitis (**Fig. 1**). Clear cell chondrosarcoma is an important differential diagnosis to consider and is difficult to differentiate on imaging. However, chondroblastomas tend to be in a younger age group (mean age 22.3 years compared with clear cell chondrosarcomas mean age 36.6 years), smaller and confined to the epiphysis compared with clear cell chondrosarcomas.[4]

Metaphyseal lesions demonstrating nonaggressive features include simple bone cysts, aneurysmal bone cysts (ABCs), nonossifying fibromas and osteochondromas. Simple (unicameral) cysts are central well defined lucent lesions. In the lower limb, they favor the proximal femur. They maybe multiloculated and may demonstrate slight expansion. On the contrary, aneurysmal bone cysts are eccentric, expansile lytic lesions that may have a "soap bubble" appearance. They classically demonstrated multiple fluid–fluid levels on cross-sectional imaging. In the lower limb, they favor the distal femur tibia and fibula. ABC may be primary or secondary to other lesions such as giant cell tumor (GCT), fibrous dysplasia, chondroblastoma and telangiectatic osteosarcoma. Primary ABC can demonstrate aggressive features however, rapid progression, clinical symptoms like pain and

soft-tissue swelling should raise the suspicion of a secondary ABC in an aggressive lesion like telangiectatic osteosarcoma. On imaging, noncystic, nodular/solid enhancing areas should be identified, which would suggest an underlying primary tumor and these areas should be targeted during biopsy (**Fig. 2**). Nonossifying fibromas and fibrous cortical defects are the commonest benign bone lesion seen in children and should not be considered in patients over the age of 30 years. They are eccentric cortical elongated lucent lesions. They are usually seen in the distal femur, proximal and distal tibial. They are painless, incidental, do not demonstrate periosteal reaction in the absence of a fracture and heal by sclerosis starting peripherally. Healed lesions may however be seen after 30 years of age. Possible differential diagnoses include osteoid osteomas and cortical desmoids (Bufkin lesions). The latter has a classic location in the posterior aspect of the medial distal femoral metaphysis and thought to be due to repetitive stress at the attachment of the medial head of gastrocnemius. On the contrary, osteoid osteomas are painful lesions, typically at night, demonstrate thick cortical sclerosis, a nidus which may only be appreciated on computed tomography (CT) and marked surrounding marrow/soft-tissue edema or synovitis if intra-articular (**Fig. 3**). If a painful lucent cortical lesion was encountered in the anterior tibial diaphysis with surrounding sclerosis the differential diagnosis should include a stress fracture and infection/Brodies abscess in addition to an osteoid osteoma. There is usually history of repeated stress from activity and sports in stress fractures. CT can usually differentiate stress fracture from osteoid osteoma nidus. In infection,

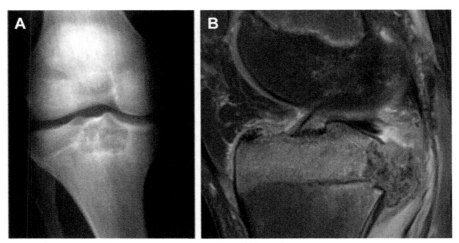

Fig. 1. Chondroblastoma: (*A*) AP radiograph demonstrating a well-defined lucent lesion in the proximal tibial epiphysis with internal mineralization. (*B*) Sagittal PD FS MR image in a different skeletally immature patient demonstrating a posterior proximal tibial epiphyseal lesion with marked surrounding marrow and soft-tissue edema.

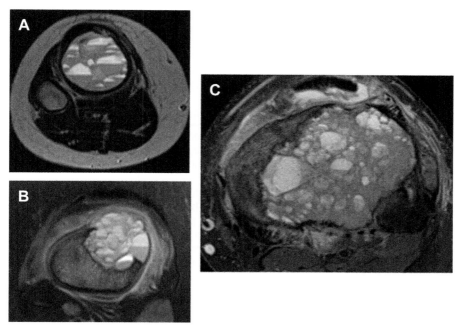

Fig. 2. (A) ABC tibia with multiple fluid–fluid levels. (B): Aggressive appearances with cortical thinning, marrow and soft-tissue edema in a primary ABC. (C) Secondary ABC in GCT. Note the soft-tissue component of the GCT with the secondary ABC formation and some fluid–fluid levels.

there might be clinical and biochemical evidence of infection like skin erythema, tenderness, induration, fever and raised inflammatory markers.

Osteochondromas are very common surface metaphyseal lesions which can be sessile or pedunculated. The vast majority are solitary, but they can be multiple in hereditary multiple exostoses (HME). They classically grow away from the joint and demonstrate cortical and medullary continuity with the parent bone. They should cease to

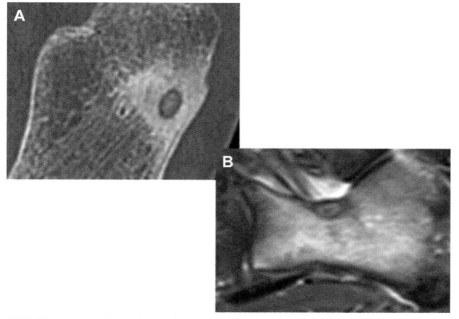

Fig. 3. (A): Axial CT: demonstrating a lucent focus in the lateral aspect of the calcaneum with surrounding sclerosis and central focus of mineralization. (B) sagittal PD FS images demonstrating the lesion in abutting the sinus tarsi with surrounding marrow and soft-tissue edema. Appearances are in keeping with an osteoid osteoma.

grow following skeletal maturity. Tug lesions may be mistaken for osteochondromas on radiography. CT can be helpful where it will show the cortical and medullary continuity in osteochondromas, whereas tug lesions appear as focal periosteal thickening at muscular attachments.

Enchondromas are other commonly encountered medullary metaphyseal or metadiaphyseal benign cartilaginous tumors mostly encountered in the second decade but may persist into adulthood. They are more common in the small bones of the hands and feet but are also seen in long bones with the femur being the most common followed by the humerus and tibia. Plain radiographs may show well defined lucent lesions with the characteristic "rings and arcs" chondroid mineralization. However, the most important differential diagnosis to consider is low-grade chondrosarcoma. Clinical and radiological differentiation is important as histopathological differentiation can often be difficult. History of pain and clinically palpable swelling should raise the suspicion for chondrosarcomas which tend to favor a metaphyseal location compared with enchondromas which tend to be diaphyseal. Murphy and colleagues[5] showed that when compared with enchondromas, chondrosarcomas demonstrate endosteal scalloping that involves more than two-thirds of the cortical thickness and extends more than two-thirds of the length of the lesion as well as cortical remodeling, thickening or destruction, periosteal reaction and extraosseous soft tissue (Fig. 4).

Bone infarcts are other lesions that may present with intramedullary calcification. These tend to have serpiginous morphology and on MR imaging, the central part of the lesion retains a normal marrow fat signal. Chondroid-type mineralization may also be seen in fibrous dysplasia (Fig. 5). These lesions are commonly monostotic but can be polyostotic. It can affect any bone in the body although the femur is a commonly affected bone in both types. Whole body MR imaging is useful to rule out polyostotic involvement. They may be lucent or sclerotic and classically demonstrate "ground glass matrix" on plain radiographs. They may demonstrate endosteal scalloping and secondary ABC formation. Malignant transformation is rare.

Giant cell tumors (GCTs) are locally aggressive, intermediate metaepiphyseal tumors commonly seen after closure of the growth plate. They are well defined, lucent lesions reaching the subchondral region. They maybe expansile and may demonstrate secondary ABC changes in 10%[6] (see Fig. 2). GCTs are commonly seen around the knee (50% to 60% of all cases) with the distal femur being the most common site followed by the proximal tibia (Fig. 6). Local recurrence can occur in up to 35% to 40% of cases.[7] Distant metastasis occurs to the lungs in 3% of cases. This is particularly in high risk patients with high-grade tumors, recurrences, tumors in the spine, proximal femur, and distal radius.[8]

Radiographically Nonaggressive Tumors

Patients older than 40 years

Nonaggressive bone lesions (lucent and sclerotic) are not expected to develop or progress after the age of 40 and indeed, any known preexisting nonaggressive lesion should either consolidate and heal or remain static. Any new osseous lesion in a patient after the age of 40 years should be viewed with high suspicion of malignancy. Of course, there are degenerative changes that will start to manifest in those patients. Geodes or intraosseous cysts are not uncommonly referred to the bone tumor team as a lucent lesion of concern especially in patients with history of malignancy. These lesions are subchondral with associated degenerative changes in the relevant joint and demonstrate fluid signal characteristics on MR imaging. It may have surrounding marrow edema like signal. CT would be helpful in identifying a communication between the joint and the intraosseous cyst to confirm the diagnosis. Occasionally, there might be some synovial tissue within these lesions that will give an atypical heterogenous signal on MR imaging. In these cases, biopsy or follow-up MR imaging may be required in high risk individuals.

Radiographically Aggressive Tumors

Patients younger than 40 years

In this age group, the commonest primary bone malignancy is osteosarcoma. In the lower limb, it is commonly seen in the distal femur and proximal tibia. Skip lesions are seen in around 15% of cases and hence imaging of the whole bone is recommended[9] Radiographically, osteosarcomas may be lytic, blastic or mixed with cortical destruction, aggressive periosteal reaction and an ossifying soft-tissue mass (Fig. 7). Cross-sectional imaging will better assess the true extent of the lesion, presence of skip lesions and may demonstrate certain features that aid in classifying the subtype like the presence of a secondary ABC in telangiectatic osteosarcoma.

The main differential diagnosis on imaging in this age group is osteomyelitis. In neonate, this tends to be in the epiphysis and metaphysis, in the metaphysis in children and epiphysis and subchondral regions in adults. They can have aggressive features on imaging. The patient may have

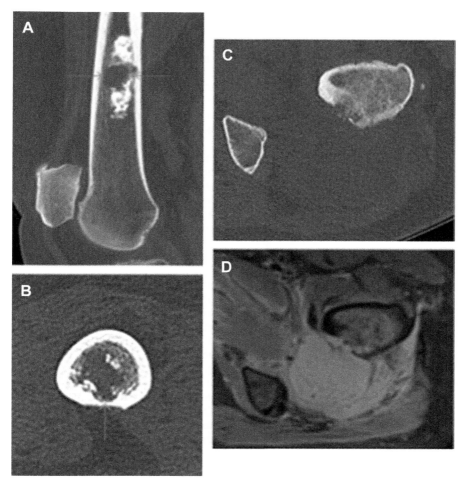

Fig. 4. Chondorsarcoma. (*A*) and (*B*) Sagittal and axial CT. Lucent focus in the center of mature medullary mineralization in a chondroid lesion. Note the endosteal scalloping posteriorly. Appearances are concerning for chondrosarcoma. (*C*) Axial CT images demonstrating ill-defined sclerosis in the proximal femur of a different skeletally mature individual at the level of the lesser trochanters with cortical destruction. (*D*) Axial PD FS MR image in the same patient demonstrating a large extraosseous soft-tissue component posteromedially. Note the marked marrow and surrounding soft-tissue edema. Biopsy proved a chondorsarcoma.

constitutional symptoms like fever and pain with elevated hematological and biochemical inflammatory markers. However, these clinical features are not unique to osteomyelitis but can also be seen in Ewing's sarcoma, Langerhans cell histiocytosis and chronic recurrent multifocal osteomyelitis (CRMO) (**Fig. 8**). The latter two may show multiple lesions on whole body imaging but ultimately, biopsy may be required for a definitive diagnosis.

Adamantinoma is a low-grade malignant tumor usually seen in the second and third decade of life with a typical location in the anterior tibial diaphysis. It appears as lytic cortical lesions that can be multiloculated and separated by areas of normal bone. It can be difficult to differentiate from osteomyelitis which some regard

as being on the opposite ends of the pathological spectrum. Aggressive changes in serial radiographs should raise the suspicion and biopsy may ultimately be required (**Fig. 9**).

Radiographically Aggressive Tumors

Patients older than 40 years
Metastases are the commonest bone tumors in adults above 40 years of age. They may be single or multiple, with a predilection to areas of red marrow due to increased blood supply in these areas and therefore seen as medullary metadiaphyseal lesions. Loss of the normal yellow marrow in the epiphysis of skeletally mature individuals is always abnormal and usually points to a hematological problem that will require further

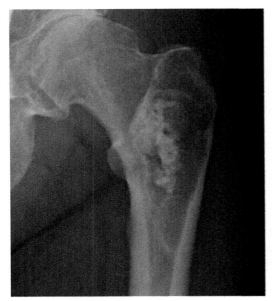

Fig. 5. A: AP radiograph demonstrating a well-defined lucent lesion in the proximal femoral metadiaphysis with internal mineralization in a skeletally mature individual. The main differential diagnoses include a chondroid lesion or FD.

investigations. Commonly encountered scenario in clinical practice is the presence of metadiaphyseal medullary foci of altered marrow signal on MR imaging in patients with history of a known primary neoplasm. Differentiating hematopoietic red marrow from metastases is essential. Hematopoietic red marrow tends to have an intermediate soft T1 signal and intermediate to subtly high signal on the fluid sensitive sequences and lacks any significant surrounding edema. From our experience, this is a particularly common finding in the proximal femoral metaphysis. CT to assess the osseous architecture and chemical shift MR imaging to look for intracellular fat, which is seen in benign but not malignant lesions, can be used as problem solving tools. Yet, biopsy may still ultimately be required. Metastatic lesions may be sclerotic, lytic, or mixed. Sclerotic metastases are seen in prostate, breast, and bronchogenic carcinoma. Lytic lesions are seen in renal cell carcinoma and thyroid cancer and tend to be expansile and vascular in both cases. Breast and lung cancers may show mixed lytic sclerotic lesions. Cortical metastases are rare but have also been reported, usually from lung, breast, renal, pancreas and larynx primaries.[10] Multiple lucent cortical lesions classically described as "punched out lesions" are seen in multiple myeloma. Bone metastases are very rare in the pediatric population but can be seen in neuroblastomas, clear cell sarcoma of the kidney and as skip lesions from osteosarcomas and Ewing's sarcomas.

Osteosarcomas may be seen in the older population secondary to Paget's disease, fibrous dysplasia and irradiation. Other possibilities

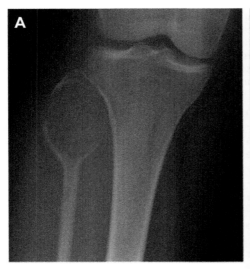
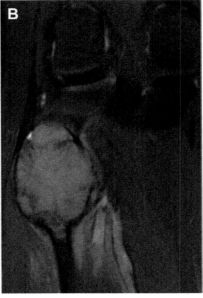

Fig. 6. GCT proximal fibula. (*A*) AP radiograph demonstrating an expansile epiphyseal lucent lesion in a skeletally mature individual with septations and cortical thinning. (*B*) Coronal PD FS MR imaging image demonstrating the expansile lesion with cortical thinning in keeping with a GCT of bone.

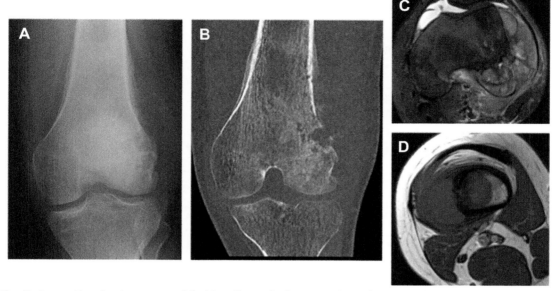

Fig. 7. Conventional osteosarcoma (*A*) AP radiograph demonstrating sclerosis in the distal metaphysis with aggressive lamellated periosteal reaction and extraosseous ossification. (*B*) Coronal CT image demonstrating the ill-defined sclerosis, cortical destruction and aggressive periosteal reaction. (*C*) Axial PD FS MR image demonstrating the large extraosseous component with surrounding marrow edema. (*D*) Axial T1-weighted image in a different patient with osteosarcoma in the distal femur with large extraosseous soft tissue. Note that the vessels are separated from the tumor with a preserved fat plane.

include hematological malignancy such as multiple myeloma and lymphoma. Infection can also be seen in this age group.

Soft-tissue tumors and tumor-like conditions

Soft-tissue masses are commonly encountered in the lower limbs in routine clinical practice. The vast majority of these lesions are nonneoplastic lesions secondary to trauma like hematomas and Morel Lavalee lesions, degenerative like ganglia especially when close to joints or tendon sheaths, inflammatory like synovial thickening, post-surgical like seromas or infectious like cellulitis and abscesses. True neoplastic lesions can be seen and the vast majority are benign and indeed, lipomas represent the most common soft-tissue tumor accounting for up to 50% of all soft-tissue tumors.[11] Malignant primary soft-tissue tumors are rare and even in the presence of previous malignancy, a malignant soft-tissue lesion is more likely to represent a primary soft-tissue sarcoma than a metastatic deposit[12] Soft-tissue metastases are usually from lung primaries or melanomas.

Ultrasound is the initial and main imaging modality used to assess these lesions and will be able to achieve the diagnosis in the majority of cases. It is able to establish whether the lesion is cystic or solid, assess its vascularity and can occasionally demonstrate focal calcifications.

MR imaging can be used if the sonographic features are non-specific or there is suspicion of malignancy. MR imaging of soft-tissue tumors should always include skin markers to localize the lesion. MR imaging protocols should at least include axial T1- and T2-weighted images without fat saturation along with T1 and STIR images in a longitudinal plane. MR imaging is more sensitive in depicting soft-tissue edema associated with aggressive lesions. It can also establish the relation of the lesion to adjacent anatomic structures, demonstrate the true extent of the lesion providing more accurate local staging, and with the opportunity to use contrast, can highlight areas of necrosis so areas of viable tissue can be targeted for biopsy. Contrast can also confirm whether a lesion that demonstrates fluid signal characteristics is indeed cystic or solid as in the case of myxomas. Contrast is also useful in postoperative patients to assess for local recurrences. The majority of soft-tissue lesions will have nonspecific appearances on MR imaging but the anatomical relationship of the lesion to the adjacent structures can suggest the most likely diagnosis despite the non-specific appearances. Lesions intimately associated with the neurovascular bundle may be neurogenic like

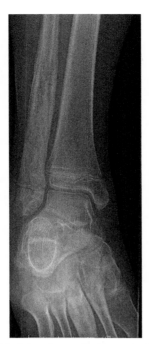

Fig. 8. CRMO: AP radiograph demonstrating osseous expansion and thick periosteal reaction in the distal fibula in a skeletally immature individual. Appearances are in keeping with osteitis and infection should be considered. However, also note similar changes in the 3rd metatarsal. Multiplicity suggests CRMO although infection remains a possibility although less likely. Full body imaging may demonstrate further lesions.

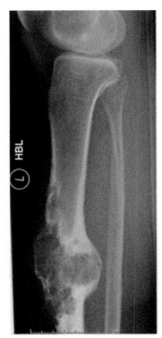

Fig. 9. Adamantinoma: Lateral radiograph of the tibia demonstrating the expansile "bubbly" lucent lesion in the tibial diaphysis, classic location for an adamantinoma. Osteofibrous dysplasia is on the other end of the spectrum and any changes or aggressive features on serial radiograph should raise the suspicion of adamantinoma.

benign or malignant nerve sheath tumors or of vascular origin like leiomyosarcomas from the vessel wall. Enhancing lesions centered on the fascia with surrounding soft-tissue edema are suggestive of myxofibrosarcomas. MR imaging signal can also give an idea of the histological components of the lesion and hence aid in their diagnoses. High T1 may be due to fat, blood, melanin or proteinaceous contents. Low T2 signal maybe due to fibrous tissue, hemosiderin or calcification. The latter two can result in blooming artefact on gradient echo sequences (GREs).

Plain radiography can depict calcifications seen in vascular malformations, myositis ossificans, soft-tissue chondromas and more sinister lesions like synovial sarcomas. CT may be utilized to illustrate more subtle calcification and also assess for any osseous involvement of the adjacent bones.

High T1 lesions

Lipomas as mentioned are the most commonly seen soft-tissue tumors. Most are small (<5 cm) and superficial and are easily diagnosed on ultrasound.[11] However, lesions that are larger, deeper and inhomogeneous on ultrasound with abnormal internal vascularity will warrant further assessment with MR imaging. Intramuscular and intermuscular lipomas are more frequently seen in the lower extremity.[13] Simple lipomas will completely suppress on fat suppressed images (**Fig. 10**). The main differential diagnosis for such lesions is well differentiated liposarcoma. Certain features would favor a malignant pathology such as large size (>10 cm), thick septations (>2 mm), globular areas of nonfatty signal and lesions that contain less than 75% fat.[14] Largely, the distinction between the two can be confidently made. However, there are certain points that make the differentiation challenging such as that around 25% of lipomas will have sufficient non-adipose tissue and intramuscular lipomas may have traversing muscle fibers that may be difficult to distinguish from septations. Calcification is nonspecific and can be seen in both but is more prevalent in malignant lesions. The foci of nonadipose tissue and calcification in lipomas is thought to be secondary to avascular necrosis.[15] In

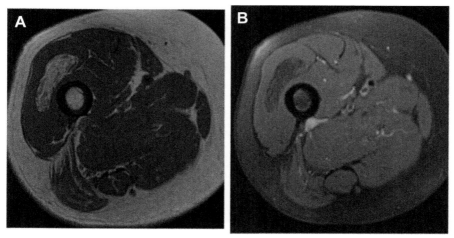

Fig. 10. IM lipoma. (*A, B*) Axial T1 and PD FS demonstrating an intramuscular lesion of fat signal that completely suppresses on the fat suppression images in keeping with a lipoma. Note the traversing muscle fibers.

doubtful circumstances, biopsy with MDM2 testing can be performed for differentiation. Myxoid liposarcoma is the second most common subtype of liposarcoma that has predilection to the lower limb especially the thigh. It tends to be deep intermuscular and has a myxoid component which may demonstrate cystic signal characteristics (**Fig. 11**). Contrast enhancement will differentiate between the two as cysts will have thin peripheral enhancement, whereas solid tumors will have variable intrinsic contrast enhancement. Other myxoid containing lesions should be considered in the differential including intramuscular myxomas, which are benign tumors which appear as well define lesions of homogenous fluid signal characteristics and variable contrast enhancement (**Fig. 12**). Myxomas can be associated with fibrous dysplasia, usually in an adjacent bone, in Mazabraud syndrome.

Hemorrhage can manifest as high T1 signal. Commonly encountered scenario in clinical practice is a mass with signal characteristics of hemorrhage. The question arises as to whether this is a hematoma or hemorrhage within a preexisting lesion. History of anticoagulation and/or trauma or surgical intervention is important. Such lesions will require follow-up clinically or with ultrasound in 3 to 6 weeks to ensure reduction in size. However, follow-up MR imaging might still be required and some lesions may ultimately require biopsy especially if there is no evidence of resolution over time (**Fig. 13**).

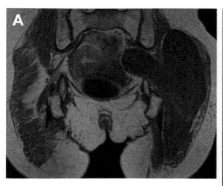
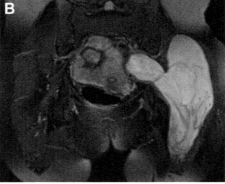

Fig. 11. Myxoid Liposarcoma: (*A, B*) coronal T1 and STIR images demonstrating a large lesion in the posterior aspect of the proximal left thigh that demonstrated largely low to isointense signal on T1-weighted images with some areas of high T1 signal within that do suppress of the fat suppression images confirming fat in the corresponding areas, whereas the remainder of the lesion demonstrates high signal on the STIR sequences. Biopsy confirmed a myxoid liposarcoma.

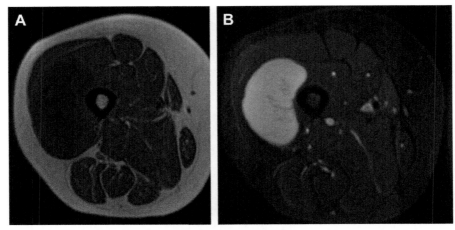

Fig. 12. IM Myxoma: (*A, B*) Axial T1 and STIR images. Note the large intramuscular lesion which demonstrates hypointense signal on the T1-weighted image and high signal on the fluid sensitive sequences. There is some heterogeneity within on the STIR sequences. Ultrasound or contrast enhanced MR imaging are sometimes needed to assess whether the lesion is solid or cystic. Biopsy proved an intramuscular myxoma.

Hemangiomas are other common lesions that usually present as masses in young individuals which on ultrasound may have areas of fat echogenicity. The overlying skin may show discoloration. Ultrasound will also demonstrate prominent vascular channels and may depict the post acoustic shadowing of phleboliths that can be confirmed on radiography (**Fig. 14**). Hemangiomas can rarely be intra-articular as is the case of synovial hemangioma. The knee joint is the most common location and tends to affect children and young adults. They may present as painful swollen joint. MR imaging will demonstrate intra-articular soft tissue, which may be focal or more frequently diffuse, of intermediate to low signal on T1-weighted images and high signal on fluid sensitive sequences. It may contain areas of high T1 signal due to slow moving blood or hemorrhage and low GRE signal due to hemosidirin from chronic haemorrhage.[16,17]

Lipoma aroborescens is another rare pathology of a frond like intra-articular mass arising from the synovium that demonstrate fat high T1 signal that is most commonly encountered in the knee but can be seen at other joints like the hip, wrist, elbow and shoulder.[18] (**Fig. 15**).

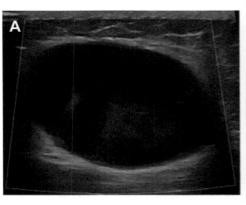
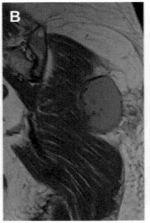
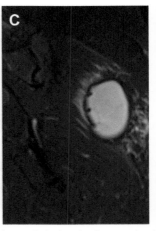

Fig. 13. Hematoma: (*A*) ultrasound image demonstrating a well-defined hypoechogenic lesion in the proximal thigh with internal echogenicites in a 74-year-old woman. Note the absence of vascularity on Doppler ultrasound. (*B, C*) Coronal T1 and STIR demonstrates the largely homogenous high T1 signal with a low-signal rim on all sequences and within suggesting hemosidirin. Follow-up ultrasound in 3 to 6 weeks is required to ensure reduction in size.

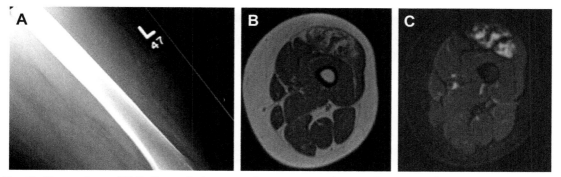

Fig. 14. Hemangioma. (*A*) Radiograph demonstrating a mass on the anterior aspect of the thigh with areas of fatty density and several pheboliths. (*B*, *C*) Axial T1 and STIR images demonstrating a large lesion in the anterior thigh with areas of fat signal that suppress on the fat-suppressed images and areas of vascular flow void. The phleboliths are better appreciated in the radiograph.

Low T2 lesions

Pigmented villonodular synovitis should always be considered in the differential diagnosis of intra-articular soft-tissue lesions especially in the knee joint (**Fig. 16**). Pigmented villonodular synovitis (PVNS) is a benign proliferative disease that represents the diffuse form of tenosynovial giant cell tumor (TGCT) and affects the knee in 80% of the cases.[11] The localized form is known as localized GCT of the tendon sheath most commonly affecting the hands and feet with about 17% affecting the foot and ankle.[14] Both entities are histologically identical. They demonstrate intermediate to low signal on T1- and T2-weighted images due to their fibrous content that can be seen as hypoechogenicity with post acoustic shadowing on ultrasound. The fibrous content may result in core needle biopsies proving challenging due to the tough fibrous tissue and this should be considered when planning for the procedure in terms of choice of caliber and type of the needle used. GRE images may show blooming artefact due to hemosiderin. There are usually erosions in the adjacent bones. Calcification is extremely unusual, and when seen, an alternative diagnosis should be considered.

Plantar fibroma is a commonly seen lump in the sole of the foot as a well-defined hypoechogenic oval or rounded mass on ultrasound intimately associated with the plantar fascia.

Desmoid fibromatosis or deep fibromatosis are rare locally invasive but non metastatic tumors with a peak incidence between 25 and 35 years of age. In the lower limbs, the most common location is the anterior quadriceps musculature of the thigh (12%), the popliteal fossa in the knee (7%) and the lower leg (5%). These lesions demonstrate low signal on T1- and T2-weighted images especially in the final stages of the disease when there is increase in the fibrous component and reduction in the cellular component.[19]

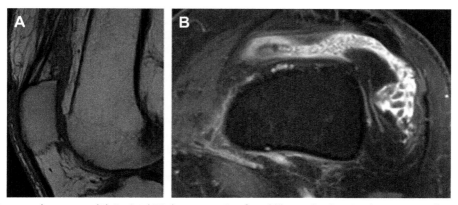

Fig. 15. Lipoma arborescens: (*A*) Sagittal T1 demonstrating frond like projections in the suprapatellar recess with signal characteristics similar to subcutaneous fat. (*B*) Axial PD FS showing that the signal suppresses on fat suppressed images confirming their fatty compositions. Note that these are better appreciated in the presence of a joint effusion.

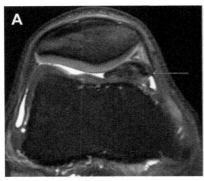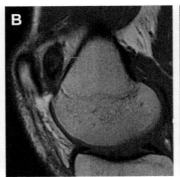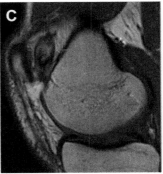

Fig. 16. PVNS: (*A*) axial PD FS: note the lesion in the suprapatellar recess (*arrow*). (*B, C*) Sagittal T1 pre- and post-contrast demonstrating enhancement of the lesion with low-signal foci on all sequences. Appearances are of PVNS.

Calcification

Synovial sarcoma should always be considered when soft-tissue masses, especially with calcification, are encountered particularly in the popliteal fossa and foot and ankle. Calcification is seen in around 33% of cases, which is usually punctate, eccentric, or peripheral. The challenge with these lesions is their indolent slow progression as juxta articular masses that slowly grow in size over a long period.

Myositis ossificans can be mistaken for a soft-tissue sarcoma and frequently referred to the Sarcoma team. It presents as a soft-tissue mass that demonstrate non-specific aggressive features on MR imaging. There is usually a history of trauma or neuropathic disease as in patients with spinal cord injuries and involuntary severe muscle spasms that may result in muscular tears and hematomas. Follow-up with radiograph and/or CT will demonstrate ossification and follow-up MR imaging will demonstrate resolution of the initial aggressive soft-tissue changes. However, an important differential to consider is parosteal osteosarcoma where the bone formation is central progressing peripherally compared with the peripheral rim ossification in myositis ossificans that progress centrally. Rare cause of calcification within soft tissue is extraskeletal chondromas. These have predilection to the hands and feet, may show mineralization on radiography and remodeling of the adjacent bones due to their indolent nature.[20]

SUMMARY

This article was written with particular emphasis on the practical approach to bone and soft-tissue tumors that are common to the lower limbs. Knowledge of the patient's age, location of the lesion and its relationship to the adjacent structures are pivotal in providing a reasonable diagnosis. Uncertainty about the diagnosis or atypical presentation and features should prompt referral to the Sarcoma Team.

CLINICS CARE POINTS

- The value of clinical history and clinical examination should never be underestimated.
- Radiography remains essential in the diagnosis of bone lesions. Aggressive features do not necessarily indicate a neoplastic process.
- Some neoplastic lesions have indolent course such as synovial sarcoma.
- Uncertainty or atypical features should prompt referral to the Sarcoma Team.

REFERENCES

1. Miller SL, Hoffer FA. Malignant and benign bone tumors. Radiol Clin North Am 2001. https://doi.org/10.1016/S0033-8389(05)70305-5.
2. Xu H, Ding Y, Niu X, et al. Chondroblastoma of bone in the extremities: a multicenter retrospective study. J Bone Jt Surg - Am 2014. https://doi.org/10.2106/JBJS.N.00992.
3. Motamedi K, Seeger LL. Benign bone tumors. Radiol Clin North Am 2011;49(6):1115–34.
4. Kaim AH, Hügli R, Bonél HM, et al. Chondroblastoma and clear cell chondrosarcoma: Radiological and MRI charactersistics with histopathological correlation. Skeletal Radiol 2002. https://doi.org/10.1007/s00256-001-0450-3.
5. Murphey D. Enchondroma Versus Chondrosarcoma in the appendicular skeleton: differerntiating features. Radiographics 1998;18(5):1213–37.
6. Murphey MD, Nomikos GC, Flemming DJ, et al. Imaging of giant cell tumor and giant cell reparative

granuloma of bone: radiologic-pathologic correlation. Radiographics 2001;21(5):1283–309.

7. Mavrogenis AF, Igoumenou VG, Megaloikonomos PD, et al. Giant cell tumor of bone revisited. SICOT-J 2017. https://doi.org/10.1051/sicotj/2017041.

8. Muheremu A, Niu X. Pulmonary metastasis of giant cell tumor of bones. World J Surg Oncol 2014. https://doi.org/10.1186/1477-7819-12-261.

9. Sajadi KR, Heck RK, Neel MD, et al. The incidence and prognosis of osteosarcoma skip metastases. In: Clinical orthopaedics and related research. 2004. https://doi.org/10.1097/01.blo.0000141493.52166.69.

10. Hendrix RW, Rogers LF, Davis TM. Cortical bone metastases. Radiology 1991. https://doi.org/10.1148/radiology.181.2.1924781.

11. Bancroft LW, Peterson JJ, Kransdorf MJ, et al. Soft tissue tumors of the lower extremities. Radiol Clin North Am 2002. https://doi.org/10.1016/S0033-8389(02)00033-7.

12. Abed R, Grimer RJ, Carter SR, et al. Soft-tissue metastases: their presentation and origin. J Bone Joint Surg Br 2009. https://doi.org/10.1302/0301-620X.91B8.21680.

13. Burt AM, Huang BK. Imaging review of lipomatous musculoskeletal lesions. SICOT-J 2017. https://doi.org/10.1051/sicotj/2017015.

14. Hochman MG, Wu JS. MR imaging of common soft tissue masses in the foot and ankle. Magn Reson Imaging Clin N Am 2017;25(1):159–81.

15. Kransdorf MJ, Bancroft LW, Peterson JJ, et al. Imaging of fatty tumors: distinction of lipoma and well-differentiated liposarcoma. Radiology 2002. https://doi.org/10.1148/radiol.2241011113.

16. Abdulwahab AD, Tawfeeq DN, Sultan OM. Intra-articular synovial hemangioma: a rare cause of knee pain and swelling. J Clin Imaging Sci 2021. https://doi.org/10.25259/JCIS_129_2020.

17. Larbi A, Viala P, Cyteval C, et al. Imaging of tumors and tumor-like lesions of the knee. Diagn Interv Imaging 2016. https://doi.org/10.1016/j.diii.2016.06.004.

18. De Vleeschhouwer M, Van Den Steen E, Vanderstraeten G, et al. Lipoma arborescens: review of an uncommon cause for swelling of the knee. Case Rep Orthop 2016. https://doi.org/10.1155/2016/9538075.

19. Mark D. AFIP ARCHIVES From the Archives of the AFIP Musculoskeletal Fibromatoses: radiologic-Pathologic Correlation 1 LEARNING OBJECTIVES FOR TEST 6. RadioGraphics 2009;29:2143–76.

20. Benradi L, El Haissoufi K, Haloui A, et al. Soft tissue chondroma of the plantar foot in a 14-year-old boy: a case report. Int J Surg Case Rep 2022. https://doi.org/10.1016/j.ijscr.2021.106688.

MR Imaging of the Lower Limb: Pitfalls, Tricks, and Tips

Julia Daffinà, MD[a], Riccardo Monti, MD[a], Francesco Arrigoni, MD[b], Federico Bruno, MD[b,*], Pierpaolo Palumbo, MD[b], Alessandra Splendiani, MD[a], Ernesto Di Cesare, MD[a,c], Carlo Masciocchi, MD[a], Antonio Barile, MD[a]

KEYWORDS

- MR imaging • Knee • Ankle • Foot

KEY POINTS

- MR imaging is one of the most widely used imaging tools to assess several pathologic conditions in the lower limb.
- Several anatomic variants and imaging artifacts can show unusual appearance and mimic pathologic entities.
- Knowledge of the possible imaging pitfalls encountered in MR imaging of the lower limb, and the available tips and tricks to recognize them, is essential to avoid significant diagnostic errors.

INTRODUCTION

Among imaging modalities, MR imaging is one of the most used techniques to evaluate acute and chronic disorders affecting the lower limb, from traumatic to inflammatory and tumoral diseases.[1–8]

This imaging technique carries an excellent diagnostic accuracy thanks to its high-intrinsic spatial and contrast resolution; however, there are different kinds of anatomic variants and artifacts that can be confused with pathologic entities.[6,7,9–15]

Our aim is to discuss most common diagnostic pitfalls of the lower limb with specific attention to the knee, ankle, and foot joints.

The knowledge of normal anatomic variants, correlation with age, symptoms, and medical history together with these potential MR imaging pitfalls is fundamental for an accurate interpretation of the imaging findings of the lower limb.

KNEE

MR imaging of the knee joint is considered a useful tool that can even be compared with arthroscopy, in the diagnosis of knee acute or chronic pain, mechanic limitation, and after trauma.[7,11,12,16–19]

Apart from radiography, which maintains its role in evaluating bone lesions in a trauma center and computed tomographic scan that can be indicated to reveal occult fractures, an MR imaging taken in a second place is fundamental to evaluate not only soft-tissue damages but also occult fractures.[9,20]

Standard MR imaging of the knee should include the evaluation of the cruciate ligaments, collateral ligaments, the menisci, the extensor system in addition to bones, chondral surfaces, and remaining soft tissues.[3]

According to several studies, the difference in evaluating the cruciate ligaments and menisci by using different magnetic field strength is minimal and mainly given by the higher resolution of the obtained images.[9,20]

Although the introduction of 3.0 T MR imaging scanners has allowed a more adequate study of knee lesions with increased signal-to-noise ratio, it is also more prone to artifacts compared with 1.5 T scanners.[9,20]

Generally, T1-weighted and proton density images are used to assess bone and ligaments anatomy but also bone marrow. It is crucial in evaluating the presence of osteophytes, intra-

[a] Department of Biotechnological and Applied Clinical Sciences, University of L'Aquila, L'Aquila, Italy; [b] San Salvatore Hospital, Via Lorenzo Natali 1, L'Aquila 67100, Italy; [c] Department of Life, Health and Environmental Sciences, University of L'Aquila, L'Aquila, Italy
* Corresponding author.
E-mail address: federico.bruno.1988@gmail.com

Radiol Clin N Am 61 (2023) 375–380
https://doi.org/10.1016/j.rcl.2022.10.010
0033-8389/23/© 2022 Elsevier Inc. All rights reserved.

radiologic.theclinics.com

articular loose bodies, and bone tumors. T2 with fat suppression or short tau inversion recovery (STIR) images are mandatory to evaluate bone marrow edema. T2 GRE is sometimes used because of its high efficiency in identifying blood and calcifications. There are many different but equally acceptable MR imaging protocols but generally given by a combination of these sequences in the 3 planes: axial, sagittal, and coronal.

Contrast is generally waived although it could be useful in the evaluation of patients with suspect meniscal tear after a meniscal repair (in this case, in fact, after intra-articular injection of gadolinium the presence of contrast within the meniscal repair or in a new location is highly suggestive a retear or new tear) or osteochondritis dissecans, which can be suspected in some ossification variants of the femoral condyles. Osteochondritis dissecans or fractures could also be misdiagnosed in cases of irregular epiphyseal ossification in pediatric patients.[21]

Sources of MR imaging pitfalls are mainly given by anatomic variants and technique-related artifacts.

Among variants, the dorsal defect of the patella and sulcus terminalis may be mistaken for pathologic condition. Regarding the case of bipartite patella, when symptomatic, there might be bone marrow edema, which should not be confused with a fracture. Another benign defect is the cortical avulsive irregularity of the femur, and this should not be confused with a neoplastic lesion.[17,22]

Starting with meniscal tear identification, this can often be difficult. Studying menisci on T1-weighted images can be misleading mistaking tears with an intrameniscal degeneration.[11]

Furthermore, some anatomic structures may be misinterpreted more commonly as lateral meniscus tears; for example, the gap between the anterior transverse meniscal ligament and the anterior horn, the space between the peripheral posterior horn of the lateral meniscus and popliteus tendon, meniscofemoral ligaments (Humphrey and Wrisberg), which may look like loose bodies or vertical or oblique tears of the posterior horn of the lateral meniscus known as "Wrisberg pseudo-tear" **Fig. 1**.

Moreover, some meniscal variants, such as meniscal flounce, most frequently seen in medial meniscus when the knee is flexed disappearing with full extension may resemble a lesion. These pitfalls can be avoided by following the meniscus and ligament structures on more than one sequence.[9,10,20]

Both the oblique meniscomeniscal ligament and the so-called ring meniscus variant can mimic a bucket-handle tear.[23]

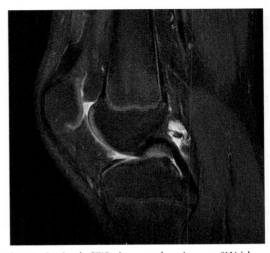

Fig. 1. Sagittal STIR image showing a "Wrisberg pseudo-tear".

The difference in signal intensity given by the interwining between the anterior cruciate ligament (ACL) collagenous fibers at its tibial extremity and the anterior fibrocartilagineous fibers of the lateral meniscus may also look like an anterior meniscal tear, which is a rare founding especially if alone.

Another important phenomenon that must be recognized is vacuum; this term used to identify air within the joint, and it can be a challenging differential diagnosis and generally requires 3T scanners.[24]

MR imaging artifact that can lead to pitfalls are mainly magic angle, truncation or Gibbs artifact, and motion artifacts.

Magic angle is an artifact given by the horizontal orientation of the magnetic field, which determines a focal elongation of images miming meniscal degeneration. It is maximum on short-TE sequences (such as T1 and GRE) and when the structure that we are studying has an orientation at 55° angle of the magnetic field. The truncation effect is defined by the presence of linear artifacts parallel to the articular surface that can generally be reduced by increasing the matrix size or by using smoothing filters.[25]

Finally, other common pitfalls that involve the meniscal articular surface mimicking a meniscal tear are intrasubstance mucoid degeneration of menisci, meniscal contusions, and in children, it is common to see a peripheral high-signal intensity (probably due to peripheral vascularization) within the meniscus.[7,20,23]

Concerning cruciate ligaments, many factors could mislead in the evaluation of ACL and posterior cruciate ligament (PCL's) state. The presence of ACL or PCL ganglion but also the anteromedial meniscofemoral ligament is rare.

The infrapatellar and intermeniscal plica, which on sagittal images can be seen anteriorly at ACL, may mimic ACL fibers when instead there is a tear but it could also look like a partial tear of the anteromedial bundle of ACL.

A complete ACL tear that created a scar or thickening could be erroneously mistaken for an intact ligament[4,11,16,20,22] **Fig. 2.**

The evaluation of postsurgery knee is much more complex, and the imaging criteria for the evaluation of menisci and ligaments are not always reliable. Knowing the acceptable postsurgical findings is fundamental in the evaluation of MR imaging because these might be routinely visualized after surgery while considered pathologic in the preoperative knee.[8,10–12]

ANKLE AND FOOT

MR imaging of the ankle and foot has a fundamental role in detecting abnormalities because of its ability to display superior soft tissue contrast compared with radiography.[3–6,8,14,26]

As for the knee, there are many accepted MR imaging protocols that always include a fat-saturated T2 or STIR sequence for bone marrow edema evaluation in the suspect of fractures or overuse injuries. Apart from bone marrow edema, T1 sequence is useful in the study of the Achilles tendon and of the plantar fascia.[2]

The field of view should be the smallest possible, centering the examination to the specific clinical question (ankle or foot) to ensure the best spatial resolution possible.

Apart from ligaments and tendons, a correct ankle MR imaging should evaluate the sinus tarsi, the tarsal tunnel, and the plantar fascia. When studying the foot, hindfoot, midfoot, and forefoot should be studied with a tailor-made protocol, if possible.

The magic angle artifact can apply to the ankle as well; in fact, it generally affects the posterior tibial tendon at his navicular insertion, the peroneal tendons posterior to the lateral malleolus but also the anterior tendons of the ankle joint. To avoid (or at least reduce) this effect, patient should be positioned supine or with a 20° plantar flexion decreasing the angle between tendons and the main magnetic vector[5] **Fig. 3.**

Another common pitfall is failure in fat suppression, and this generally seems to be caused by the contact with the coils and an inhomogeneous static magnetic field. Using inversion recovery images and multichannel phase array coils can help reduce this defect[3,4,27] **Fig. 4.**

The presence of multiple insertional slips of the anterior tibial tendon, inserting into the base of the first metatarsal and medial cuneiform bone, is a normal variant that can seem like a longitudinal tear.[28]

Considering the posterior compartment of the ankle, a normal variant, which can sometimes mimic a pathologic condition of the Achilles tendon, is the incomplete fusion of gastrocnemius and soleus tendons forming the tendon. Xanthomatous of the Achilles tendon also should be carefully diagnosed with the help of the patient's medical history.

Furthermore, the striated aspect of the posterior talofibular and deltoid ligament that can be seen especially in young patients must not be confused with a tear or sprain.

The talofibular and posterior intramalleolar ligaments that have a transverse course on the sagittal plane and should not be confused with intra-articular bodies.[3–5]

Accessory bones are well-corticated structures that result from unfused ossification center; they can be found in various locations and are a major issue to be considered in the foot and ankle.[29]

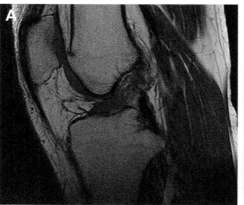
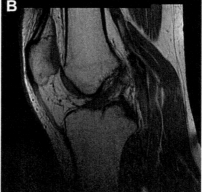

Fig. 2. MRI sagittal image of ACL (*A*) and PCL (*B*) tears.

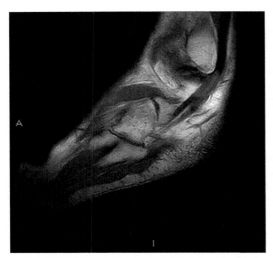

Fig. 3. T2 sagittal image showing Magic angle artifact of the peroneal tendons.

They are typically asymptomatic but when associated with pain, there could be hyperintensity on T2 sequences and therefore, in such cases, it is important to look for surrounding soft tissue swelling or metatarsal malalignment to distinguish them from fractures or loose bodies. For example, an intratendinous accessory navicular bone can alter the posterior tibial tendon insertion on the navicular bone.[27,29,30]

The most frequent are os naviculare, os peroneum, os trigonum, os intermetatarseum, os subfibulare, os vesalianum, and os sustentaculum.[3,27,29] The os intermetatarseum can be symptomatic and associated to bone marrow and soft tissue edema, which can makes it difficult to distinguish with a Lisfranc fracture and dislocation of the second metatarsal bone.[4,5]

The hallux sesamoids are considerably variable in size, shape, and number. The correct diagnosis of acute or chronic pathologic conditions can be a diagnostic challenge. A common pitfall is mistaking a bipartite sesamoid for a fractured sesamoid.[27,29]

Among causes of heel pain in the pediatric population, the posterior calcaneal apophysis development is common and should be distinguished from diseases such as Sever disease, infection, avascular necrosis, or fractures. This can be challenging because of frequent fragmentation and increased density of the calcaneal apophysis.

Considering different causes of bone marrow edema, which can be caused by unmobilization or diabetic foot, we should keep in mind that in adolescents there might be hyperintense foci in T2 sequences that represent normal red marrow islands[3,4,31] **Fig. 5.**

Also for the ankle's evaluation, contrast is generally waived. It can sometimes become helpful like in the diagnosis of osteomyelitis or, with intra-articular injection, for example, to evaluate the presence of a recess in the talocalcaneonavicular joint (between the medial plantar oblique and the inferior plantar longitudinal fibers) that could look like a spring ligament tear.[5]

Muscle variants are also frequent incidental MR imaging findings in the ankle. These variants are often asymptomatic but may cause mass effect with palpable swelling and therefore compression and pain.

The most frequent muscle variants are the flexor accessorious digitorum longus (within the tarsal

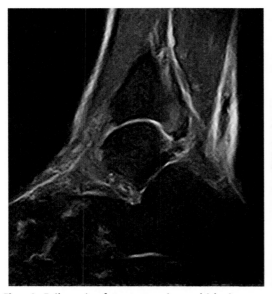

Fig. 4. Failure in fat suppression which is more evident in those areas of contact with the coil.

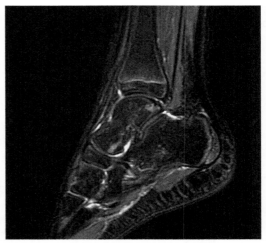

Fig. 5. Bone marrow edema of a young patient representing normal red marrow islands.

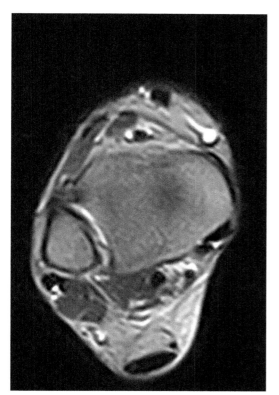

Fig. 6. Axial image of accessory soleus, a frequent muscle variant.

tunnel), the peroneus quartus (within the peroneal tunnel), and the accessory soleus (that inserts on the calcaneus separately from the Achilles tendon)[32,33] (**Fig. 6**).

Because of the vast variety of surgical procedures that can be used for traumatic and degenerative pathologic conditions treatment, access to surgical documentation is often necessary for an adequate interpretation of postoperative changes and eventually postoperative complications. In fact, many surgeries involve tendon transfers; therefore, images could be confounding.[6]

CLINICS CARE POINTS

- MRI of te lower limb, with its high-intrinsic spatial and contrast resolution, has an excellent diagnostic accuracy.
- anatomic variants can mimic pathologic entities.
- MRI artifacts can be a cause of diagnostic pitfall.
- anatomic variants can sometimes cause painful syndromes.

DISCLOSURE

The authors have nothing to disclose.

REFERENCES

1. Cekdemir YE, Mutlu U, Karaman G, et al. Evaluation of computed tomography images of calcaneus for estimation of sex. Radiologia Med 2021;126(8):1064–73.
2. Albano D, Bonifacini C, Zannoni S, et al. Plantar forefoot pain: ultrasound findings before and after treatment with custom-made foot orthoses. Radiologia Med 2021;126(7):963–70.
3. Tall MA, Thompson AK, Greer B, et al. The pearls and pitfalls of magnetic resonance imaging of the lower extremity. J Orthop Sports Phys Ther 2011;41(11):873–86.
4. Bencardino JT, Rosenberg ZS. Normal variants and pitfalls in MR imaging of the ankle and foot. Magn Reson Imaging Clin N Am 2001;9(3):447–63, x.
5. Gyftopoulos S, Bencardino JT. Normal variants and pitfalls in MR imaging of the ankle and foot. Magn Reson Imaging Clin N Am 2010;18(4):691–705.
6. LiMarzi GM, Scherer KF, Richardson ML, et al. CT and MR Imaging of the Postoperative Ankle and Foot. Radiographics 2016;36(6):1828–48.
7. Barile A, Conti L, Lanni G, et al. Evaluation of medial meniscus tears and meniscal stability: weight-bearing MRI vs arthroscopy. Eur J Radiol 2013;82(4):633–9.
8. Bruno F, Arrigoni F, Palumbo P, et al. Weight-bearing MR Imaging of Knee, Ankle and Foot. Semin Musculoskelet Radiol 2019;23(6):594–602.
9. Oei EH, Ginai AZ, Hunink MG. MRI for traumatic knee injury: a review. Semin Ultrasound CT MR 2007;28(2):141–57.
10. Mohankumar R, White LM, Naraghi A. Pitfalls and pearls in MRI of the knee. AJR Am J Roentgenol 2014;203(3):516–30.
11. Naraghi A, White L. MRI evaluation of the postoperative knee: special considerations and pitfalls. Clin Sports Med 2006;25(4):703–25.
12. Bruno F, Goderecci R, Barile A, et al. Comparative evaluation of meniscal pathology: MRI vs arthroscopy. J Biol Regul Homeost Agents 2019;33(2 Suppl. 1):9–14. XIX Congresso Nazionale S I C O O P Societa' Italiana Chirurghi Ortopedici Dell'ospedalita' Privata Accreditata.
13. Masciocchi C, Barile A, Lelli S, et al. Magnetic resonance imaging (MRI) and arthro-MRI in the evaluation of the chondral pathology of the knee joint. Radiol Med 2004;108(3):149–58.
14. Barile A, Bruno F, Arrigoni F, et al. Emergency and Trauma of the Ankle. Semin Musculoskelet Radiol 2017;21(3):282–9.

15. Masciocchi C, Barile A. Magnetic resonance imaging of the hindfoot with surgical correlations. Skeletal Radiol 2002;31(3):131–42.

16. Huang M, Li Y, Li H, et al. Correlation between knee anatomical angles and anterior cruciate ligament injury in males. Radiologia Med 2021;126(9):1201–6.

17. Vanhoenacker F, De Vos N, Van Dyck P. Common Mistakes and Pitfalls in Magnetic Resonance Imaging of the Knee. J Belg Soc Radiol 2016;100(1):99.

18. Bruno F, Barile A, Arrigoni F, et al. Weight-bearing MRI of the knee: a review of advantages and limits. Acta Biomed 2018;89(1-S):78–88.

19. Mariani S, La Marra A, Arrigoni F, et al. Dynamic measurement of patello-femoral joint alignment using weight-bearing magnetic resonance imaging (WB-MRI). Eur J Radiol 2015;84(12):2571–8.

20. Oei EH, Nikken JJ, Verstijnen AC, et al. MR imaging of the menisci and cruciate ligaments: a systematic review. Radiology 2003;226(3):837–48.

21. Laloo F, De La Hoz Polo M, Haque S. Imaging Pitfall in the Pediatric Knee: Irregular Epiphyseal Ossification at the Femoral Condyle. J Belg Soc Radiol 2021;105(1):84.

22. Liu YW, Skalski MR, Patel DB, et al. The anterior knee: normal variants, common pathologies, and diagnostic pitfalls on MRI. Skeletal Radiol 2018;47(8):1069–86.

23. Bolog NV, Andreisek G. Reporting knee meniscal tears: technical aspects, typical pitfalls and how to avoid them. Insights Imaging 2016;7(3):385–98.

24. Sakamoto FA, Winalski CS, Schils JP, et al. Vacuum phenomenon: prevalence and appearance in the knee with 3 T magnetic resonance imaging. Skeletal Radiol 2011;40(10):1275–85.

25. Turner DA, Rapoport MI, Erwin WD, et al. Truncation artifact: a potential pitfall in MR imaging of the menisci of the knee. Radiology 1991;179(3):629–33.

26. Albano D, Cortese MC, Duarte A, et al. Predictive role of ankle MRI for tendon graft choice and surgical reconstruction. Radiol Med 2020;125(8):763–9.

27. Shortt CP. Magnetic resonance imaging of the midfoot and forefoot: normal variants and pitfalls. Magn Reson Imaging Clin N Am 2010;18(4):707–15.

28. Mengiardi B, Pfirrmann CW, Vienne P, et al. Anterior tibial tendon abnormalities: MR imaging findings. Radiology 2005;235(3):977–84.

29. Vora BMK, Wong BSS. Common accessory ossicles of the foot: imaging features, pitfalls and associated pathology. Singapore Med J 2018;59(4):183–9.

30. Szaro P, Polaczek M, Swiatkowski J, et al. How to increase the accuracy of the diagnosis of the accessory bone of the foot? Radiol Med 2020;125(2):188–96.

31. Rossi I, Rosenberg Z, Zember J. Normal skeletal development and imaging pitfalls of the calcaneal apophysis: MRI features. Skeletal Radiol 2016;45(4):483–93.

32. Ekstrom JE, Shuman WP, Mack LA. MR imaging of accessory soleus muscle. J Comput Assist Tomogr 1990;14(2):239–42.

33. Yu JS, Resnick D. MR imaging of the accessory soleus muscle appearance in six patients and a review of the literature. Skeletal Radiol 1994;23(7):525–8.

Imaging of the Peripheral Nerves of the Lower Extremity

Yoshimi Endo, MD[a,b],*, Theodore T. Miller, MD[a,b], Darryl B. Sneag, MD[a,b]

KEYWORDS

- Peripheral nerve • Neuropathy • MR neurography • Ultrasound • Nerve entrapment • Neuroma

KEY POINTS

- Lower extremity peripheral neuropathy is common but physical examination and electrodiagnostic testing for its workup may not be accurate.
- Magnetic resonance (MR) neurography and ultrasound have become indispensable tools for imaging peripheral nerves.
- High spatial resolution of ultrasound allows detailed anatomic evaluation particularly of superficial nerves.
- MR neurography also affords high spatial resolution but its superior soft tissue contrast may identify subtle nerve abnormalities and muscle denervation more reliably than ultrasound.
- Familiarity with normal and abnormal appearances of peripheral nerves, as well as normal anatomy, anatomic variations, and common sites of entrapment is important for effectively evaluating peripheral nerves on imaging.

INTRODUCTION

Lower extremity peripheral neuropathy is a common condition encountered in clinical practice, seen in at least 26% of those aged 65 years or older and with a higher prevalence in patients with certain comorbidities such as diabetes, nutritional deficiencies, and autoimmune disease.[1] Peripheral nerve evaluation begins with a clinical assessment and physical examination but these may not be accurate in identifying the type or specific location of nerve injury. Electrodiagnostic testing, comprising nerve conduction studies and electromyography, is usually indicated when nerve injury is suspected but its accuracy depends on time from injury and operator experience.[2]

Following continued technical advancements during the past 20 years, imaging studies, particularly magnetic resonance (MR) neurography and ultrasound, have become indispensable tools for the evaluation of peripheral nerves. Both imaging modalities are also operator dependent; firm grasp of the anatomy of the nerves of interest and radiologist experience will determine the accuracy of these studies for identifying and characterizing peripheral nerve abnormalities.

TECHNICAL CONSIDERATIONS

Before the study is begun, any relevant history of prior surgery or penetrating trauma should be obtained from the patient, and the skin should be inspected for scars because these are sites for potential iatrogenic or traumatic nerve injury.

MR neurography of the lower extremities is ideally performed on a 3.0 T magnet, rather than 1.5 T, to maximize signal-to-noise ratio (SNR) and spatial resolution for a given acquisition time. Exceptions are made if there are contraindications to 3.0 T, such as implantable devices that may only be conditionally approved at 3.0 T, or if susceptibility artifact from metal obscures relevant anatomy despite the

[a] Hospital for Special Surgery, 535 East 70th Street, New York, NY 10021, USA; [b] Weill Medical College of Cornell University, Weill Cornell Medicine, 1300 York Avenue, New York, NY 10065, USA
* Corresponding author. Hospital for Special Surgery, 535 East 70th Street, New York, NY 10021.
E-mail address: endoy@hss.edu

Radiol Clin N Am 61 (2023) 381–392
https://doi.org/10.1016/j.rcl.2022.10.011

use of metal artifact reduction sequences.[3] High channel count surface array flexible coils that conform to the regional anatomy (e.g., thigh, lower leg) should be used to also maximize SNR.

Recommended MR neurography protocols vary depending on the peripheral nerve(s) in question but typically comprise a combination of high in-plane spatial resolution two-dimensional (2D) axial intermediate-weighted (~0.2–0.5 mm in-plane) and fat-suppressed fluid-sensitive (~0.4–0.8 mm in-plane) sequences usually obtained with slice thicknesses of 2.5 to 3.5 mm (Table 1). For fat-suppression, 2-point, 2D axial Dixon fat-water separation techniques are favored for 2 reasons: (1) maximize SNR (compared with short-tau inversion recovery) and (2) ensure robust fat saturation (compared with chemical fat-suppression, particularly when imaging the limb off-isocenter or curved anatomy such as the ankle region), which is needed to maximize contrast resolution between nerves and background soft tissues and also to depict active denervation of muscle that manifests as diffusely increased T2-weighted signal intensity. Dixon imaging provides both fluid-sensitive "water" and "fat" images, the latter being useful for evaluating fatty infiltration of muscle seen in chronic denervation states. For some lower extremity nerves (eg, saphenous and deep peroneal) that run alongside blood vessels that may confound interpretation due to their similar size and signal intensity, a fat-suppressed three-dimensional (3D) gradient-echo–based technique, known as reversed free-induction steady-state precession (PSIF),[4,5] may be helpful. Finally, additional oblique coronal and sagittal imaging planes can be obtained depending on the body region and course of the nerve.

On ultrasound, high-frequency linear transducers of 15 MHz or higher are used to visualize most nerves of the lower extremity. For small-caliber nerves such as sensory nerves in the subcutaneous fat, a high-frequency hockey stick probe often provides optimal visualization. Nerves that course in deeper tissues, such as the sciatic nerve, may require a lower frequency (eg, 9 or 11 MHz) linear transducer for better sound penetration. All nerves should be evaluated in both longitudinal and transverse planes; the fine

Table 1
Example protocol for lower extremity MR neurography at 3.0 Tesla

	Sequence Types		
	2D Intermediate-Weighted FSE	2D T2-Weighted FSE	3D T2w Gradient Echo (PSIF)[a]
Sequence Parameters			
TR/TE (ms)	3500–6000/35	3500–6000/80	9.5/5
FOV (cm) (variable depending on size of extremity)	8–18	10–20	10–12
Matrix size (FExPE)	512 × 352	320 × 224	320–224
Number of slices	54–70	30–40	90
Slice thickness (mm) (no gap)	2.5–3.5	2.5–3.0	2.0
Echo train length	10–15	12–16	1
Bandwidth (Hz/pixel)	195	391	122
Fat suppression technique	None	Dixon	Dixon
#Excitations (phase oversampling)	1.5–2	1.5–2	1
Parallel imaging factor	1.75	1–1.5	2
Imaging plane(s)	Axial	Axial; longitudinal (sagittal or coronal)	Axial
Acquisition time (minutes)	3–5	4–6	6

[a] PSIF: reversed free-induction steady-state precession (prototype sequence, on GE Healthcare platforms, courtesy of Daehyun Yoon from Stanford University), FE, frequency encoding; FOV, field of view; FSE, fast spin echo; PE, phase encoding; SE, slice encoding; TR/TE, repetition time/echo time.

architecture of the individual fascicles and the intervening internal epineurium/perineurium is best assessed in the transverse plane, whereas subtle caliber change or segmental structural abnormality is often more conspicuous when imaged longitudinally. The ultrasonographer should also note any symptoms elicited while scanning over the nerve (sonopalpation). Paresthesia in the distribution of a sensory nerve during sonopalpation, mimicking the Tinel sign, increases diagnostic confidence that the nerve is abnormal. If the ultrasonographer is uncertain whether a particular nerve is enlarged, scanning the same nerve in the contralateral lower extremity for comparison can be valuable.

General Imaging Features of Peripheral Nerve Injury

Normal peripheral nerves, with the combination of multiple fascicles, intervening internal epineurium/perineurium, and surrounding outer epineurium, are said to have a "honeycomb" appearance in cross section on ultrasound, which is also appreciable on MR neurography for larger nerves. Abnormal nerves, such as those with neuritis or extrinsic compression, will be enlarged and their internal architecture disrupted; enlargement of the individual fascicles and effacement of the perineurium such that the fascicles seem as a single conglomerate of or cluster of fascicles will be visible on both ultrasound and MR neurography. Ultrasound may show the abnormality with greater anatomic detail because it has higher spatial resolution for superficial nerves compared with MR imaging. The major advantage of MR neurography is its superior soft tissue contrast. Demyelination of peripheral nerves without axonal damage may manifest as signal hyperintensity of all or one or a few fascicles of the nerve on T2-weighted and fat-suppressed sequences without change in size or morphology, which may not be appreciable on ultrasound.

In a compressive neuropathy, the nerve will be small in caliber at the compression site and enlarged immediately more proximally as well as be hyperintense on T2-weighted, fat-suppressed sequences. Both MR imaging and ultrasound should be able to characterize the source of extrinsic compression but fibrous bands implicated in various nerve compression syndromes are often thin and imperceptible on either imaging modality.

Nerve lacerations secondary to penetrating trauma or iatrogenic injury may be complete, involving all the fascicles and the surrounding epineurium, or partial, involving only one or a few fascicles. In a lacerated nerve, both ultrasound and MR neurography will detect the disrupted fascicle(s) as an abnormal segment of the nerve but a discrete discontinuity of the fascicle(s) may not be confidently detected as there is usually laceration scar that obscures the anatomy of the nerve.[6] In the chronic phase, a posttraumatic neuroma may develop, composed of nonneoplastic disorganized neuronal elements and fibrous tissue.[7] On imaging, neuromas present as heterogeneously enlarged segments at the end of (endbulb neuroma) or along (neuroma-in-continuity) the nerve, which are of variable signal intensity on MR imaging but hypoechoic on ultrasound.

Muscle denervation is a secondary sign of injury for nerves providing motor innervation. In the acute phase, denervated muscle exhibits diffuse hyperintensity reflecting edema on fluid-sensitive sequences as early as 1 to 2 days after injury.[8] Edema will progress to fatty atrophy in the chronic phase, manifesting as a combination of strands of T1-hyperintensity and loss of bulk. On ultrasound, acute denervation results in patchy areas hyperechogenicity while chronic denervation results in homogeneous hyperechogenicity and loss of bulk.

IMAGING OF SPECIFIC NERVES
Sciatic Nerve

The sciatic nerve (L4-S3) provides motor innervation to the hamstrings before dividing into tibial and common peroneal nerves in the distal thigh. The sciatic nerve exits the pelvis usually antero-inferior to the piriformis, courses between the ischial tuberosity and the greater trochanter posterior to the obturator internus, superior and inferior gemelli, and quadratus femoris muscles, and descends distally in the posterior compartment of the thigh.

Given its large size, the sciatic nerve is easily visible throughout its course on MR neurography. On ultrasound, the nerve distal to the piriformis is visible in most patients (**Fig. 1**) but may be difficult to see in heavy patients. Deep and proximal to the piriformis, the nerve is usually not visible on ultrasound.

Close proximity to the hip joint makes the sciatic nerve vulnerable to iatrogenic injury, particularly during hip replacement; instruments used to cut the bone or screws placed in the bone can lacerate the sciatic nerve[9] (**Fig. 2**), postoperative hematomas can compress the nerve, and suture can result in tethering of the nerve. Hip dislocation or fractures can traumatize the nerve, and proximal hamstring tears can cause compression either directly by the torn tendon or indirectly by hematoma[10,11] (**Fig. 3**).

In piriformis syndrome, irritation of the sciatic nerve by an abnormality of the piriformis muscle is thought to result in sciatic neuropathy. Muscle strain, hematoma, or hypertrophy may cause

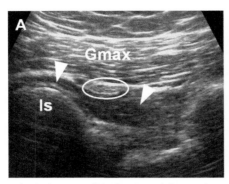
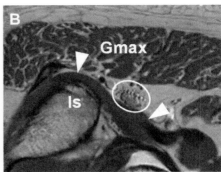

Fig. 1. Normal sciatic nerve. (*A*) Ultrasound short axis to the sciatic nerve and (*B*) axial intermediate-weighted fast spin echo (FSE) image oriented upside down show the normal anatomy of the nerve (circle) coursing posterior to the obturator internus (*arrowheads*) and deep to the gluteus maximus (Gmax), lateral to the ischium (Is).

sciatic nerve compression on MR imaging.[12] Variations in the course of the sciatic nerve have been described, with the entire nerve exiting the pelvis antero-inferior to the piriformis being the most common and the peroneal division coursing through the piriformis muscle while the tibial division courses antero-inferior to the piriformis being the second most common, seen in approximately 14% of cadavers.[13] Although controversial, this anatomic variation has also been implicated in piriformis syndrome.

Femoral Nerve

The femoral nerve (L2-L4) courses through or posterior to the psoas major muscle and then between the psoas and iliacus muscles in the retroperitoneum, exiting the pelvis deep to the inguinal ligament. Distal to the inguinal ligament, the femoral nerve traverses the femoral triangle together with the femoral artery and vein and splits into anterior and posterior divisions. The femoral nerve provides motor branches to the psoas major and iliacus muscles in the pelvis. The anterior division provides motor innervation to the pectineus and sartorius muscles and sensory innervation to the anteromedial thigh. The posterior division provides motor branches to the quadriceps muscles, articular branches to the hip and knee, and a sensory nerve, the saphenous nerve, which innervates the medial leg.

The femoral nerve may be entrapped by the inguinal ligament due to prolonged lithotomy position.[14,15] Injury to the femoral nerve may occur during surgery in the groin area, particularly herniorrhaphy, or during hip surgery (**Fig. 4**). Psoas hematomas, such as in anticoagulated patients, can compress the femoral nerve.[14]

On ultrasound, the femoral nerve is poorly visualized proximal to the level of the inguinal ligament due to its deep pelvic location.[16] The nerve is visible at the level of the inguinal ligament immediately lateral to the femoral artery but more distally,

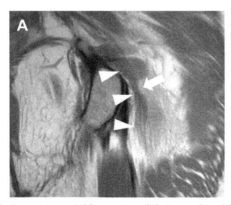
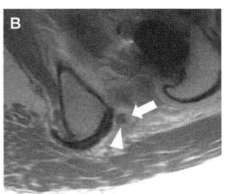

Fig. 2. Sciatic nerve partial laceration. (*A*) Coronal and (*B*) axial intermediate-weighted FSE images in a 29-year-old woman with acute foot drop after hip replacement earlier on the same day show gap of the lateral (peroneal) fascicles (*arrows*) while the medial (tibial) fascicles (*arrowheads*) are spared, reflecting a partial laceration from osteotome used to cut the femoral neck.

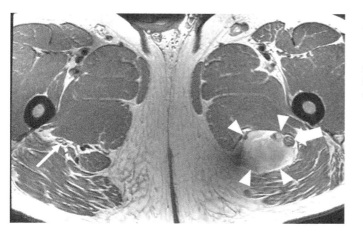

Fig. 3. Sciatic nerve irritation by hematoma. Axial intermediate-weighted FSE image in a 42-year-old man with acute left hamstring tear shows swollen left sciatic nerve (*thick arrow*) surrounded by hematoma (*arrowheads*) (*thin arrow* = normal right sciatic nerve).

the nerve will again be difficult to see.[16] MR neurography is preferred especially in these segments of the femoral nerve not well assessed by ultrasound.[17]

Saphenous Nerve

The saphenous nerve is the largest cutaneous branch of the femoral nerve. It descends with the superficial femoral artery and vein in the adductor canal in the midthigh, then courses away from the superficial femoral vessels anterolateral to the sartorius and pierces the deep fascia between the sartorius and gracilis in the distal thigh to enter the subcutaneous tissues where it gives off an infrapatellar branch, innervating the medial aspect of the knee, lower leg, and foot.[18,19]

Saphenous nerve entrapment caused by fibrous bands or as the nerve crosses the fascia

has been described but most saphenous neuropathies are iatrogenic. Knee surgery, particularly in the setting of hamstring tendon harvesting for anterior cruciate ligament reconstruction, can injure the saphenous nerve or its infrapatellar branch[20] (**Fig. 5**). Due to its proximity to the superficial femoral vessels, vascular surgery can also injure the nerve.[14]

Lateral Femoral Cutaneous Nerve

The lateral femoral cutaneous nerve (L2-L3) emerges lateral to the psoas major and courses anterior to the iliacus muscle before it exits the pelvis usually 1 cm medial to the anterior superior iliac spine.[21] Anatomic variations in how the nerve exits the pelvis relative to the inguinal ligament and the anterior superior iliac spine have been reported.[22] Distal to the inguinal ligament, the nerve

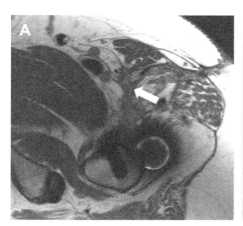
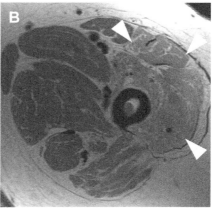

Fig. 4. Femoral nerve transection. (*A*) Axial intermediate-weighted FSE image of the proximal left thigh in a 53-year-old man with quadriceps weakness after hip replacement shows postoperative scar (*arrow*) along the expected course of the posterior division of the femoral nerve. (*B*) Axial intermediate-weighted FSE image slightly more distal shows denervation edema in the quadriceps muscles (*arrowheads*), which is a secondary sign of nerve injury.

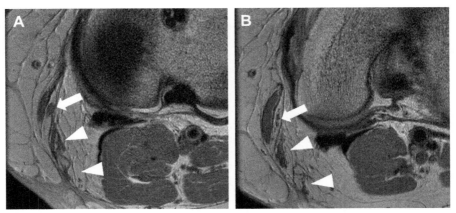

Fig. 5. Saphenous nerve neuroma. (A) Axial intermediate-weighted FSE image of the knee in a 46-year-old woman with anterior knee pain after ACL reconstruction with hamstring autograft shows thickening of the saphenous nerve (*arrow*) posterior to the sartorius muscle reflecting a neuroma-in-continuity, secondary to injury during graft harvesting. (B) Axial intermediate-weighted FSE image immediately more proximal to (A) shows normal fascicular architecture of the saphenous nerve (*arrow*). The gracilis and semitendinosus are attenuated (*arrowheads*) secondary to harvesting for the ACL graft.

branches into anterior and posterior divisions, which provide sensory innervation to the anterior and lateral thigh, respectively.

Entrapment of the lateral femoral cutaneous nerve, known as meralgia paresthetica, presents with pain, numbness, and paresthesias of the anterolateral thigh. Entrapment most commonly occurs at the level of the inguinal ligament, and tight clothes, seatbelts, and obesity are risk factors[21] (Fig. 6).

Ultrasound can identify the lateral femoral cutaneous nerve in most patients and may be more sensitive than MR imaging in detecting abnormalities of the nerve.[23] MR neurography better evaluates the

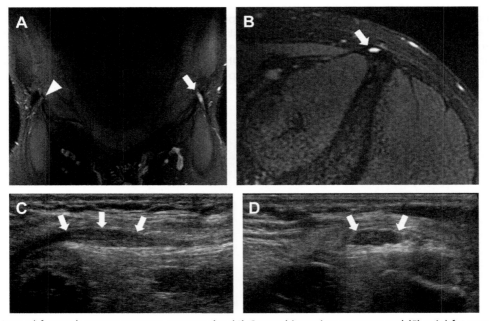

Fig. 6. Lateral femoral cutaneous nerve neuropathy. (A) Coronal inversion recovery and (B) axial fat-suppressed T2-weighted images in a 57-year-old man with meralgia paresthetica show a markedly hyperintense and enlarged left lateral femoral cutaneous nerve (*arrows*) as it courses anterior to the anterior superior iliac spine (arrowhead in (A) = normal right lateral femoral cutaneous nerve). Ultrasound (C) long and (D) short axes to the lateral femoral cutaneous nerve show segmental thickening of the nerve (*arrows*) as it exits the pelvis.

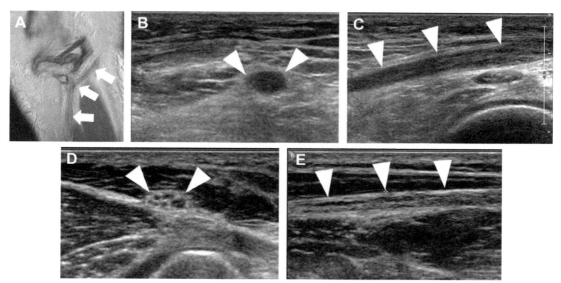

Fig. 7. Common peroneal nerve stretch injury. (*A*) Sagittal intermediate-weighted FSE image of the knee in a 21-year-old man shows tethering and kinking of the common peroneal nerve (*arrows*) at site of posterolateral corner injury. Ultrasound (*B*) short and (*C*) long axes to the common peroneal nerve 3 months later show diffuse thickening of the nerve and effacement of its perineurium (*arrowheads*). (*D, E*) Ultrasound of the normal common peroneal nerve (*arrowheads*) of the uninjured leg for comparison.

more proximal segment of the nerve before it emerges out of the pelvis.[24]

Common Peroneal Nerve

The common peroneal nerve (L4-S2) originates from the lateral fascicles of the sciatic nerve, diverging from the tibial nerve in the distal thigh and coursing laterally around the fibular neck and through the fibular (peroneal) tunnel between the peroneus longus muscle origin and fibula. At this level, the deep peroneal nerve courses anterior to and can be distinguished from the superficial peroneal nerve. A third branch, the recurrent articular branch, innervates the proximal tibiofibular joint.

Common peroneal neuropathy, frequently presenting as foot drop, is the most common mononeuropathy of the lower extremity,[25] due both to its superficial location in the knee and relatively fixed path around the fibular neck and in the fibular tunnel. Significant weight loss and prolonged cross-legged or squatting positions are known risk factors.[26,27]

Acute common peroneal neuropathy can be idiopathic or posttraumatic (**Fig. 7**). The peroneal nerve is also the most common site of intraneural ganglion cysts (**Fig. 8**); cysts that originate from the proximal tibiofibular joint dissect along the recurrent articular branch and into the common peroneal nerve, resulting in foot drop.[28]

Superficial Peroneal Nerve

The superficial peroneal branch of the common peroneal nerve courses posterolateral to the deep peroneal branch around the fibular neck. Distal to the fibular tunnel, the superficial peroneal

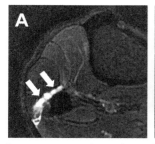
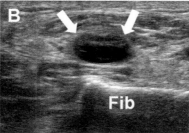
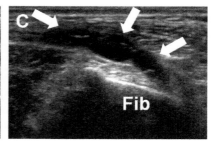

Fig. 8. Intraneural ganglion of the common peroneal nerve. (*A*) Axial fat-suppressed T2-weighted image of the proximal lower leg and ultrasound (*B*) short and (*C*) long axes to the common peroneal nerve of a 51-year-old man show ganglion cyst tracking into the nerve (*arrows*) (Fib = proximal fibula).

nerve courses anteriorly between the anterior and lateral compartments of the lower leg and pierces the deep fascia in the lower half of the lower leg to enter the subcutaneous fat.[18] The nerve then divides into the medial dorsal cutaneous and intermediate dorsal cutaneous nerves, although the exact location where this branching occurs varies. These 2 branches provide sensory innervation to the dorsal foot except for the first webspace, which is innervated by the deep peroneal nerve, and the dorsolateral aspect of the foot and fifth toe, which is innervated by the sural nerve. Proximally, the superficial peroneal nerve provides motor innervation to the peroneus longus and brevis muscles.

Superficial peroneal nerve entrapment is known to occur where the nerve pierces the deep fascia in the distal part of the lower leg, especially in dancers who perform repetitive plantar flexion of the ankle. Fascial defects, fascial thickening, muscle herniations, or scarring may be seen along the nerve in superficial peroneal nerve entrapment, or no structural abnormality may be seen but the patient may exhibit a Tinel's sign where the nerve pierces the deep fascia. The superficial peroneal nerve or its dorsal cutaneous branches are also vulnerable to iatrogenic or laceration injury (**Fig. 9**).

The superficial peroneal nerve is usually visible on ultrasound throughout its course, and because of its superficial course, ultrasound may be able to characterize its fascicular architecture to a greater detail than MR imaging. Ability to assess for the Tinel's sign and identify muscle herniations dynamically are additional advantages of ultrasound for evaluating the superficial peroneal nerve. MR imaging has the advantages of providing a more global evaluation of the lower leg and ankle, and anecdotally, more accurately detecting denervation compared with ultrasound.

Deep Peroneal Nerve

The deep peroneal nerve courses lateral to the anterior tibial artery within the anterior compartment of the leg deep to the extensor muscles. Either at the level of the ankle joint or within the anterior tarsal tunnel, which is a fibro-osseous tunnel bound superficially by the inferior extensor retinaculum and the dorsal capsule of the talonavicular joint deep to it,[29] the nerve divides into smaller lateral and larger medial branches. The deep peroneal nerve provides motor innervation to the extensor musculature. In the foot, the lateral branch provides motor innervation to the extensor digitorum brevis and sensory innervation to the sinus tarsi, ankle joint, and third through fifth tarsometatarsal joints,[30] whereas the medial branch provides sensory innervation to the first webspace.

Injury to the deep peroneal nerve in the upper half of the leg will cause weakness of the dorsiflexors of the ankle and foot (**Fig. 10**). At the level of the foot and ankle, the deep peroneal nerve can be compressed by the inferior extensor retinaculum in the anterior tarsal tunnel, presenting as anterior tarsal tunnel syndrome.

On ultrasound, the deep peroneal nerve can consistently be visualized at the level of the ankle. At the level of the proximal leg, the nerve may be more difficult to identify especially in obese patients. Identification of the anterior tibial artery is helpful because the deep peroneal nerve courses immediately lateral to it in the leg.[31] Distal to the ankle, the medial and lateral branches of the deep peroneal nerve are small in caliber but should be visible in most patients on high-resolution ultrasound. MR

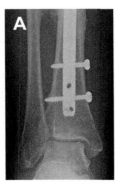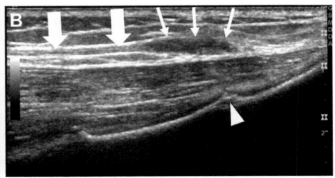

Fig. 9. Superficial peroneal nerve neuroma. (*A*) Frontal radiograph of the ankle of a 36-year-old woman shows screw tips protruding laterally from the distal tibia. (*B*) Ultrasound long axis to the superficial peroneal nerve (*thick arrows*) shows hypoechoic thickening of the nerve reflecting a neuroma-in-continuity (*thin arrows*), along the trajectory of a screw tip (*arrowhead*). The nerve had been punctured by a guidewire that was used for screw placement.

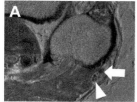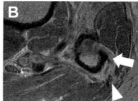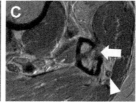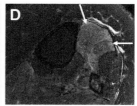

Fig. 10. Entrapment of deep peroneal nerve. (*A–C*) Axial intermediate-weighted FSE images superior to inferior in a 58-year-old woman show entrapment of the deep peroneal nerve (*thick arrows*) at the site of fibular fracture while the superficial peroneal nerve (*arrowheads*) is spared. (*D*) Axial fat-suppressed T2-weighted image shows denervation of the anterior compartment of the lower leg (*Thin arrows*).

neurography will identify the deep peroneal nerve and its medial and lateral branches in their entirety, although dedicated thin high-resolution images are required and the PSIF sequence may be helpful to suppress small vessels.

Tibial Nerve

The tibial nerve (L4-S3) is the larger, medial bundle of the sciatic nerve and descends in the popliteal fossa with the popliteal vessels. In the leg, the nerve courses anterior to the soleus muscle and posterior to the muscles of the deep posterior compartment (posterior tibial, flexor digitorum longus, flexor hallucis longus, and popliteus) and enters the tarsal tunnel in the ankle. It gives off the medial calcaneal nerve, which is a sensory nerve, and then bifurcates into the medial and lateral plantar nerves usually in the tarsal tunnel, and these latter 2 nerves provide sensory innervation to the sole of the foot and motor innervation to most intrinsic foot muscles. In the lower leg, the tibial nerve provides motor branches to the muscles of the deep posterior compartment and the superficial posterior compartment (gastrocnemius, soleus, and plantaris).

Tarsal tunnel syndrome is compression of the tibial nerve within a fibro-osseous tunnel, the boundaries of which are composed of the talus and calcaneus anterolaterally and flexor retinaculum posteromedially. The posterior tibial, flexor digitorum longus, and flexor hallucis longus tendons together with the tibial neurovascular bundle course through the tarsal tunnel, and any space-occupying lesion narrowing this space can result in tarsal tunnel syndrome. Tenosynovitis, accessory muscles, ganglion cysts, and neoplastic processes are reported causes of tarsal tunnel syndrome; gait disturbances, such as hindfoot valgus and those secondary to tarsal coalition, are also implicated.[25,32] The tibial nerve is also at risk of iatrogenic injury during ankle surgery (**Fig. 11**).

On ultrasound, the tibial nerve in the proximal leg may be difficult to assess in obese patients. The tibial nerve and the medial and lateral plantar nerves at the level of the tarsal tunnel are consistently seen. When following these nerves under ultrasound, it is helpful to remember that the medial plantar nerve courses anterior to the lateral plantar nerve in the tarsal tunnel, and distal to the tarsal tunnel, the medial plantar nerve courses immediately plantar to where the flexor digitorum longus and flexor hallucis longus tendons cross (knot of Henry). These nerves are well visualized with MR neurography.

Sural Nerve

The sural nerve is a sensory nerve that provides sensation to the posterolateral leg and the dorsolateral foot. There are anatomic variations[33] but it typically forms from "medial sural" and "lateral sural" contributions from the tibial and common peroneal nerves, respectively, in the distal thigh that join after variable distances but most

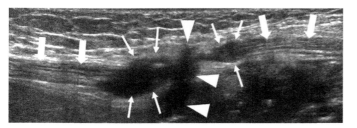

Fig. 11. Tibial nerve transection. Panoramic ultrasound long axis to the tibial nerve (*thick arrows*) at the level of the posterior ankle in a 75-year-old woman with acute numbness in the bottom of the foot after ankle replacement shows discontinuity of the nerve due to iatrogenic transection and stump neuromas (*thin arrows*) at the cut ends. Linear hypoechoic tract (*arrowheads*) at the site of transection presumably is the path of the saw used to cut the distal tibia.

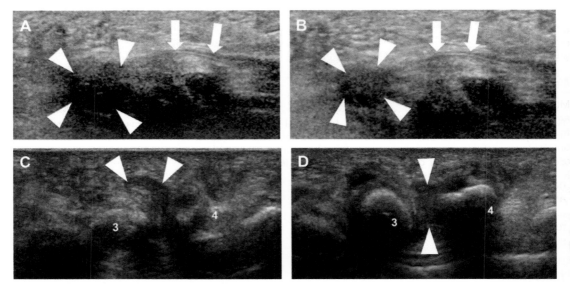

Fig. 12. Morton neuroma. (*A*) Ultrasound long axis to the plantar aspect of the third webspace shows combination of Morton neuroma and intermetatarsal bursa (*arrowheads*) in the third webspace. (*B*) Gentle compression along the dorsal surface of the webspace compresses out the fluid in the intermetatarsal bursa, and the remaining hypoechoic mass represents the neuroma (*arrowheads*) (*arrows* = interdigital nerve). (*C*) Ultrasound short axis to the plantar aspect of the third webspace shows Morton neuroma that has displaced plantarly (*arrowheads*) when the foot is squeezed, which is the sonographic equivalent of a "Mulder sign." (*D*) Without compression, the neuroma (*arrowheads*) stays between the metatarsals (3, 4 = third and fourth metatarsals, respectively).

commonly in the midposterior calf. It then descends at midline and then anterolateral to the Achilles tendon, terminating as the lateral dorsal cutaneous nerve in the foot.

The sural nerve is the most common donor for nerve grafting but it is also susceptible to injury during various types of trauma, such as distal fibular fractures, ankle sprains, and tendon tears. It can also be injured during surgery of the lower leg or ankle, including Achilles tendon repair.[34]

Because of its superficial location and its close proximity to the lesser saphenous vein, the sural

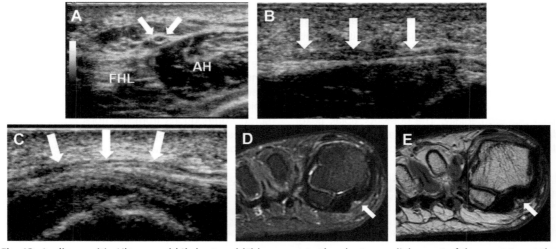

Fig. 13. Joplin neuritis. Ultrasound (*A*) short and (*B*) long axes to the plantar medial aspect of the great toe at the level of the metatarsophalangeal joint in a 31-year-old woman with prior medial sesamoidectomy show a thickened medial plantar digital nerve (*arrows*). (FHL = flexor hallucis longus tendon; AH = abductor hallucis muscle) (*C*) Ultrasound long axis to the medial plantar digital nerve of the contralateral great toe shows a normal thickness nerve for comparison (*arrows*). (*D*) Axial fat-suppressed T2-weighted and (*E*) intermediate-weighted FSE images show the nerve to be abnormally hyperintense (*arrows*).

nerve is easily seen in the distal calf on ultrasound and then can be traced proximally into the midcalf or distally into the foot as necessary. The nerve is well visualized on MR neurography.

Morton Neuroma and Joplin Neuroma

Morton neuroma is fibrotic tissue that develops around the interdigital nerve, most commonly in the third webspace but also commonly involving the second webspace. High heel shoes are thought to be contributory, and it is more common in women. On MR imaging, Morton neuromas are dumbbell-shaped masses that are isointense to muscle on T1-weighted and intermediate-weighted sequences. Because of its high fibrous content, Morton neuromas may be T2-hypointense. On ultrasound, a hypoechoic soft tissue mass will be seen in the webspace, continuous with the interdigital nerve; scanning along the plantar aspect of the webspace in long axis and applying gentle pressure on the dorsal aspect allows differentiation of intermetatarsal bursitis from the neuroma (**Fig. 12**). What has historically been interpreted as the Morton neuroma on MR imaging and ultrasound may be an overestimation of its true size because all Morton neuromas have thickened bursal tissue around it visible during surgery.[35] Ability to assess for the sonographic Mulder sign (see **Fig. 12**), a reproducible click as the neuroma is displaced plantarly when the forefoot is squeezed, and the presence of a Tinel sign, are advantages of ultrasound over MR imaging.

The medial plantar proper digital nerve to the great toe, which has a motor branch to the flexor hallucis brevis muscle and sensory innervation to the medial aspect of the great toe, is susceptible to repetitive compression and entrapment at the first metatarsophalangeal joint, resulting in Joplin neuroma or neuritis[25,36] (**Fig. 13**). Sports requiring pivoting and impact at the great toe, such as soccer and basketball, and surgery for hallux valgus are risk factors. The medial plantar proper digital nerve is visible on high-resolution ultrasound and MR neurography,[37] which may show focal enlargement or scar-encasement of the nerve at the level of the metatarsophalangeal joint.

SUMMARY

Imaging, particularly MR neurography and ultrasound, plays a critical role in the workup of patients presenting with peripheral neuropathy. Familiarity with the appearance of normal and injured peripheral nerves as well as the normal anatomic course, known anatomic variations, and common injury sites of the nerve(s) of interest is necessary for radiologists to effectively use these high-resolution imaging modalities.

CLINICS CARE POINTS

- Ultrasound has higher spatial resolution for superficial nerves but the superior soft tissue contrast of MR neurography may identify subtle nerve abnormalities as areas of signal hyperintensity.
- In a compressive neuropathy, the nerve is small at the site of compression and enlarged immediately more proximally on both ultrasound and MR neurography.
- Nerve lacerations may be partial or complete and can result in posttraumatic neuromas in the chronic phase.

DISCLOSURE

Hospital for Special Surgery has an institutional research agreement with GE Healthcare.

ACKNOWLEDGMENTS

None.

REFERENCES

1. Mold JW, Vesely SK, Keyl BA, et al. The prevalence, predictors, and consequences of peripheral sensory neuropathy in older patients. J Am Board Fam Pract 2004;17:309–18.
2. Feinberg J. EMG: myths and facts. HSS J 2006;2: 19–21.
3. Sneag DB, Zochowski KC, Tan ET. MR neurography of peripheral nerve injury in the presence of orthopedic hardware: technical considerations. Radiology 2021;300:246–59.
4. Chung YC, Merkle EM, Lewin JS, et al. Fast T(2)-weighted imaging by PSIF at 0.2 T for interventional MRI. Magn Reson Med 1999;42:335–44.
5. Gyngell ML. The application of steady-state free precession in rapid 2DFT NMR imaging: FAST and CE-FAST sequences. Magn Reson Imaging 1988;6: 415–9.
6. Endo Y, Sivakumaran T, Lee SC, et al. Ultrasound features of traumatic digital nerve injuries of the hand with surgical confirmation. Skeletal Radiol 2021;50:1791–800.
7. Murphey MD, Smith WS, Smith SE, et al. From the archives of the AFIP. Imaging of musculoskeletal neurogenic tumors: radiologic-pathologic correlation. Radiographics 1999;19:1253–80.
8. Bendszus M, Koltzenburg M, Wessig C, et al. Sequential MR imaging of denervated muscle: Experimental study. AJNR Am J Neuroradiol 2002; 23:1427–31.

9. Flug JA, Burge A, Melisaratos D, et al. Post-operative extra-spinal etiologies of sciatic nerve impingement. Skeletal Radiol 2018;47:913–21.

10. Hernesman SC, Hoch AZ, Vetter CS, et al. Foot drop in a marathon runner from chronic complete hamstring tear. Clin J Sport Med 2003;13:365–8.

11. Macdonald J, McMahon SE, O'Longain D, et al. Delayed sciatic nerve compression following hamstring injury. Eur J Orthop Surg Traumatol 2018;28:305–8.

12. Petchprapa CN, Rosenberg ZS, Sconfienza LM, et al. MR imaging of entrapment neuropathies of the lower extremity. Part 1. The pelvis and hip. Radiographics 2010;30:983–1000.

13. Pokorný D, Jahoda D, Veigl D, et al. Topographic variations of the relationship of the sciatic nerve and the piriformis muscle and its relevance to palsy after total hip arthroplasty. Surg Radiol Anat 2006;28:88–91.

14. Busis NA. Femoral and obturator neuropathies. Neurol Clin 1999;17:633–53.

15. Wilson M, Ramage L, Yoong W, et al. Femoral neuropathy after vaginal surgery: a complication of the lithotomy position. J Obstet Gynaecol 2011;31:90–1.

16. Martinoli C, Miguel-Perez M, Padua L, et al. Imaging of neuropathies about the hip. Eur J Radiol 2013;82:17–26.

17. Chhabra A, Faridian-Aragh N. High-resolution 3-T MR neurography of femoral neuropathy. AJR Am J Roentgenol 2012;198:3–10.

18. Yablon CM, Hammer MR, Morag Y, et al. US of the peripheral nerves of the lower extremity: A landmark approach. Radiographics 2016;36:464–78.

19. Hunter LY, Louis DS, Ricciardi JR, et al. The saphenous nerve: its course and importance in medial arthrotomy. Am J Sports Med 1979;7:227–330.

20. Pękala PA, Tomaszewski KA, Henry BM, et al. Risk of iatrogenic injury to the infrapatellar branch of the saphenous nerve during hamstring tendon harvesting: a meta-analysis. Muscle Nerve 2017;56:930–7.

21. Grossman MG, Ducey SA, Nadler SS, et al. Meralgia paresthetica: diagnosis and treatment. J Am Acad Orthop Surg 2001;9:336–44.

22. Aszmann OC, Dellon ES, Dellon AL. Anatomical course of the lateral femoral cutaneous nerve and its susceptibility to compression and injury. Plast Reconstr Surg 1997;100:600–4.

23. Powell GM, Baffour FI, Erie AJ, et al. Sonographic evaluation of the lateral femoral cutaneous nerve in meralgia paresthetica. Skeletal Radiol 2020;49:1135–40.

24. Chhabra A, Del Grande F, Soldatos T, et al. Meralgia paresthetica: 3-Tesla magnetic resonance neurography. Skeletal Radiol 2013;42:803–8.

25. Donovan A, Rosenberg ZS, Cavalcanti CF. MR imaging of entrapment neuropathies of the lower extremity. Part 2. The knee, leg, ankle, and foot. Radiographics 2010;30:1001–19.

26. Poage C, Roth C, Scott B. Peroneal nerve palsy: evaluation and management. J Am Acad Orthop Surg 2016;24:1–10.

27. Masakado Y, Kawakami M, Suzuki K, et al. Clinical neurophysiology in the diagnosis of peroneal nerve palsy. Keio J Med 2008;57:84–9.

28. Van den Bergh FRA, Vanhoenacker FM, De Smet E, et al. Peroneal nerve: normal anatomy and pathologic findings on routine MRI of the knee. Insights Imaging 2013;4:287–99.

29. Ferkel E, Davis WH, Ellington JK. Entrapment neuropathies of the foot and ankle. Clin Sports Med 2015;34:791–801.

30. Kennedy JG, Brunner JB, Bohne WH, et al. Clinical importance of the lateral branch of the deep peroneal nerve. Clin Orthop Relat Res 2007;459:222–8.

31. Becciolini M, Pivec C, Riegler G. Ultrasound imaging of the deep peroneal nerve. J Ultrasound Med 2021;40:821–38.

32. Trepman E, Kadel NJ, Chisholm K, et al. Effect of foot and ankle position on tarsal tunnel compartment pressure. Foot Ankle Int 1999;20:721–6.

33. Steele R, Coker C, Freed B, et al. Anatomy of the sural nerve complex: Unaccounted anatomic variations and morphometric data. Ann Anat 2021;238:151742.

34. Molloy A, Wood EV. Complications of the treatment of Achilles tendon ruptures. Foot Ankle Clin 2009;14:745–59.

35. Cohen SL, Miller TT, Ellis SJ, et al. Sonography of Morton neuromas: what are we really looking at? J Ultrasound Med 2016;35:2191–5.

36. Still GP, Fowler MB. Joplin's neuroma or compression neuropathy of the plantar proper digital nerve to the hallux: clinicopathologic study of three cases. J Foot Ankle Surg 1998;37:524–30.

37. Le Corroller T, Santiago E, Deniel A, et al. Anatomical study of the medial plantar proper digital nerve using ultrasound. Eur Radiol 2019;29:40–5.

Imaging-Guided Musculoskeletal Interventions in the Lower Limb

Domenico Albano, MD, PhD[a,1], Carmelo Messina, MD[a,b,1],
Salvatore Gitto, MD[b], Francesca Serpi, MD[b],
Luca Maria Sconfienza, MD, PhD[a,b,*]

KEYWORDS

- Ultrasound • Intervention • Guidance • Musculoskeletal • Hip • Knee • Ankle • Foot

KEY POINTS

- Ultrasound is the preferred imaging modality for guiding musculoskeletal injection procedures.
- Local anesthetics and steroids are the mostly used injectates.
- Promising results with variable evidence have been reported when using regenerative medications.

INTRODUCTION

Image-guided interventional procedures are widely used to treat musculoskeletal disorders.[1–3] Ultrasound (US) is often the preferred modality when targeting superficial structures, being also essential to confirm the diagnosis preoperatively.[4,5] Further, US ensures real-time monitoring of needle and drugs placement, avoiding neurovascular bundles, and does not use ionizing radiations.[6] Imaging guidance increases accuracy, safety, and efficacy of most musculoskeletal interventional procedures.[7–13]

In the lower limb, the most common indications for interventional procedures are degenerative joint and tendon disorders. Different technical approaches can be chosen, as well as different kind of needles and drugs. Local anesthetics (LA), steroids, and hyaluronic acid (HA) are common injectates; however, regenerative medications (ie, platelet-rich plasma [PRP]), prolotherapy, botulinum toxin type A, ethanol, and cryotherapy may be also used in selected musculoskeletal conditions.

Here, we review the evidence, indications, and technique of most image-guided musculoskeletal interventional procedures performed in the lower limb.

HIP

Hip Joint

Evidence

Generally performed in patients with hip osteoarthritis,[14–16] US guidance improves the accuracy of blinded intra-articular injections from 67% to 88% to 97%.[17] Steroid injections produce short-to-mid-term pain relief and function improvement.[14,18] Conversely, the effects of HA can last up to 6 months, despite studies showed that HA is not superior to steroids or placebo in terms of pain and function improvement.[10,19–21] A systematic review has shown similar effects of PRP and HA in hip osteoarthritis.[22] Moreover, image-guided hip injections are performed to administer contrast media before MR/CT arthrography[23,24] or to perform LA test to confirm the intra-articular origin of

[a] IRCCS Istituto Ortopedico Galeazzi, Cristina Belgioioso 173, 20157 Milano, Italy; [b] Dipartimento di Scienze Biomediche per La Salute, Università Degli Studi di Milano, Cristina Belgioioso 173, 20157 Milano, Italy
[1] Domenico Albano and Carmelo Messina share the first authorship as they contributed equally.
* Corresponding author.
E-mail address: io@lucasconfienza.it

Radiol Clin N Am 61 (2023) 393–404
https://doi.org/10.1016/j.rcl.2022.10.012

pain.[25] Finally, US-guided arthrocentesis is essential for the diagnostic workup of painful total hip arthroplasty to detect implant infection before surgery.

Technique

The patient is supine with hip in neutral rotation. Injection/aspiration of joint fluid is generally performed using in-plane caudal-to-cranial approach, placing a convex probe parallel to the femoral neck. The best target is the femoral head-neck junction where the joint capsule is wider. Joint injection leads to capsule distension and can be also followed using color-Doppler to demonstrate the correct substance distribution.[26] Arthrocentesis in patients with joint fluid can be performed using the same approach (**Fig. 1**). However, when joint infection without fluid is suspected (**Fig. 2**), samples can be collected by (1) US-guided intra-articular injection and reaspiration of saline to be used for culture and (2) US-guided periprosthetic synovial biopsy after local anesthesia.[27]

Iliopsoas Bursa

Evidence

Previous studies reported the feasibility and accuracy of image-guided iliopsoas bursa injection of LA/steroid in patients with iliopsoas tendinopathy/bursitis.[28,29] This procedure can be helpful in patients with hip pain, particularly those with iliopsoas impingement after total hip replacement. About 90% of patients with total hip arthroplasty affected by iliopsoas tendinopathy/bursitis report pain improvement after US-guided iliopsoas bursa LA/steroid injection,[30] although repeated procedures might be needed to obtain pain relief.[31]

Technique

The patient is supine with hip in neutral rotation. The injection is performed with an in-plane lateral-to-medial approach with the probe in transverse position parallel to the iliopectineal eminence (**Fig. 3**). Needle tip is advanced to reach the bursa, until the deep margin of the iliopsoas tendon. This procedure can be performed as a diagnostic test by injecting LA (ie, 10 mL of lidocaine 2%) and then evaluating pain reduction during walking after 10 minutes from injection.

Greater Trochanteric Pain Syndrome

Evidence

US-guided LA/steroid injection has shown to provide short-to-mid-term pain relief in patients with greater trochanteric pain syndrome, although similar 3 to 6 months results have been reported also without guidance.[32] US-guided injections have better results than blinded procedures when the target is the greater trochanteric bursa.[33] Other procedures can also be performed, including US-guided tendon fenestration and PRP injections, with no superiority compared with LA/steroid injections.[34,35] However, US-guided PRP injections could present more long-lasting pain relief than LA/steroid injections.[36]

Technique

The patient is in lateral decubitus position on the unaffected hip. The probe can be placed transverse on the middle trochanteric facet or sagittal along the gluteus medius tendon. With an in-plane approach, the needle is directed toward the greater trochanter, advancing the tip up to the trochanteric bursa between the gluteus medius tendon (deep) and the gluteus maximus muscle (superficial; **Fig. 4**).

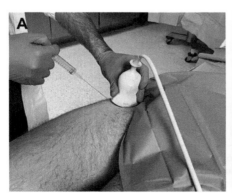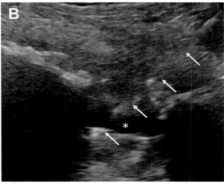

Fig. 1. Arthrocentesis of total hip arthroplasty. The patient is supine with the probe parallel to the prosthetic neck (*A*) and the needle (*arrows*) inserted with in-plane caudal-to-cranial approach (*B*) placing the tip on the prosthetic neck to aspirate joint fluid (*asterisk*).

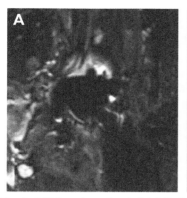
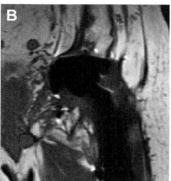
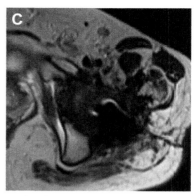

Fig. 2. MR imaging of painful failed THA. Coronal STIR (*A*), coronal T1-weighted (*B*) and axial T2-weighted (*C*) images of THA without effusion. In this case, US-guided injection of the dry THA was not feasible, thus US-guided periprosthetic synovial biopsy was performed.

KNEE
Knee Joint

Evidence
US guidance improves the efficacy of joint aspiration and injections.[37–39] US-guided intra-articular LA/steroid administration provides short-to-mid-term pain and function improvement in inflammatory arthritis, with controversial results in degenerative osteoarthritis.[40,41] US-guided HA injection might lead to better improvement than LA/steroid injection in osteoarthritis.[42,43] Moreover, US-guided injection of PRP and other regenerative substances has shown to be effective in knee osteoarthritis with clinical benefit up to 1 year.[44]

Technique
The patient is supine and his knee slightly flexed (20°–30°) to push the fluid in the suprapatellar recesses. A linear probe is positioned on the suprapatellar recess in a transverse scan. The most used technique is to insert the needle with in-plane superolateral approach, to reach the suprapatellar recess between the prefemoral fat pad (deep) and suprapatellar fat pad and quadriceps tendon (superficial; Figs. 5 and 6). However, other approaches can also be used.

Patellar Tendon

Evidence
Several treatments have been tested in patellar tendinopathy but US-guided fenestration seems to be the most effective for pain and function improvement.[45] Outcome may be further improved by associating PRP injection.[46] However, there are still controversial data concerning the use of PRP alone. Alternative options include steroid, high-volume LA/steroid and saline, hyperosmolar dextrose, and HA injections.[11]

Technique
The patient is supine with his knee slightly flexed. The linear probe is positioned on either the long

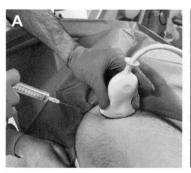
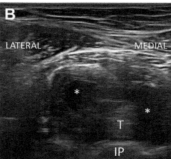
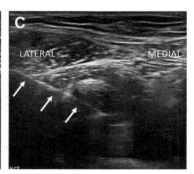

Fig. 3. Injection of iliopsoas bursitis. The patient is supine and the probe is in transverse position (*A*, *B*) parallel to the iliopectineal eminence (IP) to identify the iliopsoas tendon (T) surrounded by the distended bursa (*asterisk*). The injection (*C*) is performed with in-plane lateral-to-medial approach with the needle (*arrows*) advanced within the bursa.

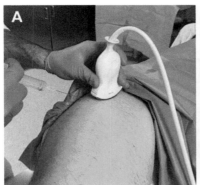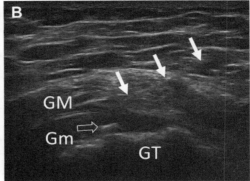

Fig. 4. Greater trochanteric pain syndrome injection. The patient is in lateral decubitus (*A*) on the unaffected hip with the probe being placed sagittal along the gluteus medius tendon. With in-plane approach (*B*), the needle (*arrows*) is directed toward the greater trochanter (GT), advancing the tip between the gluteus medius tendon (Gm) and the gluteus maximus muscle (GM). Enthesopatic calcification within the gluteus medius tendon is seen (*void arrow*).

or the short axis of the tendon, and the needle is inserted with in-plane approach to reach the target area of intratendinous degeneration or between tendon and Hoffa's fat pad (**Fig. 7**). Tendon needling can also be performed in association by puncturing repeatedly both the affected area and the normal tendon fibers.

Baker's Cyst

Evidence
Baker's cyst aspiration and LA/steroid injection is a safe procedure that can be done under US guidance for pain relief and to reduce cyst volume in the short-to-mid-term.[47] The procedure can be repeated in case of recurrence and can be associated to wall fenestration in complex cysts with loculations and septa.[48]

Technique

The patient is prone with the knee extended. The probe is in transverse position on the medial aspect of popliteal fossa, and the needle is inserted with in-plane medial-to-lateral approach to place the tip within the cyst (**Fig. 8**). After aspiration, any intracystic septa can be fenestrated and 1 mL of corticosteroid can be injected.

FOOT AND ANKLE
Ankle/Foot Joints

Evidence
Imaging guidance might increase the accuracy and clinical outcome of corticosteroid injections in both degenerative and inflammatory arthritis around foot and ankle.[49,50] Interesting data have been published also regarding US-guided

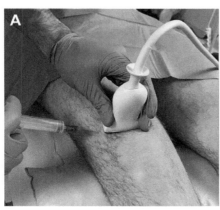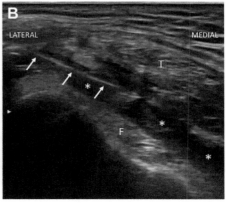

Fig. 5. Knee injection. The patient is supine and his knee slightly flexed (*A*), the needle (*arrows*) is inserted with in-plane lateral-to-medial approach (*B*) from the superolateral aspect of the knee to reach the suprapatellar recess (*asterisks*) between the prefemoral fat pad (F) and quadriceps tendon (T).

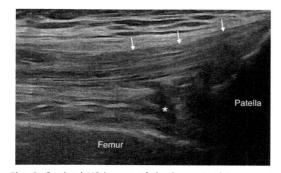

Fig. 6. Sagittal US image of the knee. In this patient, there is just a small amount of effusion in the supra-patellar recess (*asterisk*) beneath the quadriceps tendon (*arrows*). In this case, the US-guided injection of the joint can be challenging. It would be helpful to ask the patient to perform flexion-extension of the knee to push more fluid in the suprapatellar recess making the injection easier.

injection of PRP and dextrose for treating small osteochondral lesions of the talus in young patients.[51] Further, intra-articular US-guided foot/ankle injections of LA can be used as a diagnostic tool to identify the pain generator.[52]

Technique

When injecting the tibio-talar joint, the patient is supine with his foot in slight plantar flexion. Different approaches can be used to inject the joint, including in-plane distal-to-proximal anterior approach with the linear probe placed in sagittal plane or out-of-plane anterior approach with the probe in transverse plane, paying attention to avoid the extensor tendons and the anterior neuro-vascular bundle. Alternatively, the out-of-plane antero-lateral approach can be used placing the probe parallel to the anterior talofibular ligament (**Fig. 9**).

Achilles Tendon

Evidence

Several US-guided interventional procedures have been reported to treat Achilles tendinopathy, including dry needling and steroid injections, hyperosmolar dextrose, HA, and PRP or other regenerative medications, also using high-volume injections.[53,54] However, controversial results have been reported in the long-term follow-up. Moreover, meta-analysis studies demonstrated that these interventions, although being effective, are not superior to conservative treatments (ie, eccentric exercises, extracorporeal shock waves).[55,56]

Technique

Both insertional and noninsertional Achilles tendinopathy can be approached with dry needling and/or injection of PRP or other regenerative medications, placing the linear probe on the long axis and advancing the needle with in-plane caudal-to-cranial (or cranial-to caudal) approach or using the in-plane medial-to-lateral approach and positioning the tip on the most degenerated portion of the tendon. Retrocalcaneal bursa can also be injected. The patient is prone with the foot hanging over the edge of the bed. The linear probe is positioned in the short axis of the Achilles tendon identifying the bursa as a fluid layer deep to the tendon insertional portion. The needle is inserted with in-plane medial-to-lateral approach (to avoid the saphenous nerve) to reach the bursa to inject a mixture of LA/steroid (**Fig. 11**).

Plantar Fascia

Evidence

Steroid injection improves pain and function in the short-term,[57] being also more effective when guided by US than palpation.[58] Better mid-to-long-term results can be obtained injecting PRP

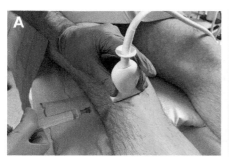
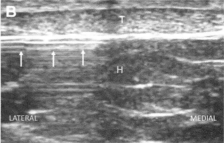

Fig. 7. Peritendinous patellar injection. The patient is supine with his knee slightly flexed and the probe aligned on the short axis of the tendon (*A*). The needle (*arrows*) is inserted with in-plane lateral-to-medial approach (*B*) to place the tip between tendon (T) and Hoffa's fat pad (H).

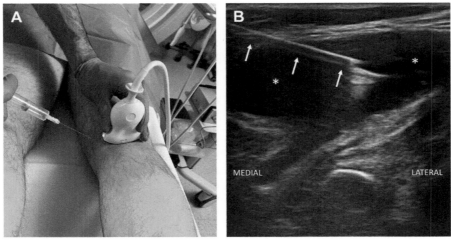

Fig. 8. Baker's cyst aspiration. The patient is prone with the probe in transverse position over the medial aspect of the popliteal fossa (*A*). The needle (*arrows*) is inserted with in-plane medial-to-lateral approach (*B*) to reach the cyst (*asterisks*).

under US guidance, with longer lasting clinical benefit.[59,60] Conversely, there is low evidence about efficacy of US-guided ozone, HA, and botulinum toxin type A injections in plantar fasciitis.[12]

Technique

The patient is prone with the foot hanging over the edge of the bed. The linear probe can be positioned in the long axis or in the short axis of plantar fascia at the insertion on the calcaneus, and the needle is inserted in-plane with proximal-to-distal approach in the former case and lateral-to-medial (to avoid the Baxter nerve in the medial aspect of the heel) in the latter. If corticosteroid is administered, the injectate should be distributed between the heel fat pad (superficial) and the fascia (deep) around fascial thickening. When using

PRP, the injectate is introduced within the fascia (**Fig. 13**). Being quite painful, a tibial nerve block within the tibial tunnel can be performed before the procedure.

Morton's Neuroma

Evidence

US-guided LA/steroid injection therapy is the most effective procedure for short-to-mid-term Morton's neuroma-related pain.[61] Procedures for Morton's neuroma treatment are more effective when guided by US than palpation, especially when LA/steroid is used.[62] Image-guided ethanol injection, radiofrequency ablation, and cryoablation have also been reported but additional studies to confirm their value are needed.[12,63]

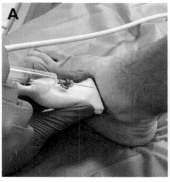
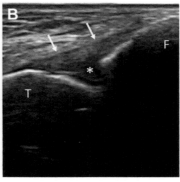
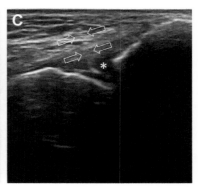

Fig. 9. Tibio-talar joint injection. The foot is slightly plantar flexed (*A*) and the probe is parallel to the anterior talofibular ligament (*B*, *arrows*) with the needle (*C*, *void arrows*) inserted with out-of-plane approach to reach the antero-lateral recess (*asterisk*). T, Talus; F, Fibula.

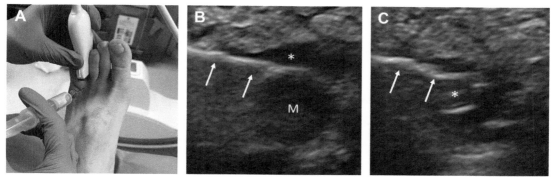

Fig. 10. Morton neuroma ethanol injection. The probe is placed in the interdigital space (*A*), and the needle (*arrows*) is inserted with in-plane dorsal-to-plantar approach (*A–C*). LA (*B*) is performed before the procedure injecting 5 mL of lidocaine 2% (*asterisk*) around Morton neuroma (M), followed by the injection of 0.5 mL of ethanol 95% (*asterisk*) within the lesion (*C*).

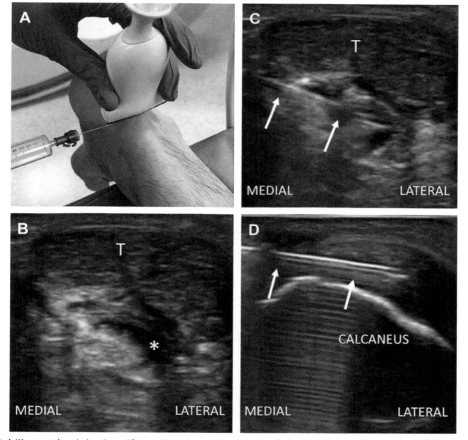

Fig. 11. Achilles tendon injection. The patient is prone with the foot hanging over the edge of the bed (*A*) and the probe placed along the short axis of the Achilles tendon (*B*) to identify the retrocalcaneal bursa (*asterisks*) as a fluid layer deep to the insertional portion of the tendon (T). The needle (*arrows*) is inserted with in-plane medial-to-lateral approach to inject the bursa (*C*) and then is advanced to reach the most degenerated portion of the tendon (*D*) to perform dry needling and/or to inject PRP or other regenerative medications.

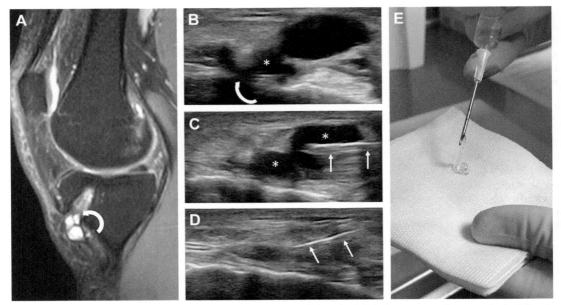

Fig. 12. Ganglion cyst aspiration. Sagittal knee MR imaging (*A*) and US (*B*) show a ganglion cyst (*asterisk*) originating from the tibial tunnel (*curved arrows*) after anterior cruciate ligament reconstruction. A 16G to 18G needle (*arrows*) is inserted with in-plane approach within the cyst (*C*) that can be easily aspirated (*D*). Note the jelly material aspirated from the cyst (*E*).

Technique

Different approaches can be used for Morton's neuroma treatment. The patient is in supine position, and a linear probe can be placed either in the interdigital space in sagittal position using an in-plane approach or in the dorsal or plantar aspect of the intermetatarsal space in transverse position using an out-of-plane approach. We prefer an in-plane dorsal-to-plantar approach with the probe

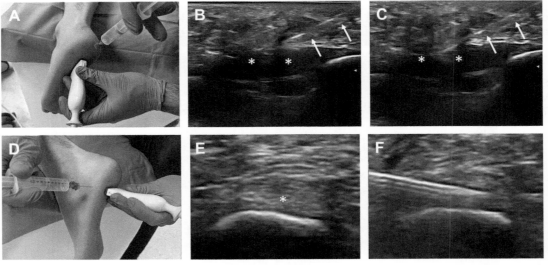

Fig. 13. Plantar fascia injection. The patient is prone with the foot hanging over the edge of the bed (*A*) and the probe placed along the long axis of the plantar fascia (*B*), which is thickened and hypoechoic (*asterisk*). The needle (*arrows*) is inserted with in-plane proximal-to-distal approach (*B, C*). Then, the procedure can involve the injection of corticosteroid between the heel fat pad and the fascia (*B*), or the injectate (in this case PRP) can be administered directly within the fascia (*C*). Alternatively, the fascia can be scanned in short axis (*D, E*) at the insertion on the calcaneus and the needle (*arrows*) can be inserted with in-plane lateral-to-medial approach (*F*).

place in the interdigital space. Then, a mixture of 1 to 2 mL LA/steroid can be injected around the lesion. In case of ethanol injection, local anesthesia should be performed before the procedure (ie, 5 mL of lidocaine 2%) followed by the injection of 0.5 mL of ethanol 95% within the lesion (**Fig. 10**).

Ganglia

Evidence

Ganglion cysts usually arise around joints and can be symptomatic due to compression of neurovascular bundles or superficially visible as lumps. US-guided aspiration/injection of ganglia has been shown to be a less invasive approach compared with surgery. The latter approach seems to have lower recurrence rate,[64] although series on US-guided treatments for knee/ankle ganglia reported immediate symptoms resolution in 90% of cases and recurrence in 20% of patients.[65]

Technique

Patient position and technical approach varies according to the location of the cyst. When possible, in-plane approach is always preferred to avoid surrounding neurovascular. A 18-G needle minimum size is required to aspirate the dense mucin-filled cysts (**Fig. 12**). Lidocaine or saline can be injected within the cyst for content dilution, making the aspiration easier. No consensus exists about the advantage of steroid injection after aspiration.

In conclusion, US-guided interventional procedures in the lower limb are very widely performed in clinical practice. They are relatively easy to perform and very effective in some cases, although for some of them, evidence is sparse.

DISCLOSURE

S. Gitto was supported by Fondazione Umberto Veronesi, Italy (Post-doctoral Fellowship 2022). The other authors have nothing to disclose.

CLINICS CARE POINTS

- US-guided interventional procedures are commonly performed to treat several musculoskeletal conditions
- Evidence is present for few of them, while others are performed more practice-based than evidence-based
- Steroids are the most powerful substances which can be used, although with relatively short duration of action and potential damage to cartilage and tendons over time

REFERENCES

1. Sconfienza LM, Chianca V, Messina C, et al. Upper Limb Interventions. Radiol Clin North Am 2019;57: 1073–82.
2. Tortora S, Messina C, Gitto S, et al. Ultrasound-guided musculoskeletal interventional procedures around the shoulder. J Ultrason 2021;21:e162–8.
3. Chan BY, Lee KS. Ultrasound Intervention of the Lower Extremity/Pelvis. Radiol Clin North Am 2018; 56:1035–46.
4. Sconfienza LM, Albano D, Allen G, et al. Clinical indications for musculoskeletal ultrasound updated in 2017 by European Society of Musculoskeletal Radiology (ESSR) consensus. Eur Radiol 2018;28: 5338–51.
5. Hall MM, Allen GM, Allison S, et al. Recommended musculoskeletal and sports ultrasound terminology: a Delphi-based consensus statement. Br J Sports Med 2022;2021:105114.
6. Sconfienza LM, Albano D, Messina C, et al. Ultrasound-Guided Percutaneous Tenotomy of the Long Head of Biceps Tendon in Patients with Symptomatic Complete Rotator Cuff Tear: In Vivo NoncontRolled Prospective Study. J Clin Med 2020;9: 2114.
7. Sconfienza LM, Adriaensen M, Albano D, et al. Clinical indications for image-guided interventional procedures in the musculoskeletal system: a Delphi-based consensus paper from the European Society of Musculoskeletal Radiology (ESSR)—part I, shoulder. Eur Radiol 2020;30:903–13.
8. Sconfienza LM, Adriaensen M, Albano D, et al. Clinical indications for image-guided interventional procedures in the musculoskeletal system: a Delphi-based consensus paper from the European Society of Musculoskeletal Radiology (ESSR)—Part II, elbow and wrist. Eur Radiol 2020;30:2220–30.
9. Sconfienza LM, Adriaensen M, Albano D, et al. Clinical indications for image guided interventional procedures in the musculoskeletal system: a Delphi-based consensus paper from the European Society of Musculoskeletal Radiology (ESSR)—part III, nerves of the upper limb. Eur Radiol 2020;30: 1498–506.
10. Sconfienza LM, Adriaensen M, Alcala-Galiano A, et al. Clinical indications for image guided interventional procedures in the musculoskeletal system: a Delphi-based consensus paper from the European Society of Musculoskeletal Radiology (ESSR) — part IV, hip. Eur Radiol 2022;32:551–60.
11. Sconfienza LM, Adriaensen M, Albano D, et al. Clinical indications for image-guided interventional procedures in the musculoskeletal system: a Delphi-based consensus paper from the European Society of Musculoskeletal Radiology (ESSR)-part V, knee. Eur Radiol 2022;32:1438–47.

12. Sconfienza LM, Adriaensen M, Albano D, et al. Clinical indications for image-guided interventional procedures in the musculoskeletal system: a Delphi-based consensus paper from the European Society of Musculoskeletal Radiology (ESSR)-part VI, foot and ankle. Eur Radiol 2022; 32:1384–94.

13. Sconfienza LM, Adriaensen M, Albano D, et al. Clinical indications for image-guided interventional procedures in the musculoskeletal system: a Delphi-based consensus paper from the European Society of Musculoskeletal Radiology (ESSR)-part VII, nerves of the lower limb. Eur Radiol 2022;32: 1456–64.

14. Atchia I, Kane D, Reed MR, et al. Efficacy of a single ultrasound-guided injection for the treatment of hip osteoarthritis. Ann Rheum Dis 2011;70:110–6.

15. Silvestri E, Barile A, Albano D, et al. Interventional therapeutic procedures in the musculoskeletal system: an italian survey by the italian college of musculoskeletal radiology. Radiol Med 2018;123: 314–21.

16. Chianca V, Orlandi D, Messina C, et al. Interventional therapeutic procedures to treat degenerative and inflammatory musculoskeletal conditions: state of the art. Radiol Med 2019;124:1112–20.

17. Hoeber S, Aly AR, Ashworth N, et al. Ultrasound-guided hip joint injections are more accurate than landmark-guided injections: a systematic review and meta-analysis. Br J Sports Med 2016;50:392–6.

18. McCabe PS, Maricar N, Parkes MJ, et al. The efficacy of intra-articular steroids in hip osteoarthritis: a systematic review. Osteoarthr Cartil 2016;24: 1509–17.

19. Liao YY, Lin T, Zhu HX, et al. Intra-articular viscosupplementation for patients with hip osteoarthritis: a meta-analysis and systematic review. Med Sci Monit 2019;25:6436–45.

20. Leite VF, Daud Amadera JE, Buehler AM. Viscosupplementation for hip osteoarthritis: a systematic review and meta-analysis of the efficacy on pain and disability, and the occurrence of adverse events. Arch Phys Med Rehabil 2018;99:574–83.e1.

21. Brander V, Skrepnik N, Petrella RJ, et al. Evaluating the use of intra-articular injections as a treatment for painful hip osteoarthritis: a randomized, double-blind, multicenter, parallel-group study comparing a single 6-mL injection of hylan G-F 20 with saline. Osteoarthr Cartil 2019;27:59–70.

22. Berney M, McCarroll P, Glynn L, et al. Platelet-rich plasma injections for hip osteoarthritis: a review of the evidence. Ir J Med Sci 2021;190:1021–5.

23. Sconfienza LM, Albano D, Messina C, et al. How, when, why in magnetic resonance arthrography: An international survey by the European society of musculoskeletal radiology (ESSR). Eur Radiol 2018;28:2356–68.

24. Bellelli A, Silvestri E, Barile A, et al. Position paper on magnetic resonance imaging protocols in the musculoskeletal system (excluding the spine) by the Italian College of Musculoskeletal Radiology. Radiol Med 2019;124:522–38.

25. Lynch TS, Steinhaus ME, Popkin CA, et al. Outcomes After Diagnostic Hip Injection. Arthroscopy 2016;32:1702–11.

26. Albano D, Chianca V, Tormenta S, et al. Old and new evidence concerning the crucial role of ultrasound in guiding intra-articular injections. Skeletal Radiol 2017;46:963–4.

27. Sconfienza LM, Albano D, Messina C, et al. Ultrasound-Guided Periprosthetic Biopsy in Failed Total Hip Arthroplasty: A Novel Approach to Test Infection in Patients With Dry Joints. J Arthroplasty 2021;36: 2962–7.

28. Blaichman JI, Chan B, Michelin P, et al. US-guided Musculoskeletal Interventions in the Hip with MRI and US Correlation. Radiographics 2020;40:181–99.

29. Payne JM. Ultrasound-Guided Hip Procedures. Phys Med Rehabil Clin N Am 2016;27:607–29.

30. Adler RS, Buly R, Ambrose R, et al. Diagnostic and therapeutic use of sonography-guided iliopsoas peritendinous injections. AJR Am J Roentgenol 2005;185:940–3.

31. Nunley RM, Wilson JM, Gilula L, et al. Iliopsoas bursa injections can be beneficial for pain after total hip arthroplasty. Clin Orthop Relat Res 2010;468: 519–26.

32. Brinks A, van Rijn RM, Willemsen SP, et al. Corticosteroid injections for greater trochanteric pain syndrome: a randomized controlled trial in primary care. Ann Fam Med 2011;9:226–34.

33. McEvoy JR, Lee KS, Blankenbaker DG, et al. Ultrasound-guided corticosteroid injections for treatment of greater trochanteric pain syndrome: greater trochanter bursa versus subgluteus medius bursa. AJR Am J Roentgenol 2013;201:W313–7.

34. Jacobson JA, Yablon CM, Henning PT, et al. Greater trochanteric pain syndrome: percutaneous tendon fenestration versus platelet-rich plasma injection for treatment of gluteal tendinosis. J Ultrasound Med 2016;35:2413–20.

35. Fitzpatrick J, Bulsara MK, O'Donnell J, et al. The effectiveness of platelet-rich plasma injections in gluteal tendinopathy: a randomized, double-blind controlled trial comparing a single platelet-rich plasma injection with a single corticosteroid injection. Am J Sports Med 2018;46:933–9.

36. Ali M, Oderuth E, Atchia I, et al. The use of platelet-rich plasma in the treatment of greater trochanteric pain syndrome: a systematic literature review. J Hip Preserv Surg 2018;5:209–19.

37. Maricar N, Parkes MJ, Callaghan MJ, et al. Where and how to inject the knee–a systematic review. Semin Arthritis Rheum 2013;43:195–203.

38. Wu T, Dong Y, Song H, et al. Ultrasound-guided versus landmark in knee arthrocentesis: a systematic review. Semin Arthritis Rheum 2016;45:627–32.

39. Sibbitt WL, Band PA, Kettwich LG, et al. A randomized controlled trial evaluating the cost-effectiveness of sonographic guidance for intra-articular injection of the osteoarthritic knee. J Clin Rheumatol 2011;17:409–15.

40. Babaei-Ghazani A, Najarzadeh S, Mansoori K, et al. The effects of ultrasound-guided corticosteroid injection compared to oxygen-ozone (O 2-O 3) injection in patients with knee osteoarthritis: a randomized controlled trial. Clin Rheumatol 2018; 37:2517–27.

41. Henriksen M, Christensen R, Klokker L, et al. Evaluation of the benefit of corticosteroid injection before exercise therapy in patients with osteoarthritis of the knee: a randomized clinical trial. JAMA Intern Med 2015;175:923–30.

42. Campbell KA, Erickson BJ, Saltzman BM, et al. Is local viscosupplementation injection clinically superior to other therapies in the treatment of osteoarthritis of the knee: a systematic review of overlapping meta-analyses. Arthroscopy 2015;31: 2036–45. e14.

43. Ma X L, Kuang M, Zhao J, et al. Efficacy and safety of intraarticular hyaluronic acid and corticosteroid for knee osteoarthritis: A meta-analysis. Int J Surg 2017;39:95–103.

44. Rahimzadeh P, Imani F, Faiz SHR, et al. The effects of injecting intra-articular platelet-rich plasma or prolotherapy on pain score and function in knee osteoarthritis. Clin Interv Aging 2018;13:73–9.

45. Chen PC, Wu KT, Chou WY, et al. Comparative effectiveness of different nonsurgical treatments for patellar tendinopathy: a systematic review and network meta-analysis. Arthroscopy 2019;35: 3117–31.e2.

46. Dragoo JL, Wasterlain AS, Braun HJ, et al. Platelet-rich plasma as a treatment for patellar tendinopathy: a double-blind, randomized controlled trial. Am J Sports Med 2014;42:610–8.

47. Bandinelli F, Fedi R, Generini S, et al. Longitudinal ultrasound and clinical follow-up of Baker's cysts injection with steroids in knee osteoarthritis. Clin Rheumatol 2012;31:727–31.

48. Köroğlu M, Çallioğlu M, Eriş HN, et al. Ultrasound guided percutaneous treatment and follow-up of Baker's cyst in knee osteoarthritis. Eur J Radiol 2012;81:3466–71.

49. Jha AJ, Viner GC, McKissack H, et al. Accuracy of talonavicular injection using ultrasound versus anatomical landmark: a cadaver study. Acta Radiol 2020;61:1359–64.

50. Protheroe D, Gadgil A. Guided intra-articular corticosteroid injections in the midfoot. Foot Ankle Int 2018;39:1001–4.

51. Akpancar S, Gül D. Comparison of platelet rich plasma and prolotherapy in the management of osteochondral lesions of the talus: A retrospective cohort study. Med Sci Monit 2019;25: 5640–7.

52. Mitchell MJ, Bielecki D, Bergman AG, et al. Localization of specific joint causing hindfoot pain: Value of injecting local anesthetics into individual joints during arthrography. Am J Roentgenol 1995;164: 1473–6.

53. Boesen AP, Hansen R, Boesen MI, et al. Effect of high-volume injection, platelet-rich plasma, and sham treatment in chronic midportion achilles tendinopathy: a randomized double-blinded prospective study. Am J Sports Med 2017;45: 2034–43.

54. Albano D, Messina C, Usuelli FG, et al. Magnetic resonance and ultrasound in achilles tendinopathy: Predictive role and response assessment to platelet-rich plasma and adipose-derived stromal vascular fraction injection. Eur J Radiol 2017;95: 130–5.

55. Kearney RS, Parsons N, Metcalfe D, et al. Injection therapies for Achilles tendinopathy. Cochrane Database Syst Rev 2015;2015:CD010960.

56. Maffulli N, Papalia R, D'Adamio S, et al. Pharmacological interventions for the treatment of achilles tendinopathy: a systematic review of randomized controlled trials. Br Med Bull 2015; 113:101–15.

57. Johannsen FE, Herzog RB, Malmgaard-Clausen NM, et al. Corticosteroid injection is the best treatment in plantar fasciitis if combined with controlled training. Knee Surg Sports Traumatol Arthrosc 2019;27:5–12.

58. Chen CM, Chen JS, Tsai WC, et al. Effectiveness of device-assisted ultrasound-guided steroid injection for treating plantar fasciitis. Am J Phys Med Rehabil 2013;92:597–605.

59. Hohmann E, Tetsworth K, Glatt V. Platelet-rich plasma versus corticosteroids for the treatment of plantar fasciitis: a systematic review and meta-analysis. Am J Sports Med 2021;49: 1381–93.

60. Alkhatib N, Salameh M, Ahmed AF, et al. Platelet-rich plasma versus corticosteroids in the treatment of chronic plantar fasciitis: a systematic review and meta-analysis of prospective comparative studies. J Foot Ankle Surg 2020;59: 546–52.

61. Matthews BG, Hurn SE, Harding MP, et al. The effectiveness of non-surgical interventions for common plantar digital compressive neuropathy (Morton's neuroma): a systematic review and meta-analysis. J Foot Ankle Res 2019;12:12.

62. Morgan P, Monaghan W, Richards S. A systematic review of ultrasound-guided and

non-ultrasound-guided therapeutic injections to treat Morton's neuroma. J Am Podiatr Med Assoc 2014;104:337–48.

63. Santos D, Morrison G, Coda A. Sclerosing alcohol injections for the management of intermetatarsal neuromas: A systematic review. Foot 2018;35: 36–47.

64. Dias JJ, Buch K. Palmar wrist ganglion: does intervention improve outcome a prospective study of the natural history and patient-reported treatment outcomes. J Hand Surg Br Eur 2003;28:172–6.

65. Ju BL, Weber KL, Khoury V. Ultrasound-guided therapy for knee and foot ganglion cysts. J Foot Ankle Surg 2017;56:153–7.

Moving?

Make sure your subscription moves with you!

To notify us of your new address, find your **Clinics Account Number** (located on your mailing label above your name), and contact customer service at:

Email: journalscustomerservice-usa@elsevier.com

800-654-2452 (subscribers in the U.S. & Canada)
314-447-8871 (subscribers outside of the U.S. & Canada)

Fax number: 314-447-8029

Elsevier Health Sciences Division
Subscription Customer Service
3251 Riverport Lane
Maryland Heights, MO 63043

Printed and bound by CPI Group (UK) Ltd, Croydon, CR0 4YY

08/05/2025

01864724-0015